Pre-Clinical Operative Dentistry and Endodontics
Including Viva Voce Questions

Narendranatha Reddy P.
Vanitha N.

Bangalore

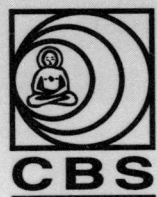

CBS

CBS PUBLISHERS & DISTRIBUTORS PVT. LTD.
New Delhi • Bengaluru • Pune • Kochi • Chennai

ISBN : 978-81-239-1529-6

First Edition : 2008
Reprint : 2011

Published by Satish Kumar Jain and produced by V.K. Jain for
CBS Publishers & Distributors Pvt. Ltd.,
CBS Plaza, 4819/XI Prahlad Street, 24 Ansari Road, Daryaganj,
New Delhi - 110002, India.   • Website: www.cbspd.com
e-mail: delhi@cbspd.com, cbspubs@vsnl.com, cbspubs@airtelmail.in
Ph.: 23289259, 23266861, 23266867   • Fax: 011-23243014

Branches:
• Bengaluru: Seema House, 2975, 17th Cross, K.R. Road,
  Bansankari 2nd Stage, Bangalore - 560070   Ph.: 26771678/79
  Fax: 080-26771680   • e-mail: bangalore@cbspd.com
• Pune: Bhuruk Prestige, Sr. No. 52/12/2+1+3/2,
  Narhe, Haveli (Near Katraj-Dehu Road by Pass), Pune-411051
  Ph.: +91-20-32404169   • Fax: 020-24464059
  e-mail: pune@cbspd.com
• Kochi: 36/14, Kalluvilakam, Lissie Hospital Road,
  Cochin - 682018, Kerala • e-mail: cochin@cbspd.com
  Ph.: 0484-4059061-65   • Fax: 0484-4059065
• Chennai: 20, West Park Road, Shenoy Nagar, Chennai - 600030
  e-mail: chennai@cbspd.com   Ph.: 044-26260666-26202620
  Fax: 044-45530020

Printed at :
Diamond Agencies Pvt. Ltd., Noida (UP)

Pre-Clinical
Operative Dentistry
and
Endodontics
Including Viva Voce Questions

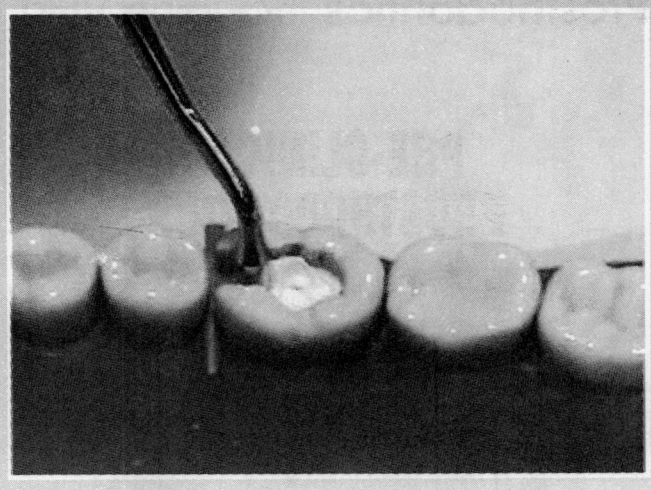

Notes on
Operative Detistry and Endodontics

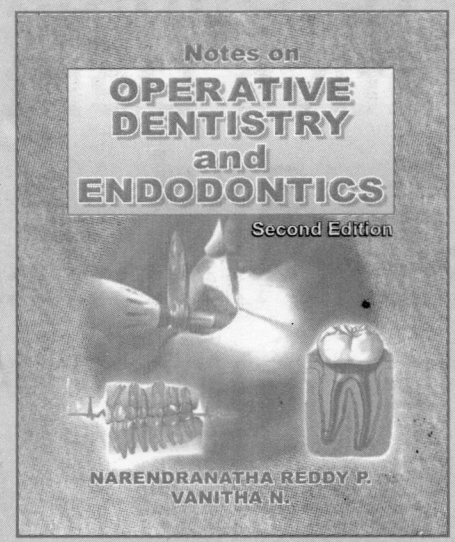

Pre-Clinical Prosthodontics Including Viva Voce Questions

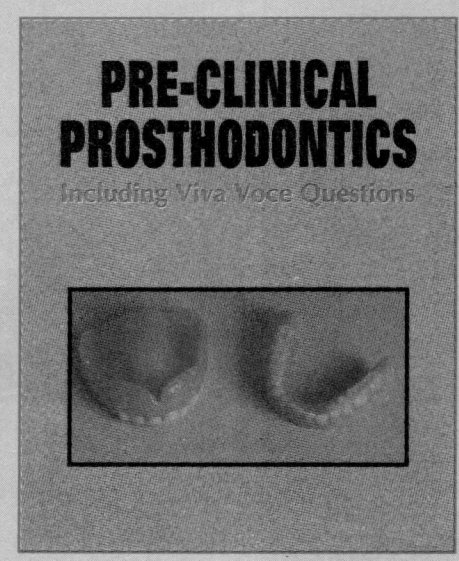

to

our

parents

PREFACE

The compilers have aimed at bringing out a comprehensive book *Pre-Clinical Operative Dentistry and Endodontics*, which should ideally be able to meet the requirements of the First and Second BDS students. Though a few Indian editions are available on this subject, most of them, unfortunately, are based on *viva voce* questions only. It is a well known fact that the students have to study from at least four to five textbooks for this speciality. And, it is also true that it is a complicated task for them in the early phase of the course. In an attempt to overcome this hazard, we have come up with the present edition which provides the students both the theory part (in a simplified logical manner) as well as *the viva* voce questions.

Although utmost care has been taken in preparing the text material, any slipups are purely coincidental and are regretted. As this is the first book of this kind, a few lapses are inevitable. We, therefore, welcome the suggestions from both the teachers as well as the students for further improvement in the latter editions. Helpful comments will be duly acknowledged.

Dr. Narendranatha Reddy P.
Dr. Vanitha N.

drpnnreddy@hotmail.com
drvanithan@hotmail.com

Acknowledgements

First and foremost, we would like to express our deep gratitude to our beloved teacher Dr. Vipool H. Malkan, Professor and Head, Department of Conservative Dentistry and Endodontics, Sri Rajiv Gandhi College of Dental Sciences, Bangalore, for his immense and constant support.

We are indebted to Dr. Yellappa G., Professor and Head, Department of P and SD; Dr. Rayeesa Saleem, Professor, Department of OD and E; and Dr. Arun Jacob Silas, Principal, SRGCDS, Bangalore; for their endless encouragement.

We are appreciative of Dr. Hari Kiran, Dr. Rajasekhara Reddy, Dr. Lokeswara Reddy, Dr. K.S.R. Prasad, Dr. Nidhi Sinha, Dr. Sashikanth, Dr. Naveen, Dr. Revanth, Dr. Rishidhar, Dr. Srinivas, Dr. Apoorva, Dr. Jenny, Dr. Siddhartha Varma, Dr. Kalyan, Dr. Rajesh and Dr. Subhash in lending their hand in the preparation of this work.

We extend our heartfelt thanks to our friend Mr. Babu Prasad, DTP operator, for his excellent typeset and graphic work.

We are obliged to Mr. Satish Kumar Jain, Managing Director, who came forward to publish this title, and also to Mr. Y.N. Arjuna, Publishing Director, and Mr. Deepak Rao, General Manager (South), CBS Publishers & Distributors, for their cooperation in this project.

Last but not least, we are grateful to our parents and family members for their tolerance of our absence and their sustained backup.

Dr. Narendranatha Reddy P.
Dr. Vanitha N.

About the Book

The main gist of the material on *Pre-Clinical Operative Dentistry and Endodontics* is presented under six sections. The brief description of each section is given here to give an overview of the topics presented.

The first and the foremost is *Section I: Operative Dentistry* which describes the topics right from the identification of teeth to the more complex issues like operating dental instruments, dental caries, principles of cavity preparation and restorations, etc.

Section II: Endodontics describes concisely the internal anatomy of the tooth, etiology of pulp and periapical diseases, rationale of endodontic therapy with an outline of RCT along with the endodontic instruments, materials used and various pulpal procedures with a feather-touch on surgical endodontics.

Section III: Dental Biomaterials provides information regarding restorative materials used in operative dentistry.

Section IV: Pre-Clinical Operative Work Area describes about the working area of conservative dentistry including the phantom head jaws and typhodont teeth, etc.

Section V: Foundation to Clinical Dentistry portraits about clinical environment by describing the infection control methods, instrument processing and sterilization and operating field along with isolation and moisture control.

And the last *Section VI: The Review* presents a set of about 500 *viva voce* questions to test the reader's ability of having fully grasped the subject.

CONTENTS

Section II
ENDODONTICS

Section III
DENTAL BIOMATERIALS

Section IV
PRE-CLINICAL OPERATIVE WORK AREA

Section V
FOUNDATION TO CLINICAL DENTISTRY

Section VI
THE REVIEW

About the Course

Operative Dentistry and Endodontics is a branch of dentistry that explores the methods of keeping and using tooth without extracting and is a science which researches arresting disease of teeth hard tissues and restoration of failure tooth. Viewed from a much broader perspective, however, the discipline assumes much greater importance within the total spectrum of dentistry. It has often been described as "bread and butter" of dentistry since it generally comprises the largest percentage of the clinical work load of most general practitioners. Coming to the academic perspective, this is one of the two subjects that will be studied throughout the BDS course from first to the final year, although the theory examination will be given in the last year (the other subject being *prosthodontics,* which deals with the replacement of missing teeth). The clinical part of the course will commence in the third year. To get accustomed to the clinical environment, a laboratory curriculum called *Pre-Clinical Operative Dentistry and Endodontics* is designed and is followed for the first two years of the BDS programme. It introduces the student to the fundamental principles of operative dentistry techniques, focusing on various cavity preparation designs (will be learning on extracted teeth or artificial teeth), indications, correct manipulation and utilization of numerous restorative materials. It has only University practical examination (no theory examination) which will be held at the end of the second year. The University examination consists of *Spotters identification* (of various instruments and materials commonly used), *Preparation of Class II Conventional Cavity for Silver Amalgam in Maxillary or Mandibular I or II Molar tooth* (Typhodont/ Natural Tooth) and a *Viva Voce* test. This course is intended to prepare you as fully as possible for your introduction to clinical operative dentistry. With successful completion of your laboratory training, you should now be prepared to apply those basic principles and techniques in clinical practice. Your admittance into the clinic is an implied departmental trust that you possess the requisite baseline skills necessary to treat patients.

Section I
Operative Dentistry

CHAPTER 01

INTRODUCTION

– Historically, Operative Dentistry has been the primary nucleus of the dental practice. It includes everything from the prevention of caries and reminerlization of initial carious attacks to complex restorative treatments. More than a century of clinical experience has provided tradition for the treatment that are deep rooted in the dental profession.

DEFINITION OF OPERATIVE DENTISTRY

– *Operative Dentistry is the art and science of the diagnosis, treatment, and prognosis of defects of teeth that do not require full coverage restorations for the correction. Such treatment should result in the restoration of proper tooth form, function, and esthetics while maintaining the physiologic integrity of the teeth in a harmonius relationship with the adjacent hard and soft tissues, all of which should enhance the general health and welfare of the patient.*

AIMS AND OBJECTIVES

1. Diagnosis of the extent and location(s) of the lesions.

2. Prevention of the disease.

3. Interruption, i.e. prevention of further loss of the tooth structure.

4. Preservation of the vitality and important anatomy of the remaining sound tooth structure.

5. Restoration of health.

6. Preservation of esthetics.

"Father of Modern Operative Dentistry" and "The Grand Old Man of Dentistry"
                                        – Dr. G.V. Black

In this chapter, you will learn the names and location of various types of teeth in the human dentition with their functions and how they relate to each other in the same dental arch and to the teeth in the opposing arch. In preparation for learning dental charting for clinical examination, you will also learn the common systems of teeth numbering.

CHAPTER 02

DENTITIONS AN OVERVIEW

DENTITION PERIODS

- During a lifetime, people have two sets of teeth, the *Primary Dentition* and the *Permanent Dentition*.

- *Dentition* describes the natural teeth in the dental arch.

- Although there are only two sets of teeth, there are *Three Dentition Periods*, i.e. *Primary, Mixed and Permanent*.

1. PRIMARY DENTITION PERIOD

- The first set of 20 primary teeth is called the *Primary Dentition*.

- It is also referred to as deciduous dentition or milk teeth or baby teeth.

- Only primary teeth are present in the mouth during this period.

- This period occurs between approximately six months and six years of age.

- Primary dention period begins with the eruption of the primary mandibular central incisors and ends when the first permanent mandibular molar erupts.

2. MIXED DENTITION PERIOD

- During this period, children will have both primary and permanent teeth in their mouth.

- It occurs between the ages of about 6 to 12 years.

- In this period, children will lose their primary teeth and the permanent teeth begin to erupt.

- This period begins with the eruption of the first permanent tooth and ends with the shedding of the last primary tooth.

3. PERMANENT DENTITION PERIOD

- Permanent dentition refers to the 32 secondary teeth or adult teeth.

- Permanent teeth that replace the primary teeth are called *succedaneous teeth*, meaning that these teeth "succeed " (come after) deciduous teeth.

– Because there are 20 primary teeth, there are also 20 seccedaneous teeth. Molars are *not* succedaneous teeth because the premolars replace the primary molars.

– This period begins at about 12 years of age when the last primary tooth is shed.

– After eruption of the permanent canines and premolars, and the eruption of the second permanent molars, the permanent dentition is completed at about age of 14 to 15 years, except for third molars which are not erupted until about the age of 18 to 25 years.

DENTAL ARCHES

– In human mouth, there are *two* dental arches, the *Maxillary* and the *Mandibular*.

– Sometimes it may refer to the Maxillary arch as the *Upper Jaw / Upper Arch* and the Mandibular arch as the *Lower Jaw / Lower Arch*.

1. Maxillary arch

– Which is actually part of the skull and is not capable of movement.

– The teeth of the upper arch are set in the maxilla (the maxillary bone).

2. Mandibular arch

– Movable through the action of the temporomandibular joint.

– Applies force against the immovable maxillary arch.

– When the teeth of both arches are in contact, then the teeth are said to be in *Occlusion*.

QUADRANTS

– When the maxillary and mandibular arches are each divided into halves, the resulting four sections are called *Quadrants* and the dental arch is expressed by a cross (Fig. 2.1 A and B).

– They are as follows,

1. Maxillary Right Quadrant

2. Maxillary Left Quadrant

3. Mandibular Left Quadrant

4. Mandibular Right Quadrant

MAXILLARY RIGHT	MAXILLARY LEFT
MANDIBULAR RIGHT	MANDIBULAR LEFT

– Sometimes it is simplified to denote *maxillary right* as ⌋, *maxillary left* as ⌊, *mandibular right* as ⌐ and *mandibular left* as ⌐.

– Each quadrant of permanent dentition contains eight permanent teeth ($4 \times 8 = 32$) and a quadrant of Primary dentition contains five teeth ($4 \times 5 = 20$).

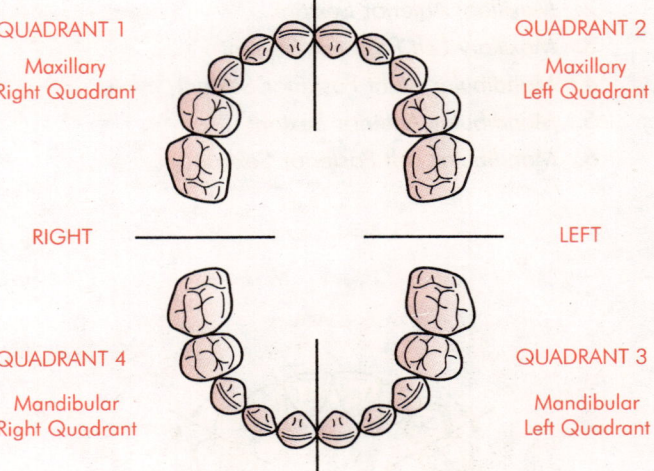

QUADRANT 1
Maxillary Right Quadrant

QUADRANT 2
Maxillary Left Quadrant

RIGHT　　　LEFT

QUADRANT 4
Mandibular Right Quadrant

QUADRANT 3
Mandibular Left Quadrant

Fig. 2.1A Primary dentition seperated into quadrants

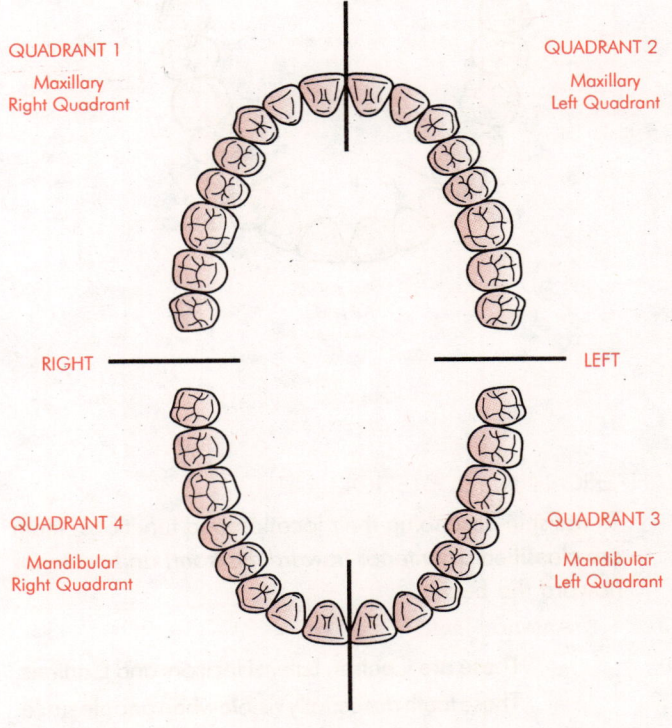

QUADRANT 1
Maxillary Right Quadrant

QUADRANT 2
Maxillary Left Quadrant

RIGHT　　　LEFT

QUADRANT 4
Mandibular Right Quadrant

QUADRANT 3
Mandibular Left Quadrant

Fig. 2.1B Permanent dentition seperated into quadrants

SEXTANTS

– Each arch can also be divided into sextants rather than quadrants.
– A sextant is one sixth of the dentition.
– There are three sextants in each arch (Fig. 2.2).
– They are as follows,
  1. *Maxillary Right Posterior Sextant*
  2. *Maxillary Anterior Sextant*
  3. *Maxillary Left Posterior Sextant*
  4. *Mandibular Right Posterior Sextant*
  5. *Mandibular Anterior Sextant*
  6. *Mandibular Left Posterior Sextant*

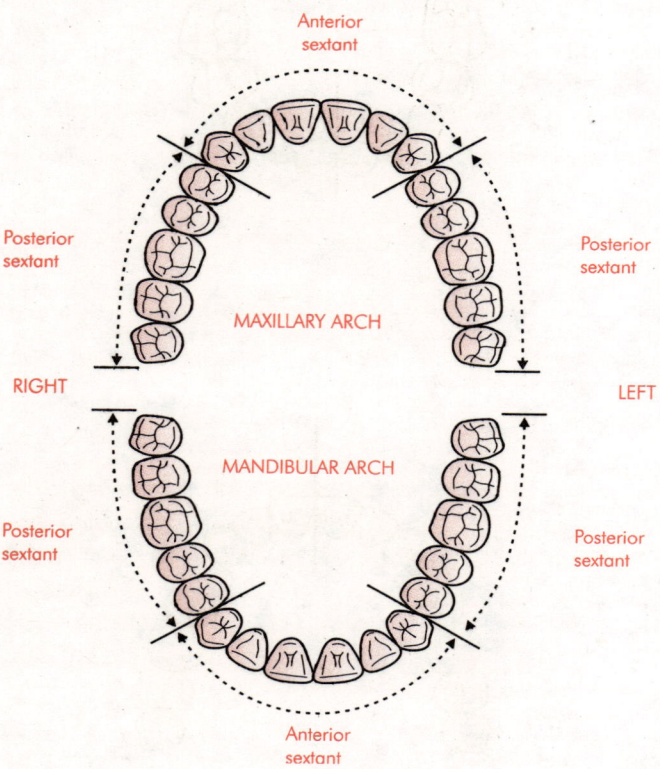

Fig. 2.2 Permanent dentition seperated into sextants

ANTERIOR AND POSTERIOR TEETH

– To assist in describing their location and functions, teeth are classified as *anterior (toward the front)* and *posterior (toward the back)*.

1. Anterior Teeth

– These are Central, Lateral Incisors and Canines.
– These teeth are usually visible when people smile.
– Anterior teeth are aligned in gentle curve.

2. Posterior Teeth

– These are Premolars and Molars.
– These teeth are aligned with little or no curvature and appear to be in an almost straight line.

TEETH—TYPES and FUNCTIONS

– Humans are omnivorous, which means they eat both meat and plants.
– To occomodate this variety in diet, human teeth are designed for cutting, tearing and grinding different types of food.

TYPES OF TEETH

– The permanent dentition is divided into four types of teeth, i.e. Incisors, Canines, Premolars and Molars.
– The primary dentition has Incisors, Canines and Molars. There are no Premolars in the primary dention.

1. Incisors

– These are single-rooted teeth with a relatively sharp, thin edge.
– They are located at the front of the mouth and are designed to cut the food without the application of heavy forces.
– The lingual surface (tongue side) is shaped like a shovel to aid in guiding the food into the mouth.

2. Canines

– They are also known as "cuspids".
– They are located at the "corner" of the dental arch.
– They are designed for cutting and tearing the food which require the application of force.
– Canines are the *longest teeth* in the human dentition.
– They are also some of the best-anchored and most stable teeth because of their longest route.
– They usually the last teeth to be last.
– Because of its sturdy crown, long route and location in the dental arch, it is refered to as the "corner stone" of the dental arch.

3. Premolars

– There are four maxillary and four mandibular premolars.
– Occasionally, the premolars are also refered to as *bicuspids*, which is inaccurate term because it refers to *two* (bi) cusps and some premolars have three cusps. Therefore, the newer term *premolar* is prefered.

– The pointed buccal cusps hold the food while the lingual cusps grind it.

– They also have a broader surface for chewing the food.

– There are no premolars in the primary dentition.

4. **Molars**

– These are much larger than premolars, usually having four or more cusps.

– Their function is to chew or grind up the food.

– Maxillary and mandibular molars differ greatly from each other in shape, size, number of cusps and roots.

TOOTH SURFACES

– The coronal portion of each tooth is divided into surfaces that are named according to related anatomic landmarks, i.e. (Fig. 2.3 A).

Mesial	-	*toward the anterior midline.*
Distal	-	*away from the anterior midline.*
Buccal	-	*toward the cheek. [Facial (refers to either buccal or labial)]*
Labial	-	*toward the lip [facial (refers to either buccal or labial)]*
Lingual	-	*toward the tongue.*
Occlusal	-	*masticating surface of a bicuspid or molar.*
Incisal	-	*functional edge of anterior tooth.*
Cervical	-	*related to cervix or neck of tooth.*
Gingival	-	*close to or in proximity of gingiva.*

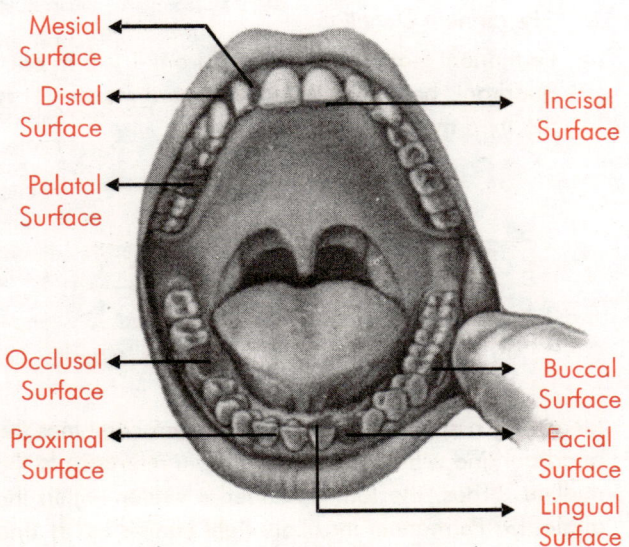

Mesial Surface
Distal Surface
Palatal Surface
Occlusal Surface
Proximal Surface
Incisal Surface
Buccal Surface
Facial Surface
Lingual Surface

Fig. 2.3 A

– The naming is further simplified by representing by the first letter of the surface or by numbering as follows (Fig. 2.3 B).

Surface	Letter	Numerical exponent
Mesial	1	M
Distal	2	D
Labial/Buccal (Facial)	3	F
Lingual	4	L
Occulusal/Incisal	5	O/I

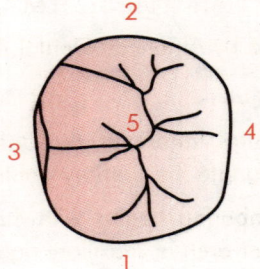

Fig. 2.3 B

– The occlusal surfaces of some teeth are divided by an oblique or transverse ridge of enamel extending from buccal to lingual surface. Ex: Maxillary first molar, Maxillary second molar and Mandibular first bicuspid. The numerical exponent 5 is used to indicate the mesial occlusal surface and the exponent 6 indicates the distal occlusal surface (Fig. 2.3 C).

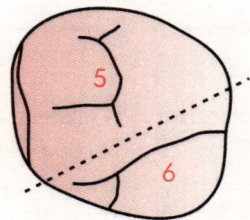

Fig. 2.3 C

– Combining the tooth number and the surface exponent or letter is used to designate the location of the carious lesion. Ex: A mesial proximal carious lesion of the mandibular left first molar is indicated by 19^1 or 19M.

The site of the proposed cavity preparation is therefore designated as 19^{1-5} or 19 MO. When the buccal groove of this tooth involved as an extension of the occlusal it is indicated as 19^{1-5-3} or 19 MOB.

TOOTH NUMBERING SYSTEMS

- Numbering systems are used as a simplified means of identifying the teeth for charting and descriptive purposes.

- There are over 12 systems are available for the recording of different teeth and teeth surfaces. Different notations are used for the permanent and deciduous dentition.

- Currently, three numbering systems are more popular in dentistry. They are described below,

1. UNIVERSAL / NATIONAL SYSTEM

- Approved by American Dental Association (ADA).

A. Primary Dentition

- Capital letters 'A' through 'T' are used to designate the primary dentition.

- Numbering begins with the right side of the upper arch at maxillary right second molar as 'A', following the arch to the maxillary left second molar (J) and then continuous to the mandibular left second molar (K), following the arch to the right side and terminates at the second molar as 'T'.

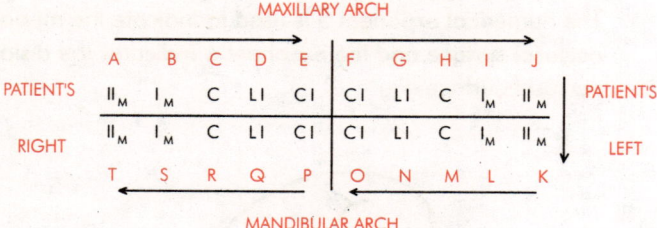

CI - Central Incisor , LI - Lateral Incisor, C - Canine, I_M - First Molar, II_M - Second Molar.

B. Permanent Dentition

- Teeth are numbered from 1 to 32 starting with the third molar (1) on the right side of the upper arch, following around the arch to the third molar (16) on the left side, descending to the lower third molar (17) on the left side and following that arch to the lower right third molar (32).

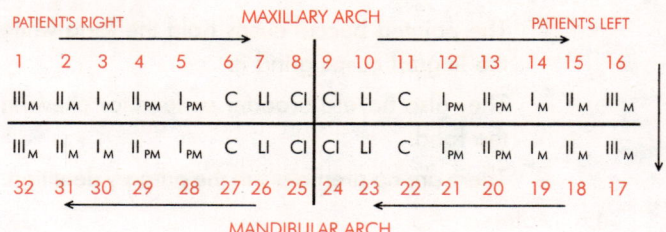

CI - Central Incisor , LI - Lateral Incisor, C - Canine, I_PM - First Premolar, II_PM - Second Premolar, I_M - First Molar, II_M - Second Molar, III_M - Third Molar.

2. ZSIGMONDY/PALMER SYSTEM

- Oldest and most widely used method.

- This notation designates each tooth based on its location in a quadrant.

- A horizontal line separates the maxillary and the mandibular arches.

- A vertical midline separates the patient's right and left side of the mouth.

A. Primary Dentition

- Deciduous teeth are designated with the capital letters beginning with the central incisor (A) to the second molar (E) in each quadrant.

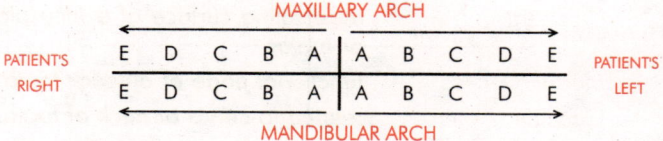

B. Permanent Dentition

- Permanent teeth are numbered from 1 – 8 in each quadrant, beginning with the central incisor (1) to the third molar (8).

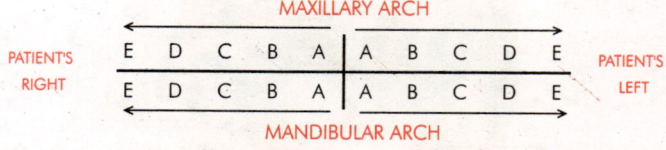

- Identifying a specific tooth by this system combines the quadrant grid with the tooth number in reference to the midline. Thus, the tooth number is written within the angle. Ex: Permanent maxillary right canine as $\underline{3|}$ and deciduous mandibular left second molar as $\overline{|E}$.

3. FEDERATION DENTAIRE INTERNATIONAL (FDI) / INTERNATIONAL NUMBERING SYSTEM / TWO DIGIT SYSTEM / ISO SYSTEM

- In this system 2 digits are used for each tooth.
- First digit indicates the quadrant, i.e.

Permanent teeth		Deciduous teeth	
Maxillary right	- 1	*Maxillary right*	- 5
Maxillary left	- 2	*Maxillary left*	- 6
Mandibular left	- 3	*Mandibular left*	- 7
Mandibular right	- 4	*Mandibular right*	- 8

- Second digit indicates the specific tooth within the quadrant (1 to 8 for permanent teeth, 1 to 5 for deciduous teeth).

- Thus, in this system combination of numbers from 11 through 48 represent permanent teeth and numbers from 51 through 85 represent deciduous teeth.

- The digits should be pronounced separately, i.e. permanent cuspids are teeth one-three, two-three, three-three and four-three.

A. Primary Dentition

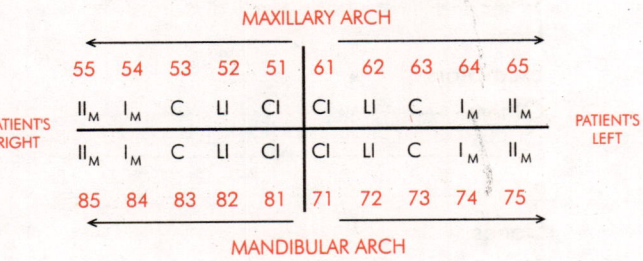

B. Permanent Dentition

MAXILLARY ARCH

PATIENT'S RIGHT ← → PATIENT'S LEFT

18	17	16	15	14	13	12	11	21	22	23	24	25	26	27	28
III$_M$	II$_M$	I$_M$	II$_{PM}$	I$_{PM}$	C	LI	CI	CI	LI	C	I$_{PM}$	II$_{PM}$	I$_M$	II$_M$	III$_M$
III$_M$	II$_M$	I$_M$	II$_{PM}$	I$_{PM}$	C	LI	CI	CI	LI	C	I$_{PM}$	II$_{PM}$	I$_M$	II$_M$	III$_M$
48	47	46	45	44	43	42	41	31	32	33	34	35	36	37	38

MANDIBULAR ARCH

Advantages

1. Simple to understand and to teach.

2. Easy to pronounce during conversation.

3. Easy to translate into computer.

4. Easy to adapt to standard charts used in general practice.

THE SAFEST METHOD

- Out of the existing systems for noting the dentition, there is no system which is poll proof.

- The safest method is to write full description of the teeth. Ex: Upper left first permanent molar.

SUPERNUMERARY TEETH DESIGNATION

- The symbol 'S' is used to dentoe the supernumerary tooth, noting the nearest normal adjacent tooth.

CHAPTER 03

OPERATIVE DENTAL INSTRUMENTS

A wide variety of dental instruments are used in dentistry today. This chapter describes the design and purpose of the dental instruments that are most commonly used by the dentist for general restorative procedures. Dental supply companies manufacture many variations of instruments in order to accomodate personel preferences. While studying the instruments in this chapter, you will learn that each instrument is designed for specific areas of a tooth as well as for the specific needs of the dentist.

CLASSIFICATION OF OPERATIVE DENTAL INSTRUMENTS

- Operative dental instruments are classified into the following types based on their functions,

1. Diagnostic Instruments
   - Mouth mirrors
   - Explorer
   - Periodontal probe
2. Cutting Instruments
   i. *Hand*
      - Hatchets
      - Chisels
      - Hoes
      - Excavators
      - Others
   ii. *Rotary*
      - Burs
      - Stones
      - Discs
      - Others
3. Condensing Instruments
   Pluggers
      - Hand
      - Mechanical
4. Plastic Instruments
   - Spatulas
   - Carvers
   - Burnishers
   - Packing instruments
5. Finishing and Polishing Instruments
   i. *Hand*
      - Orange wood sticks
      - Polishing points
      - Finishing strips

ii. *Rotary*

Finishing burs

Mounted brushes

Mounted stones

Rubber cups

Impregnated disks and wheels

6. **Isolation Instruments**

Rubberdam

Saliva ejector

Cotton roll holder

Evacuation tips and equipment

7. **Accessory Instruments**

Tweezers

Scissors

Howe pliers

Dappen dish

Others

DIAGNOSTIC INSTRUMENTS

These instruments allow the operator to thoroughly examine the health status of the oral cavity.

1. MOUTH MIRROR

– Designed to have a straight handle, a slight handle to the shank and a working end with a round metal disc and a mirror on one side (Fig. 3.1).

– The mirror can have a flat or concave surface.

– Concave surfaced ones are used to magnify the image.

– Double-sided mirrors also available which are used to retract the tongue ar cheek and view intraoral cavity simultaneously.

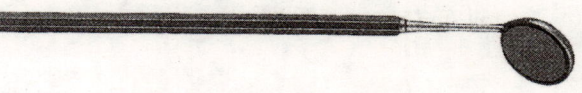

Fig. 3.1

Uses (Fig. 3.2 A to D)

1. **Indirect vision** allows the operator to see areas of the mouth that are not visible with direct vision.

2. **Light reflection** directs light into the areas of the mouth that are not directly accessible with the operating light.

3. **Retraction** maintains a clear operating field by keeping the tongue or cheek out of the way during the procedure.

4. **Tissue protection** helps guard the tongue or cheek against accidental injury from a dental bur.

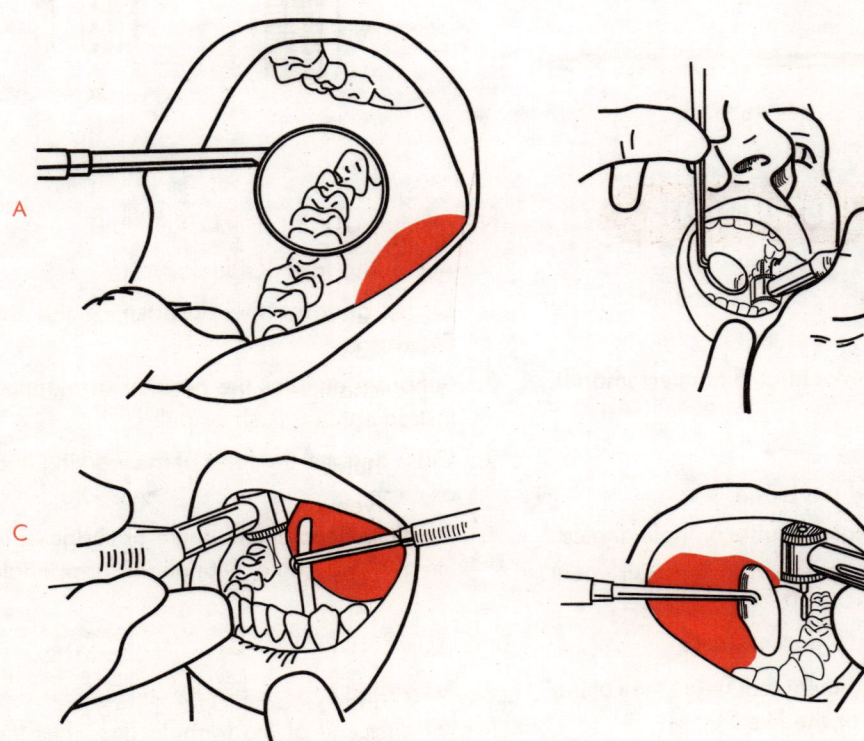

Fig. 3.2

2. EXPLORERS

– Are multifunctional instruments that are used to examine the teeth for caries, calculus, furcations or other abnormalities (Fig. 3.3).

– Many shapes of explorers available but all will have thin, flexible, wire like working end with a sharp point at the tip.

– This thin tip enables the operator to use *tactile* sensitivity to distinguish areas of decay or calculus from discrepancies on the surface of the teeth.

– Common types of explorers are the right angle, pig tail and shepherd's hook.

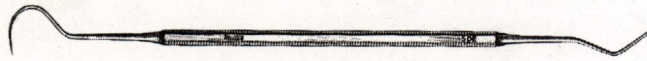

Fig. 3.3 Shepherd's hook

3. PERIODONTAL PROBE

– Used to measure the sulcus or pocket depth of the periodontium of each tooth (Fig. 3.4).

– This measurement provides the cilinician with the overall gingival health of that area.

– The working end of the instrument has calibrated markings in millimeters, which are easier to read. Some probes are colour-coded to enhance reading.

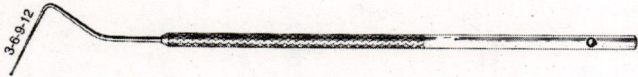

Fig. 3.4

HAND CUTTING INSTRUMENTS

PARTS OF AN INSTRUMENT (Fig. 3.5 A and B)

1. Handle/Shaft

– It may be small, medium or large diameter; smooth, knarled or serrated.

2. Shank

– Connects the shaft and the blade.

– It may be straight or single, double or triple angled.

– It is here where any angulation in the instrument can be placed.

3. Blade / Nib

– It is that part of the instrument that bears the cutting edge, condenser face or the like.

– It is the functional end of the instrument.

– It begins at the angle that terminates the shank (last angle if there is more than one).

– The blade ends in the cutting edge.

4. Cutting edge

– It is the working part of the instrument.

– It is usually in the form of a bevel with different shapes.

5. Blade angle

– It is the angle between the long axis of the blade and the long axis of the shaft.

6. Cutting edge angle

– It is an angle between the margin of the cutting edge and the long axis of the shaft.

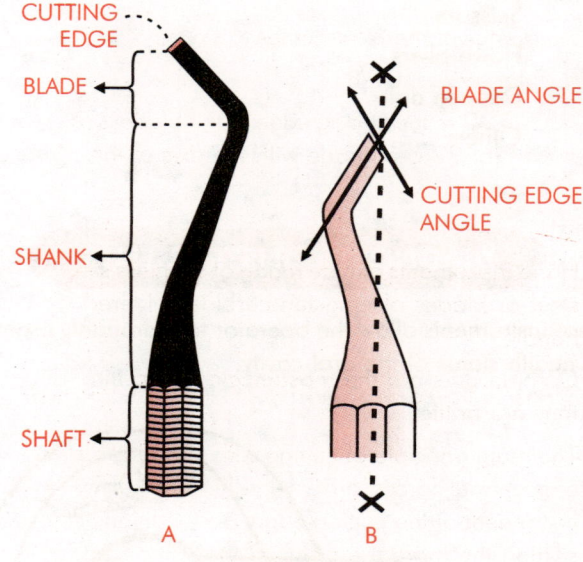

Fig. 3.5

NOMENCLATURE OF INSTRUMENT

– **According to G.V. Black,**

1. *Order* denotes the purpose of the instrument. Ex: Excavator.

2. *Suborder* denotes the position or manner of use of the instrument. Ex: Push or pull.

3. *Class* denotes the form of the working end. Ex : Hatchet or chisel.

4. *Subclass* denotes the angle or shape of the shank. Ex : Staight - no angle, Monangle - one angle.

INSTRUMENT FORMULA

– **According to G.V. Black,**

1. *The first unit* of the formula describes *the width of the blade in tenths of a millimeter*.

2. *The second unit* describes *the length of the blade in millimeters.*

3. *The third unit* describes *the angle the blade forms with the axis of the handle.* This angle is expressed in "hundredths" of a circle or in centigrades.

   Ex : *Binangle hatchet : (15-8-12)*

   – 15 = blade width 1.5 millimeters.

   – 8 = blade length 8 millimeters.

   – 12 = blade angled 12 centigrade from axis of handle or shaft.

4. *A fourth unit* is added to the basic instrument formula and is expressed in centigrades which represents the *angle formed between cutting edge and central axis of the shaft.* It is placed in the second position of the formula.

   Ex : *Gingival margin trimmer (distal):*

   12 - 92 - 10 - 8

   – 92 = the cutting edge of the blade is at an angle of 92 centigrade with the axis of the shaft.

INSTRUMENT DESIGN

– Hand instruments can be made of stainless steel, carbon steel or blades of tungsten carbide soldered to a steel handle.

– Carbide burs are the most efficient in cutting although they are brittle.

– The main principle of cutting with hand instruments is to concentrate forces on a very thin cross-section of the instrument at the cutting edge. So the thinner the cross-section the more the pressure that is concentrated and the more efficient the instrument will be.

1. Direct Cutting and Lateral Cutting Instruments

– *Direct cutting instrument is the one in which the force is applied in the same plane as to the blade and handle. It is called as a 'Single-planed' instrument. It can be used in direct and lateral cutting.*

– *Lateral cutting instrument is the one in which the force is applied at a right angle to the plane of the blade and handle. Usually it has a curved blade and is called as 'Double bladed' instrument. It has angle or curve in a plane at a right angle to that of the handle. It can only be used in lateral cutting.*

2. Contrangling

– In order to gain access to use many instruments, bend the shank at one or more points to angle of the blade relative to the handle.

– The extent of this depends on the length of the blade and the degree of angulation in the shank.

– Accordingly the working point is moved out of line with the axis of the handle. If this occurs to more than 3 mm from the handle axis (its imaginary continuation), the instrument will be out of balance in lateral cutting motions, and force will be required to keep the instrument from rotating in the hand.

– To overcome this modern operative instruments are designed to possess one or more angles in the shank, placing the working point with in 3 mm from the axis of the handle. *This principle of design is called `Contrangling'.*

– A short blade and small blade angle requires only binangle contrangling, while longer blades and greater blade angles require triple angle contrangling.

3. Right and Left Instruments

– Direct cutting instruments can be made into right or left by placing a bevel on one side of the blade. *Identification of right and left of the instrument: If the instrument is held with the cutting edge down and pointing away from the operator and the bevel is on the right side, it will be a right instrument. If the bevel is on the left it will be a left instrument.* For cutting, the non beveled side of the blade should be in contact with the wall being cut.

– Lateral cutting instruments can be made into right or left by placing the curve or angle either on the right or on the left side. *Identification of right and left of the instrument: Holding the instrument with its blade down and cutting pointing away, the instrument having that curve of the blade directed to the right is a right instrument and vice versa for the left.*

– Both right and left instruments can be used in the same cavity and in any tooth.

4. Single Bevelled Instruments

– These are single planed instruments with the cutting edge is at a right angle to the long axis of the shaft. *Identification of mesial and distal of the instrument:* If they are bevelled on the side away from the shaft, they are called *distally bevelled.* If they are bevelled on the side of the blade towards the shaft, they are called *mesially bevelled.*

– If these instruments have no angle in the shank, or an angle of 12° or less, they can be used in push (direct cutting) and scraping motions (bevelled to non-bevelled side).

- If the angle in the shank exceeds 12° the instrument could be used in pull (distally bevelled) and push (mesially bevelled) motions.

5. Bibevelled Instruments

- Only hatchets and straight chisels are bibevelled.
- The blade is equally bevelled on the both sides.
- They cut by pushing them in the direction of the long axis of the blade.

6. Triple Bevelled Instruments

- They are made by bevelling the blade laterally, along with the end, which results in three distinct cutting edges.
- Most modern single planed instruments (especially the small ones) are of triple bevelled which can increase cutting efficiency.

7. Circumferentially Bevelled Instruments

- A circumferential bevel is produced by bevelling the blade at all its peripheries.
- It is usually found in double planed instruments.

8. Single-ended and Double-ended instruments

- Single ended instruments are confined to those types of instruments having only one specific function.
- Most modern instruments are double ended which incorporates the right and left or the mesial and distal form of the instrument in the same handle.

CLASSIFICATION

- Hand cutting instruments are classified into,
  I. Excavators
  II. Chisels
  III. Special forms of chisels

I. EXCAVATORS

- Designed for the excavation of the carious dentin and for the shaping of the internal portions of the cavities.
- They are of five types

  1. *Hatchet Excavators*

     - Have the edge of the blade in parallel with the handle.
     - Usually single-planed, bibevelled instruments.
     - They cut by pushing and pull motion in the direction of the blade.
     - Use: For cleaving the enamel in incisors.
     - Instrument Formula: 6 - 2 - 12; 6 - 2 - 23.

2. *Hoe Excavators*

   - Bevel is at a right angle to the shaft (Fig. 3.6).
   - They are available in distally bevelled and mesially bevelled types.
   - Are single planed instruments with the possibility of four types of movements, i.e. vertical, pull (push), right and left.
   - Use: For cutting mesial and distal walls of premolars and molars.
   - Instrument Formula: 6 - 2 - 10; 12 - 6 - 10.

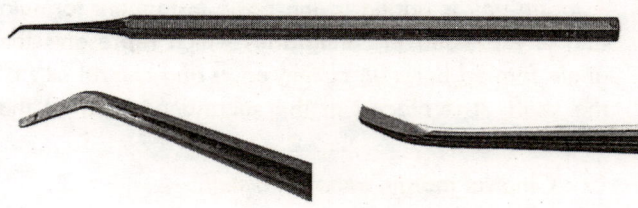

Fig. 3.6

3. *Spoon Excavators*

   - Available in pairs, i.e. left and right (Fig. 3.7).
   - Cutting edge is a semi-circular circumferential bevel and is sharpened to a thin edge.
   - It is a double planed instrument with the possibility of right or left cutting movements only.
   - Use: For the excavation of caries.
   - Instrument Formula: 8 - 6 - 12 (L)
     8 - 6 - 12 (R)
     13 - 8 - 12 (L)
     13 - 8 - 12 (R)

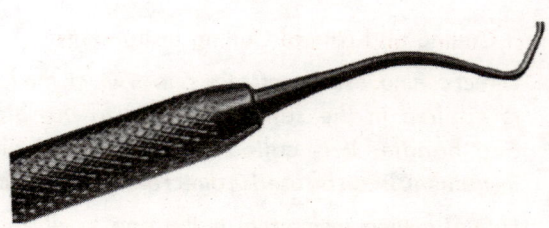

Fig. 3.7

4. *Discoid (Disc like) Excavators*

   - Have a circular blade, with a cutting edge extending around the periphery except where it joins to the shank (Fig. 3.8).
   - It is a double planed instrument with the possibility of right or left cutting movements only.

– **Use:** For the excavation of caries.

For carving metallic restorations.

– Instrument Formula: 2 0 - 2 - 12.

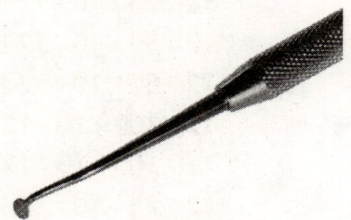

Fig. 3.8

5. Cleoid (Claw like) Excavators

– It resembles a 'claw', so the name 'cleoid' (Fig. 3.9).

– Use: In amalgam carving, burnishing and finishing of cohesive and cast gold restoration and in excavation of caries from the areas of difficult access.

– It is a double planed instrument with the possibility of lateral cutting movements only.

– Instrument Formula: 10 - 2 - 12.

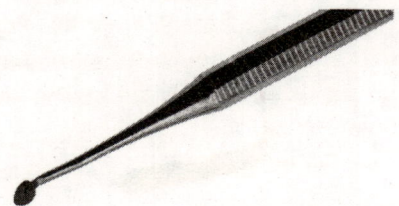

Fig. 3.9

II. CHISELS

– Are used for the cutting of enamel.

– Are usually bevelled on one side only.

– They are of four types.

1. Straight Chisels

– Have a straight blade in line with the handle and shank (Fig. 3.10).

– Bevel of the blade is at right angle to the shaft.

– Are single planed instruments with the possibility of five types of cutting movements, i.e. vertical, right, left, push and pull.

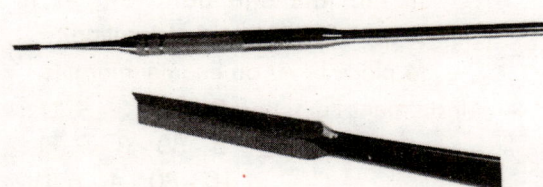

Fig. 3.10

2. Monangle Chisels

– Has a single angle between the shaft and the blade.

– Are similar to straight chisels but the blade is at an angle to the shaft.

– It may be mesially or distally bevelled.

3. Binangle Chisels

– As the name implies, there are two angles between the shaft and the blade (Fig. 3.11).

– Blade is at a right angle to the shaft as in the Hoe.

– It may be mesially or distally bevelled.

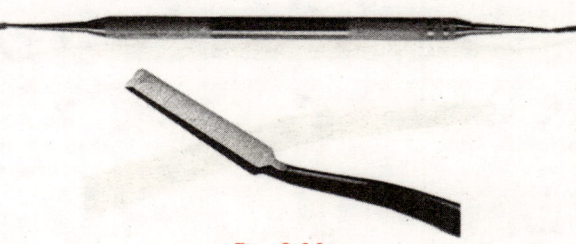

Fig. 3.11

– Use: The above mentioned three types of chisels are used for the cutting of undermined enamel.

4. Triple Angle Chisel

– Has three angles in its shank.

– It may be mesially or distally bevelled.

– Use: Usually used to flatten pulpal floors.

– Monangle, Binangle and Triple angle chisels are single planed instruments with the possibility of three cutting movements, i.e. vertical, right and left.

– Mesially bevelled chisels cut in push movements and distally bevelled ones cut in pull movements.

III. SPECIAL FORMS OF CHISELS

– Are designed to perform specific functions.

1. Enamel Hatchets

– The shank has one or more angles or curves (Fig. 3.12).

– The blade is in the same plane as with angle or angles.

– The cutting edge is parallel to the shaft.

– They may be paired, i.e. right or left or may be bibevelled.

– Uses: For cleaving undermined enamel in proximal cavities and on buccal and lingual walls where it is not possible to use a chisel.

- The smaller sizes are primarily used in anterior teeth, although are useful in bicuspids and molars.
- Larger sizes are mainly used in posterior teeth.
- Are single planed instruments with the possibility of four types of movements, i.e. vertical, push, pull and either right or left lateral cutting.
- Instrument Formula: 15 - 8 - 12 (L)
  15 - 8 - 12 (R)
  20 - 9 - 12 (L)
  20 - 9 - 12 (R)

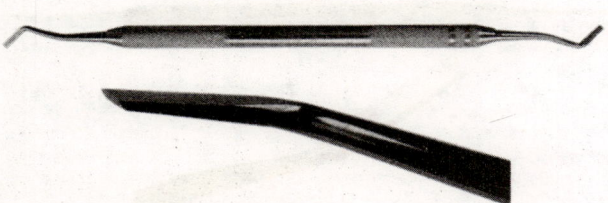

Fig. 3.12

2. *Gingival Margin Trimmers*

- Are similar to spoon excavators in both of their angles and the dimensions of their blades.
- Available in two pairs constituting a set of four.
- In a given size each pair has a right and a left bevelled instrument.
- If the cutting edge of the other pair makes an acute angle with that edge of the blade nearer to the handle, those are *Mesial GMTs* (Fig. 3.13).
- If the cutting edge of one pair makes an acute angle with that edge of the blade away from the handle, those are *Distal GMTs* (Fig. 3.14).
- Mesial GMT is used for removing the unsupported enamel rods from the gingival cavosurface margin of any mesial cavity and the buccal box.
- Distal GMT is used for removing the unsupported enamel rods from the gingival cavosurface margin of any distal cavity and the lingual or palatal box.
- *Uses*
  i. For trimming the margins of the various walls of the cavity preparation.
  ii. For bevelling gingival floor.
  iii. For forming sharp angles in the cavity preparation.

- They are primarily lateral cutting instruments.
- Instrument Formula
  i. *Amalgam:* 12 - 95 - 10 - 12 (L) ⎤ D
     12 - 95 - 10 - 12 (R) ⎦
     12 - 80 - 10 - 12 (L) ⎤ M
     12 - 80 - 10 - 12 (R) ⎦
  ii. *Inlay:* 12 - 100 - 10 - 12 (L) ⎤ D
     12 - 100 - 10 - 12 (R) ⎦
     12 - 75 - 10 - 12 (L) ⎤ M
     12 - 75 - 10 - 12 (R) ⎦

L - Left; R - Right; D - Distal; M - Mesial.

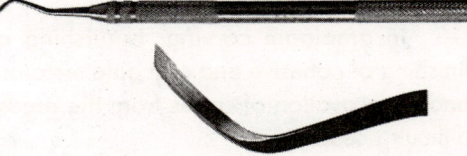

Fig. 3.13 GMT - Mesial

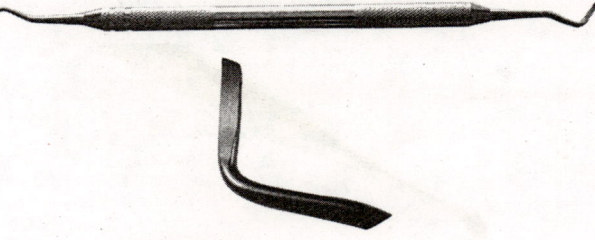

Fig. 3.14 GMT - Distal

3. *Angle Formers*

- Bevel is at angle of 80° with the shaft (forming an acute angle with the long axis of the blade) with a pointed and linear cutting edge (Fig. 3.15).
- It is considered as a combination of GMT and chisel.
- Are single planed instruments with right or left bevelling.
- They has three cutting movements, i.e. vertical, push and pull.
- *Uses*
  - to cut line and point angles in the preparation for gold restoration.
  - to place bevel on enamel margins.
- Instrument Formula: 8 - 80 - 3 - 9 (L)
  8 - 80 - 3 - 9 (R)
  10 - 80 - 4 - 6 (L)
  10 - 80 - 4 - 6 (R)

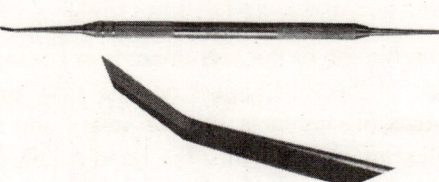

Fig. 3.15

4. Wedelstaedt Chisels (Curved Chisel)

- Resembles a straight chisel, but with a slight vertical curvature in its shank (Fig. 3.16).
- Bevelled on one side of the blade only.
- If the bevel is on the side toward the curvature of the shank, it is *mesially bevelled*; if it is on the side of the blade away from the curvature, it is *distally bevelled*.
- They are single planed instruments, with three cutting motions, i.e. vertical, right and left.
- The mesially bevelled one can be used in push movements and the distally bevelled one can used in pull movements.
- *Use:* For cleaving undermined enamel and for shaping walls.
- Instrument Formula : 15 - 15 - 3.

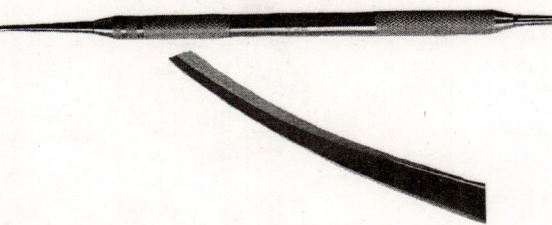

Fig. 3.16

5. Off-Set Hatchets

- It resembles the regular hatchet, except that the whole blade is rotated a quarter of a turn forward or backward around its long axis.
- These are single planned instruments with the same cutting efficieny as regular hatchets.
- They available as right or left instruments.
- However, there are two for both the right and left—one with the whole blade rotated forward and the other with the whole blade rotated backward.
- *Use:* For creating and shaping specific angulations for cavity walls, especially in areas of difficult access.
- Instrument Formula : 15 - 8 - 14 - 7.

6. Triangular Chisel

- It has a triangular blade with the base of the triangle away from the shaft.

- It has a terminal cutting edge like the straight chisel.

7. Hoe Chisel

- Resembles the hoe-excavator, but with the sturdier blade.

ADVANTAGES OF HAND CUTTING INSTRUMENTS

1. They are self-limited in cutting enamel, i.e. they will not cut sound enamel, but will cut only undermined enamel.
2. Can remove large pieces of undermined enamel quickly thus saves time and effort.
3. No vibration or heat is produced during cutting.
4. Are the most efficient way for precise intricate cutting.
5. Can create the smoothest surface of all cutting instruments.
6. Have the longest life span provided if they are resharpened.

INSTRUMENT GRASPS, RESTS AND GUARDS

1. PEN GRASP

- Instrument will be held like a pen between the thumb and first two fingers and the second finger should apply the pressure on to the instrument but not the index finger (Fig. 3.17).
- This method provides very accurate control.
- Used for lower arch instrumentation.
- The action of the instruments with the pen grasp is down and away from the operator.
- Pengrasp involves the action in the wrist of the hand.

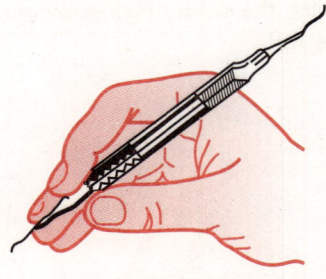

Fig. 3.17

1. Inverted pen grasp

- Similar to pen grasp but the hand is rotated to that the palm faces upwards.
- Used for upper arch instrumentation.
- Action of the instrument is up and toward the operator.

2. Modified pen grasp

- Here, the fingers and the thumb engage the instrument like a grappling hook. The base of the index finger and the tip of the middle finger reciprocates each other and the thumb is placed in the middle of these two (Fig. 3.18).

- It involves the action in the fore arm of the hand.

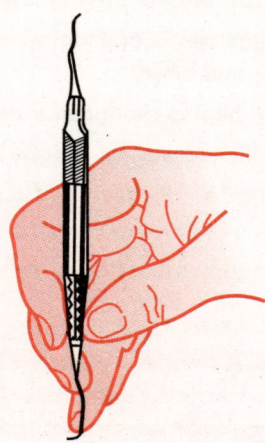

Fig. 3.18

2. PALM AND THUMB GRASP

- The instrument is held in such a way to that is used to hold a knife to whittle a piece of wood (Fig. 3.19).

- The handle of the instrument is held in the palm of the hand and is grasped by the four fingers with the thumb resting on an adjoining surface.

- Useful on maxillary teeth especially on the right side when working from the right rear chair position.

- Useful for the rotary instrumentation on anterior platalal surface.

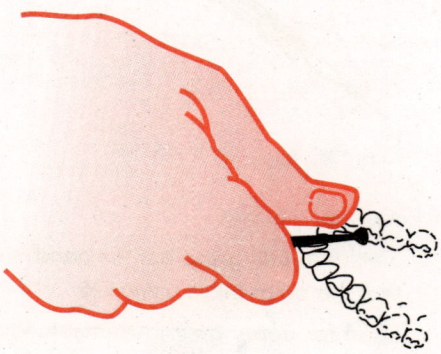

Fig. 3.19

3. MODIFIED PALM AND THUMB GRASP

- The handle of the instrument is in contact with the tips of the four fingers on one side, opposed to which are contacts with the mesial end of the first phalanx of the thumb. The hand is only about half closed, instead of fully closed as in usual palm thumb grasp. The end of the thumb is used as rest (Fig. 3.20).

- This method permits greater freedom and ease of movements and also gives a delicacy of control compared to pen grasp while preventing instrument slipping during a thrusting stroke.

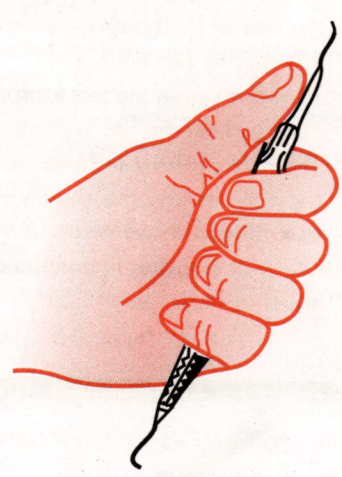

Fig. 3.20

RESTS

- Rests are used to stabilize the hand, confine the instrument to the working area and prevent injury.

- Rests are made with the fingers that do not engage the instrument.

- Rests should be placed on tooth or bony support and never on soft tissues.

GUARDS

- These are hand instruments other items such as interproximal wedges that are used to protect soft tissues from contact with the sharp instruments.

ROTARY INSTRUMENTATION

- Rotary instruments are most widely used instruments for gross removal of tooth structure.

CHARACTERISTICS

1. Speed

– Refers to the surface feet per unit time of contact that the tool has with the work to be cut or revolutions per minute.

– Speeds in dentistry are classified into,

i. According to Marzouk,

1. Ultra low speed : 300–3000 RPM
2. Low speed : 3000–6000 RPM
3. Medium high speed : 20,000–45,000 RPM
4. High speed : 45,000–1,00,000 RPM
5. Ultra high speed : > 1,00,000 RPM

ii. According to Charbenau,

1. Conventional or low speed: below 10,000 RPM.
2. Increased or high speed: 10,000–1,50,000 RPM.
3. Ultraspeed: above 1,50,000 RPM

iii. According to Sturdevant,

1. Low or slow speeds (below 12,000 RPM).
2. Medium / Intermediate speeds (12,000 to 2,00,000 RPM).
3. High / Ultrahigh speeds: (above 2,00,000 RPM).

2. Pressure (P)

– Pressure is defined as the force per unit area.

$$P = \frac{F\,(Force)}{A\,(Area)}$$

– Using the same force F, smaller tools (burs or stones) will apply more pressure to the point of contact than larger tools.

– Clinical osbservation shows, low speed requires 2–5 pounds of force, high speed requires 1 pound of force and ultra high speed requires 1-4 ounces of force for efficient cutting.

3. Heat Production

– Heat is directly proposed to the Pressure, RPM (Revolutions per minute) and area of tooth in contact with the tool, hence if any of the above factors is increased, heat production also increases.

– Heat production of 113° F temperature can cause pulpitis and pulp necrosis. Temperature of 130°F results in the permanent damage of pulps.

– To reduce the heat production coolants (such as flowing water, water-air spray or air) must be used during rotary instrumentation.

4. Vibration

– It is the product of the equipment (hand pieces and cutting tools) used and the speed of the rotation.

– Excess vibration causes annoyance to the patient, operator fatigue and excessive wear of instruments.

5. Patient Reaction

– The use of coolants, intermittent application of a tool to the tooth, sharp instruments, etc. aid in minimal patient discomfort.

6. Operator Fatigue

– High speed rotary instrumentation minimises fatigue by decreasing vibrations and the time of operation.

7. Source of Power

– Air turbine is the main power source in dental practice.

ROTARY INSTRUMENT DESIGN

– It is evaluated under two headings,

I. Dental hand piece.

II. Tools for the removal of tooth structure (bur, stone, etc.).

I. DENTAL HAND PIECE

– It is a device to hold rotating instruments, transmitting power to them and for intraoral positioning.

– They are available as *straight, contra* and *right angled*.

– These are the most frequently used devices in restorative dentistry.

– These are classified into two types based on the speed at which they rotate, i.e. *Low Speed* and *High Speed* hand pieces.

– The dental unit provides the power to the hand piece and which rotates the bur.

– They will retain the cutting tool by a screw in latch or friction grip type of attachment.

1. Low-Speed Hand Piece

– It is available in the speeds ranging from 10,000 to 30,000 RPM (Fig. 3.21).

– The rotatory instrument (bur) can be positioned to operate with a forward or backward movement.

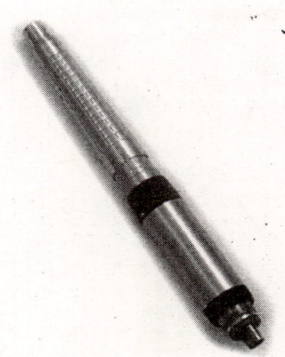

Fig. 3.21

– To adapt the low-speed handpiece for clinical and laboratory procedures, a variety of attachments or sleeves are used that fit onto the handpiece.

A.   Straight Attachment

   – It slides onto the low-speed motor and locks into place (Fig. 3.22).

   – It is most commonly used for laboratory procedures or for trimming removable prostheses outside of the mouth.

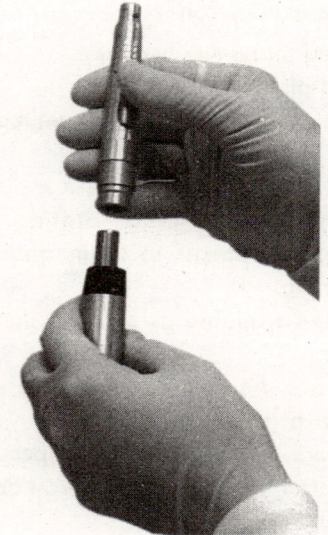

Fig. 3.22 Straight attachment slides onto the slow-speed motor

B.   Contra-Angle Attachement

   – It slides directly onto the low-speed motor and locks into place (Fig. 3.23).

   – The angle of this attachment allows easier adaptation to tooth surfaces.

   – It holds latch-type rotary instruments, endodontic files, prophylaxis cups and mandrels.

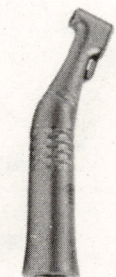

Fig. 3.23 Contra-angle attachment

2.   High-Speed Handpiece

   – It operates from air pressure and reaches speeds up to 4,50,000 RPM (Fig. 3.24).

   – Unlike the low-speed handpiece, the high-speed hand piece does not have attachments.

A.   Water Coolant System

   – The extreme high speed of the bur or stone attached to the high-speed handpiece generates frictional heat on the tooth and which may leads to pulpal damage.

   – So, to protect from the pulpal damage, it is equipped with a water coolant system.

   – The tooth and bur are constantly sprayed with cool water during use.

   – The water spray also helps to remove debris from the tooth preparation and allows for the better visibility to the operator.

B.   Bur Adaptation

   – High-speed handpieces operate with a friction-grip device.

C.   Fiberoptic Lighting

   – Some high-speed handpieces are equipped with a fiberoptic light mounted in the head of the handpieces.

   – Light ports near the bur deliver the proper amount of light directly onto the operating site.

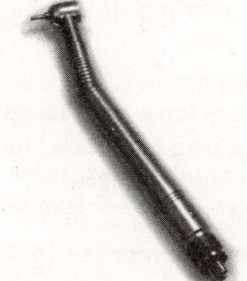

Fig. 3.24 High-speed handpiece

Evaluation Criteria

   – The following criteria are used in the evaluation of handpieces.

1.   Friction

   – It occur in the moving parts of the handpiece especially the turbine.

   – Handpiece is unsuitable to use if the frictional heat is not prevented or counteracted.

– Friction is reduced by equipping the handpiece with ball bearings, needle bearings, glass and resin bearings, etc.

2. Torque

– Refers to the ability of the handpiece to withstand lateral pressure on the revolving tool without decreasing its speed or reducing its cutting efficiency.

– It is depend upon the bearing type used and the amount of energy supplied to the handpiece.

3. Vibration

– Excessive wear of the turbine bearings will cause centric running which creates substantial vibration.

– So it is advised to follow the manufacturer's recommendations for the use and maintenance of handpieces to minimise turbine wear.

II. TOOLS FOR THE REMOVAL OF TOOTH STRUCTURE

– These are the units responsible for the removal of tooth structure.

They are of two types, i.e.

A. Dental Cutting Burs

B. Dental Abrasive Stones

A. DENTAL CUTTING BURS

– The dental bur is a small milling (cutting) instrument (Fig. 3.25).

CHARACTERISTICS

1. Composition and Manufacture

– Dental burs are of two types according to their composition, i.e. *steel burs* and *tungsten carbide burs*.

– Steel burs are made from a blank steel stock by a rotary cutter that cuts parallel to the long axis of the bur. The bur is then hardened and tempered until its Vicker's hardness number is 800 (appox) is reached.

– Tungsten carbide burs are made from powder metallurgy technique which is a process of alloying in which only the partial fusion of the constituents will occur. The tungsten carbide powder is mixed with powdered cobalt under pressure and heated in a vacuum, so that a partial sintering of the metals takes place. A blank is then formed and the bur is cut from it with a diamond tool.

– Sometimes, only the cutting head is tungsten carbide which is welded or soldered to a steel shank.

– Vicker's hardness of number of tungsten carbide type of bur is in the range of 1650 to 1700.

– Steel burs are used for regular speed instruments which are effective only for cutting dentin. Tungsten carbide burs are used for ultra speeds.

2. Classification

i. According to Composition

1. Steel burs
2. Tungsten carbide burs

ii. According to mode of attachment to handpiece

1. Latch type
2. Friction grip type

iii. According to the handpiece they are designed for

1. Contrangle bur
2. Straight handpiece bur

iv. According to the direction of rotation

1. Clockwise (right)-most common.
2. Anticlockwise (left).

v. According to length of the head

1. Long
2. Short
3. Regular

vi. According to shape and size,

1. Round burs
2. Wheel burs
3. Inverted cone burs
4. Cylindrical fissure burs
5. Tapered fissure burs
6. Pear shaped burs
7. End cutting burs

vii. According to purpose,

1. Cutting burs
2. Finishing and polishing burs

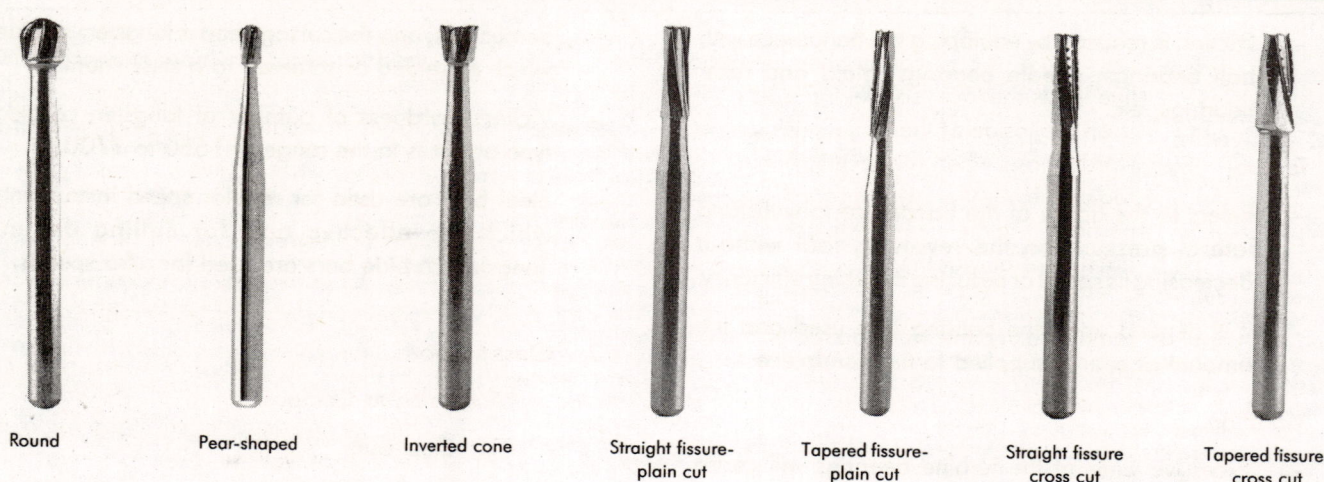

| Round | Pear-shaped | Inverted cone | Straight fissure-plain cut | Tapered fissure-plain cut | Straight fissure cross cut | Tapered fissure-cross cut |

Fig. 3.25

3. *Parts of a Bur*

– Every bur will have three parts (Fig. 3.26).

   i. *Head:* The portion which carries the cutting blades.

   ii. *Shank:* The portion connecting the head to the attachment part of handpiece.

   iii. *Shaft / Attachment Part:* The portion which is engaged with in the handpiece, which connects the shank to the head of the bur.

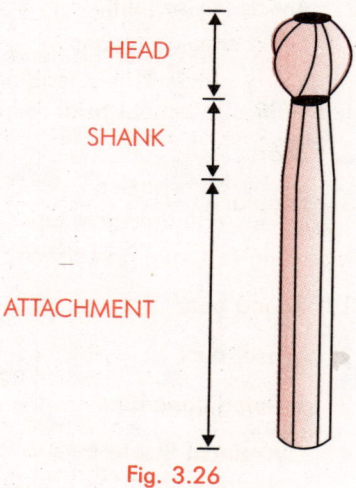

HEAD

SHANK

ATTACHMENT

Fig. 3.26

4. *General Design of Dental Bur*

   i. *Bur tooth*

– This terminates in the cutting edge or blade (Fig. 3.27).

– It has two surfaces *1. Tooth face*, which is the side of the tooth on the leading edge.

2. *Back or flank of the tooth,* which is the side of the tooth on the trailing edge.

– The number of teeth in dental cutting burs is usually 6-8.

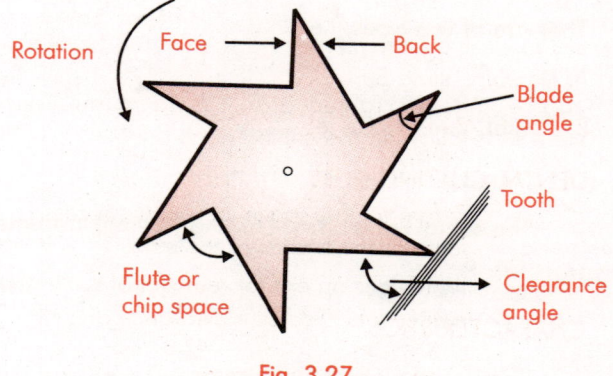

Fig. 3.27

   ii. *Rake angle*

– Refers to the angle that the face of the bur tooth makes with the radial line (refers to direction of rotation) from the center of the bur to the blade (Fig. 3.28).

– It is divided into three types, i.e.

1. *Negative rake angle* forms when the face is beyond or leading the radial line, in other words forms when the face is infront of the radial line. Most of the burs are made with negative rake angle. Advantages are longer bur life and less clogging. Disadvantage is less cutting efficiency compared to a positive rake angle.

2. *Positive rake angle* forms when the radial line leads the face, so that the rake angle is on the inside of the radial line, in other words forms when the face is behind the radial line. Advantage is its greater cutting efficient. Disadvantage is the possibility for fracture of bur tooth.

3. *Radial / zero rake angle* forms when the radial line and the tooth face coincide with each other.

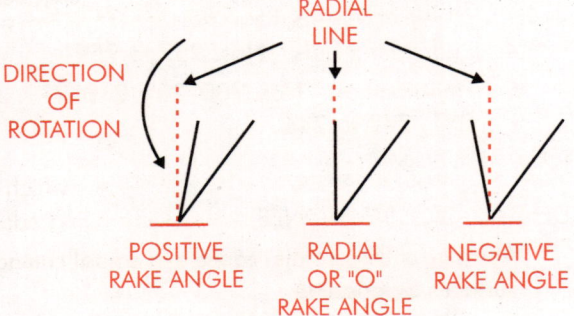

Fig. 3.28

iii. *Land*

   – Refers to the plane surface immediately following the cutting edge.

iv. *Flute / Chip space*

   – Refers to the space between successive bur teeth or the blades of the bur.

   – It provides an exit for removal of the fractured matter and creates a clearance angle.

v. *Clearance angle*

   – Refers to the angle between the back of the bur tooth and the work, in other words angle between the back of the blade and the tooth surface.

   – If a land is present on the bur, it can be divided into three types, i.e.

   1. *Primary clearance angle* is the angle the land will make with work.

   2. *Secondary clearance angle* is the angle between the back of the bur tooth and work.

   3. *Radial clearance angle* is forms when the back surface of the bur tooth is curved.

5. **Common Burs**

   i. *Round burs*

   – They are round in shape.

   – Used for initial tooth penetration, for the placement of retentive grooves, smaller caries excavation, marginating restorations.

   ii. *Inverted cone burs*

   – They are inverted cone in shape.

   – Used for cavity extension, occasionally for establishing wall angulations and retention forms.

   iii. *Cylindrical fissure / straight fissure burs*

   – Used for gross cutting, cavity extension and creation of walls.

   iv. *Tapered fissure burs*

   – Are the most universally used burs in operative dentistry.

   – Used to establish and refine the tapered walls for cast gold restorations, to produce marginal bevels, to produce retention and flaring for the amalgam.

   v. *Pear shaped burs*

   – They are numbered from 229 to 333.

   – They are shaped like pears.

   – Mainly used in pedodontics.

   vi. *End Cutting burs*

   – They are numbered from 900 to 904.

   – They are cylindrical in shape, with just the end carrying blades.

   – Very efficient in extending preparations apically without axial reduction.

   viii. *Elliptical burs*

   – Are characterised by round corners and sides with a reverse taper.

6. *Factors Influencing the Cutting of the Burs*

   i. *Rake angle*

   – *Order of cutting efficiency:* Positive rake angle > Radial rake angle > Negative rake angle.

   – Burs with a radial rake angle cut more efficiently than the burs with the negative rake angle.

   – With the burs of a negative rake angle, the cut chip moves directly away from the blade edge and often fractures into small bits or dust.

   – With the burs of a positive rake angle, the chips are larger and tend to clog the chip space.

ii. **Clearance angle**

- It provides clearance between the work and the cutting edge to prevent the tooth back from rubbing on the work.

- Large clearance angle may result in less rapid dulling of the bur.

iii. **Run-out**

- Refers to the eccentricity or maximum displacement of the bur head from its axis of rotation while the bur takes.

- The average value of clinically acceptable run-out is about 0.023 mm.

iv. **Number of teeth or blades and their distribution**

- As the number of blades decreases, the magnitude of forces at each blade increases and the thickness of the chip removed by each flute correspondingly increases.

- Fewer number of bur teeth has increased space between bur teeth and thus decreases the clogging tendency.

- Fissure bur with straight flutes produces less temperature rise than one with spiral flutes.

- The fewer the number of bur teeth, the greater the tendency for vibration.

v. **Heat treatment**

- It is used to harden a bur that is made of soft steel.

- It preserves the edge placed on the bur flute by the cutter, and hardens the bur to increase its cutting life.

- This procedure is not needed for tungsten carbide burs.

vi. **Design of flute ends**

- Dental burs are formed with two different styles of end flutes.

- The *Revelation* cut, in which the flutes come together at two junctions near a diametrical cutting edge. It shows some superior cutting efficiency in direct cutting.

- The *Star cut*, in which the end flutes come together in a common junction at the axis of the bur.

- Both types have equal cutting efficiency in lateral cutting.

vii. **Influence of the Load**

- Load is the force exerted by the dentist on the tool head and not the pressure or stress induced in the tooth during cutting.

- The minimum and maximum loads for low speed are 1000 - 1500 gm and for high speed are 60 - 120 gm.

7. **ADA Numbering System for Burs**

1. Round burs - Nos. 1/4, 1/2, 1, 2, 3, 4, 5, 6, 7, 8, 9, 10 and 11.

2. Inverted cone burs - Nos. 33 1/2 to 40.

3. Straight fissure burs - Nos. 55 1/4 to 62.

4. End cutting burs - Nos. 957 to 959.

5. Finishing burs - Nos. 200, 201, 218, 219, 230, 231, 242 to 246.

B. **DENTAL ABRASIVE STONES**

- Abrasive cutting points reduce and smooth the tooth surfaces by grinding.

- Abrasives must be used with a coolant to reduce the elevated temperatures.

Characteristics

1. **Design**

- Abrasive particles are held together by means of a binder (base) of variable nature.

- Most commonly a ceramic binder is used, particularly for binding diamond chips.

- Rubber or shellac binder may be used for soft grade stones.

2. **Factors influencing the abrasive efficiency of dental stones**

i. *Shape of abrasive particles*

- An abrasive should be in irregular shape to prevent a sharp edge.

- Therefore, the more irregular the particles, the greater the abrasive efficiency of the stone.

ii. *Hardness of the abrasive material*

- The harder the abrasive material relative to the hardness of the work, the more the abrasive efficiency of the stone.

iii. *Size of the abrasive particles*

- The larger the particles, the deeper the scratches on the surface of the work and the faster the work will be worn away.

3. **Types of Dental Stones**

    – Dental stones are of two types,

       i. Mounted

         – The abrading head is permanently welded to the shank and attachment part.

         – Are available in short, regular or long lengths; latch or friction grip form.

       ii. Unmounted

         – The abrading head is supplied separately and may be mounted on an appropriate mandrel.

         – Dental stones are available in plenty of shapes, i.e. cylinder, wheel, cone, inverted cone, tapered, dough nut, round, filamentous, V-shaped, hour glass, etc.

4. **Classification**

    – *Based on the composition of the abrasive particles,*

       i. Diamond Stones

         – They are the hardest and most efficient abrasive stones for removing tooth enamel.

         – Available in either coarse or fine grits and for either high or low speed handpieces.

         – They should not be used to cut metals or unfilled acrylic resin.

         – Their use is limited to the reduction of tooth substance, backed porcelain and composite resin.

       ii. Carbides

         – They are of silicon carbides or boron carbides.

         – The carbides are sintered with a binder into grinding wheels, discs or stones.

       iii. Sand

         – Sand and other forms of quartz (cuttle) can be bounded and mounted into different shapes of discs, stones and strips.

       iv. Aluminium Oxide

         – One of the most efficient abrasives for stones in fine cutting.

       v. Garnet

         – These particles contain a number of different minerals which possess similar physical properties and crystalline forms.

         – Used for finishing and polishing of dental appliances.

       vi. Rubber Abrasives

         – Are made for polishing of metal.

       vii. Crocus Discs

         – These are paper discs charged with iron oxide.

         – They smoothen the margins of castings after the use of sand paper abrasives.

Fundamental rules for the use of Diamond Instruments

1. Require high speed for efficient cutting.

2. Are best used with light pressure.

3. Cut most rapidly when used with water.

4. Cut harder substance more efficiently than soft.

5. For better control, they are used in a dragging movement, but without pressure rather than in a pushing movement.

6. Care must be taken to keep them out of contact with surfaces outside the field of operation.

Fundamental Rules for the use of Tungsten-Carbide Burs

1. Require high speed for efficient cutting.

2. Should be used with the light pressure.

3. Do not run bur in reverse direction.

4. Bur must always be rotating before being brought into contact with the surface to be cut.

5. For better control, bur should be used in dragging motion rather than pushing.

6. Greater care must be taken to guard against contact with surfaces outside the field of operation.

USES AND LIMITATIONS OF ROTARY INSTRUMENTS

1. Rotary instruments are the most efficient tools for the gross removal of tooth structure.

2. Dental stones (especially diamonds) have the highest efficiency in removing enamel (brittle material) whereas carbide burs have the highest efficiency in removing dentin (elastic material).

3. Use of dental stones is confined to the removal of superficial 0.5–1 mm of dentin. Burs are efficient for the removal of dentin of 2 mm or more.

LOW SPEEDS

Uses

1. For cleaning teeth.
2. Occasional caries excavation.
3. Finishing and polishing procedures.

Advantages

1. Better tactile sensation.
2. Less chance for overheating of cut surfaces.

Disadvantages

1. Ineffective.
2. Time consuming.
3. Requires heavy force application.
4. Patient discomfort.
5. Burs tend to roll out of the tooth preparation.

HIGH SPEEDS

Uses

1. For tooth preparation.
2. Removal of old restorations.

Advantages

1. Faster removal of tooth structure with less pressure, vibration and heat generation.
2. Number of rotary cutting instruments needed is reduced.
3. Better control and ease of application.
4. Instruments last longer.
5. Patient comfort.
6. Several teeth can be treated in a single appointment.

Disadvantages

1. Improper care during preparation results in the slippage of the instrument and tend to injure adjacent hard and soft tissues.
2. Scarring of adjacent uninvolved tooth.
3. Excessive removal of uninvolved tooth structure.

ULTRASONIC INSTRUMENTS

– The ultrasonic dental unit consists of an ultrasonic generator separated from a magnetostrictive transducer located with in the handpiece, and a water cooling system incorporated into the equipment for controlling heat generation.

– Ultrasonic instruments are generally not used for cavity preparations, they are mostly used for calculus and stain removal from teeth and restoration surfaces.

RESTORING INSTRUMENTS

PARTS

– Each restoring instrument is composed of three parts like hand cutting instruments, i.e. Handle, Shaft and Nib.

TYPES

– These are divided into,

1. **Mixing Instruments**

   – Spatulas are employed for the purpose of mixing.
   – Spatulas have flat and wide nibs with blunt edges and straight shank.
   – They are made of stainless steel, ivorine or plastic.

2. **Plastic Instruments**

   – These are used for carrying and handling materials after mixing while the materials are still in their plastic (soft) stage. Hence, the name plastic instrument.
   – They possess a flat sided nib with blunt edges and corners.
   – They are also available in teflon coated ones which minimizes the material adhesion and facilitates easy cleaning.

3. **Condensing Instruments**

   – They differ from each other in the surface configuration of the nib face, depending upon the material they are used with, i.e. amalgam requires smooth surfaced faces, gold foil requires serrated surfaced faces.
   – The nibs are available in different shapes, i.e. rounded, triangular, rectangular, diamond, parallelogram, etc.

4. **Burnishing Instruments**

   – The nibs of the burnishers can be ball shaped egg shaped, apple shaped, beaver tail shaped, conical hour glass shaped, fish tail shaped, bullet shaped, etc.
   – The nibs are of smooth faced.
   – *Sprately burnishers* are special type of burnishers which are used for burnishing of proximal gingival margins of metallic restorations.
   – Burnishers are also available in the form of burs which possess perfectly smooth heads.

5. **Carvers**

   – Carvers are basically cutting instruments with their blades either bevelled or knife edged.
   – The most commonly used carver is Hollen beck carver which possess double sided, knife edged,

pointed edged nibs with curved monangle or binangle shanks. They are very efficient for carving of amalgam and wax.

- The discoid and cleoid excavators can be used as amalgam and gold carvers.

- There are also special forms of carvers are available with triangular nibs and diamond shaped nibs.

6. Files

- Are used less commonly.

- Used for margination of restorations if knives and carvers will not suffice.

- The nibs are in the form of foot shaped, hatched shaped or parallelogram shaped.

- The serration on the face of nib makes a file to be pulled or pushed.

7. Knives

- Nibs possess knife edged faces on one of their side only.

- The most commonly used knife is Bard-Parker knife and has several shapes.

- Black's knives have the nibs at right angle to the handle, with the cutting edge facing away from the handle in one set and towards the hand in another set.

- Wilson's knife has the nib right angle to the shaft, which can be introduced interproximally for proximal and gingival manipulation of restorative materials.

- Stein's knife has a trapezoidal nib which is mainly used for direct gold contouring and margination.

FINISHING AND POLISHING INSTRUMENTS

- Most of the instruments are of rotary type, i.e. burs, stones, paper carried abrasives, brushes, rubber (wheel cups or cones) cloth or felt, etc.

1. Finishing Burs

- It should be atleast 12 fluted and they are available up to 40 fluted.

- They are made up of stainless steel (for amalgam) or tungsten carbide (for composite resins).

- They do not grossly cut the restorative material but removes excess and thus creates smoother surface.

- Burs are available in different shapes, i.e. rounded, apple shaped, cylindrical, inverted cone, etc. and in different sizes.

2. Paper Carried Abrasives

- These are usually sand, cuttle, garnet or boron carbide glued to paper discs or strips.

- They are attached to a mandrel and used by hand in a back and forth motion similar to a shoe polishing action.

3. Brushes

- Are available in different forms, i.e. wheels, cylinders, cones, etc.

- They can be attached by a screw in the handpiece, to a mandrel or by their own frictional attachment extension.

- Available in different sizes and used with abrasives or polishing pastes.

4. Cloth

- It is carried on a metal wheel used in the final stages of polishing with or without a polishing medium.

5. Felt

- Used to obtain lustre for metallic restorations with a polishing paste.

- Has different shapes, i.e. wheels, cones and cylinders.

ACCESSORY INSTRUMENTS

- These are miscellaneous instruments and other items that are used to complete a procedure.

1. TWEEZERS

- These are used to grasp material and / or transfer it into and out of the oral cavity.

- Available as plain or serrated tips, pointed or rounded tips, locking or unlocking varieties.

2. SCISSORS

- The one most often associated restorative dental procedures is *crown and bridge* scissors, available with either curved or straight blades (Fig. 3.29).

- They are useful for many tasks such as cutting dental dam material, retraction cord and stainless steel crowns.

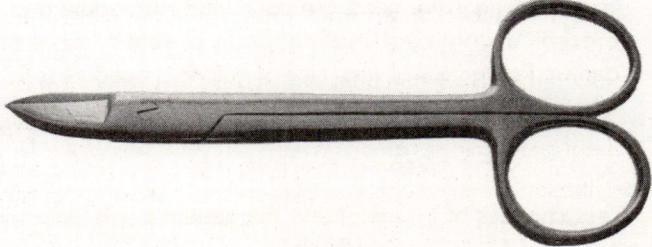

Fig. 3.29

3. HOWE PLIERS

- Also called as 110 pliers (Fig. 3.30).
- Their design is straight with beaks that have flat rounded end, making them useful for holding items.
- Are useful for carrying cotton products to and from the oral cavity, removing the matrix band, placing and removing the wedge.

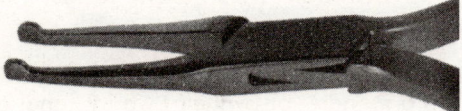

Fig. 3.30

4. DAPPEN DISH

- It is a small glass dish with different sizes of wells on either side (Fig. 3.31).
- Its primary function is to hold certain liquid dental materials during a procedure.
- The newly mixed amalgam is placed in the well, then picked up in the carrier for transfer into the prepared.

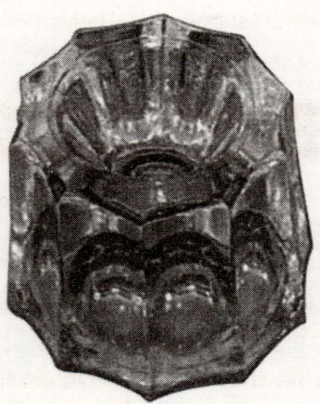

Fig. 3.31

MAINTENANCE OF CUTTING INSTRUMENTS

- Restorative procedures cannot be done adequately without proper maintenance of equipment.
- Sharp cutting instruments are particularly important and present a continual maintenance problem for the dentist. Regradless of what type of cutting procedure is to take place, it is very important to have sharp instruments.

ADVANTAGES OF SHARP INSTRUMENTS

1. Less chances of traumentizing the patient's soft tissues.
2. Decreased operator fatigue.
3. Increased operator efficiency.
4. Accurate control of instrument.

SHARPENING EQUIPMENT

It is of three types,

1. Stationary sharpening stones.
2. Mechanical sharpeners.
3. Handpiece sharpening stones.

1. STATIONARY SHARPENING STONES

- Also called as 'oilstones' because of practice of applying a coating of oil on them as an aid in the sharpening process.
- Most frequently used sharpening equipment consist of a block or stick of abrasive material called `stone'.
- Sharpening stones are available as grits, shapes and materials.

    i. Grits
    - These are available in coarse, medium and fine.
    - Fine grit stone is suitable for final sharpening of dental instruments.
    - Coarse and medium grits are used for initial reshaping of badly damaged instrument or for sharpening other dental equipment such as bench knives.

    ii. Shapes stationery stones of various shapes include,
    - Flat
    - Grooved
    - Cylindric
    - Tapered
    - Flat stones are preferred for sharpening all instruments with straight cutting edges.
    - Cylindric stones are used for sharpening instruments with concave edges.
    - Tapered stones permit using a portion of the stone with a curvature matching that of the instrument.

    iii. Materials sharpening stones are made from,
    - Natural material, synthetic material.
    - Four types of materials commonly used for sharpening stones are,
        - A. Arkansas stone
        - B. Silicon carbide

C. Aluminium oxide

D. Diamond

A. Arkansas Stone

- It is a naturally occurring material, i.e. mineral containing microcrystalline quartz.

- These are available in hard and soft varieties.

- The hard stone cut slower and is preferred because the soft stone scratches and grooves easily.

- Stones are lubricated with light machine oil because, this assists in fineness of sharpening, prevents clogging of the stone pores and avoids the creation of heat.

- When stone appears dirty, it is wiped with a clean woolen cloth soaked in oil.

- When the stone is extremely dirty, it may be wiped with a cloth soaked in alcohol.

B. Silicon Carbide (SiC)

- It is widely used as an industrial abrasive.

- It is commonly used material for grinding wheels and sandpapers, as well as for sharpening stones.

- SiC stones are available in many shapes in coarse and medium grits.

- SiC stones are normally of a dark colour, often black or greenish black.

- These stones are moderately porous and require lubrication with light oil.

C. Aluminium Oxide

- It is increasingly used to manufacture sharpening stones.

- Coarse and medium grit stones appear as speckled tan or brownish in colour.

- Fine grit stones are white.

- Water or light oil is used as lubricant.

D. Diamond

- It is hardest available abrasive and most effective for cutting and shaping hard materials.

- It is the only material capable of sharpening carbide as well as steel instruments.

- Diamond hones are small metal blocks with fine diamond particles impregnated on the surface.

- These hones include grooved, rounded and straight surfaces and are adaptable for sharpening instruments with curved blades.

- These hones are nonporous.

- Use of lubricant will extend the size of hones.

- They may be cleaned with a mild detergent and a medium bristle brush.

2. MECHANICAL SHARPENERS

- Rx Honing Machine is an example of a mechanical sharpener.

- This instrument moves a hone in a reciprocating motion at a slow speed, while the instrument is held at the appropriate angulation and supported by a rest.

- Interchangeable aluminium oxide hone of different shapes and coarseness are available to accommodate the various instrument sizes, shapes and degree of dullness.

- This type of sharpener is versatile and can fill almost all instrument sharpening needs.

3. HANDPIECE SHARPENING STONES

- Mounted SiC and aluminium oxide stones for use with both straight and angle handpieces particularly the cylindric instruments with straight sided silhouettes, are more useful for sharpening hand instruments.

PRINCIPLES OF SHARPENING

1. Sharpen the instruments only after they have been cleaned and sterilized.

2. Establish the proper bevel angle (45 degrees) and desired angle of the cutting edge to the blade before placing the instrument against the stone, and maintain these angles throughout sharpening.

3. Use a light stroke or pressure against the stone to minimize frictional heat.

4. Use a rest or guide whenever possible.

5. Remove as little metal from the blade as possible.

6. Lightly hone the unbeveled side of the blade after sharpening to remove the fine bur that may be created.

7. After sharpening sterilize the instrument.

8. Keep the sharpening stones clean and free of metal cuttings.

TECHNIQUES FOR SHARPENING INSTRUMENTS

1. MECHANICAL TECHNIQUES

- It is a quick method of sharpening hand instruments and can be easily mastered with little practice.

- Chisels, hatchets, hoes, angle formers or GMT are sharpened on a reciprocating honing sharpener.

- The blade is placed against the steady rest.
- Proper angle of the cutting edge of the blade is established before starting the motor.
- Light pressure of the instruments against the reciprocating hone is maintained with a firm grasp on the instrument.
- A trace of metal debris on the face of a flat hone along the length of the cutting edge is an indication that the entire cutting edge is contacting the hone.
- For instruments with curved blades, especially the inside curve of blades, handpiece stones are used.
- Here the instrument is held lightly against the stone with a modified pen grasp.

2. STATIONARY STONE TECHNIQUES

- The stationary sharpening stone should be at least 2 inches wide and 5 inches long.
- It should be medium grit for hand cutting instruments.
- Before the stone is used, a thin film of light oil should be placed on working surfaces.
- *Fundamental rules to be followed while using the stationary stone.*

1. Place the stone on a flat surface and do not tilt the stone while sharpening.
2. Grasp the instrument firmly, usually with a modified pen grasp, so that it will not rotate or change angles while being sharpened.
3. To ensure stability during the sharpening strokes, use the ring and little fingers as a rest, and guide along a flat surface or along the stone. This prevents rolling or dipping of the instrument which results in a distorted and uneven bevel.
4. Use a light stroke to prevent the creation of heat and the scratching of the stone.
5. Use different areas of the stone's surface while sharpening as this helps in preventing the formation of the grooves on the stone that impair efficiency and accuracy of the sharpening procedure.

SHARPENING OF INDIVIDUAL INSTRUMENTS

1. Chisels, Hatchets or Hoes

- Grasp the instrument with modified pen grasp.
- Place the blade perpendicular to the stone.
- Tilt the instrument to establish the correct bevel.
- Slide the instrument back and forth along the stone.
- The motivating force should be from the shoulder. So that the relationship of the hand to the plane of the stone is not changed during the stroke.

2. Angle Formers

- It is same as that used for chisels, hatchets except that allowance must be made for the angle of the cutting edge to the blade.

3. Gingival Margin Trimmers

- Require more orientation of the cutting edge to the stone before sharpening.
- Palm and thumb grasp is used when sharpening a trimmer with 95 or 100 centigrade cutting edge angle.
- When single bevel instruments are sharpened, a thin rough edge of distorted metal, called burr or burr edge is collected on the unbeveled side of blade.
- This side of the blade is placed flat on the stone and one short forward stroke is made.

4. Amalgam or Gold Knife

- It has a very thin blade tapering to the sharpened edge.
- In sharpening this instrument, only the edge bevels should be honed.
- To sharpen, the blade is placed on the stone with the junction of the blade and shank immediately over the edge of stone.
- The blade is then titled to form a small acute angle with the surface of stone and the stroke is straight along the stone and towards the edge of the blade.
- This method produces the finest edge and eliminates any burrs on the cutting edge.

5. Spoon Excavators and Discoids

- Spoon is placed on the far end of the stone and held so that the handle is pointing towards the operator.
- As the instrument is pulled along the stone toward the operator, the handle is rotated gradually away from the operator, until it is pointing away from the operator at the end of the stroke.
- The instrument is placed on flat surface or held in hand for this procedure.
- To hone the flat inside surface of the blade, a small cylindric stone is passed back and forth over the surface.
- Other means of sharpening spoon excavators are by grooved stone, mounted discs or stones for use with a straight handpiece.

TEST FOR SHARPNESS

The following methods of testing instruments of sharpness are available,

1. **The Light Test**

    -   This test requires you to look directly at the sharpened edge.

    -   A shiny edge indicates that the instrument is blunt while a sharp edge will appear as a black line.

    -   A sharp edge will not reflect light caused by the fine line that appears as sharpness is achieved.

2. **The Thumbnail Test**

    -   Hold the sharpened edge of the instrument at 45° angle to the nail.

    -   Using light pressure, push or pull the instrument (as dictated by the function of the instrument).

    -   If the instrument slips or glides along the nail, it is still blunt.

    -   If the instrument grabs or shaves the nail, a sharp edge has been acquired.

3. **Another method of testing sharpness** is by lightly resting the cutting edge on a hard plastic surface.

    -   Light pressure is exerted in testing for sharpness.

    -   If it slides the instrument is dull.

    -   If the cutting edge digs in during an attempt to slide the instrument forward over the surface the instrument is sharp.

CHAPTER 04

CONTACTS AND CONTOURS

- The site of actual contact between two teeth on the mesial and distal surfaces and is erroneously called a *contact point*.
- Contact areas are not present on the distal surfaces of third molars of permanent teeth and distal surfaces of second molars in deciduous teeth (which have no teeth distal to them).
- A positive relationship should exist between the contacts to resist food impaction and to protect the gingival tissue. It can be tested by passing dental floss between the teeth and observing the resistance when the floss is moved from the gingiva between the two enamel surfaces.
- The contact area in the posterior teeth is located nearer at the facial surface which causes a larger lingual embrasure.
- The contact area in anterior teeth is located nearer at the lingual surface, which causes a larger facial embrasure.
- The contact areas are usually parallel to the incisal edges of the teeth and to a line drawn through the posterior facial cusp tips.
- Contact areas are classified as rounded, broad and flat.
- The flat contact or the square shaped tooth is more difficult to clean and thus more prone to caries.
- Whenever possible a rounded contact with an open embrasure in positive relationship should be produced in the proximal restoration.

PURPOSE OF IDEAL CONTACTS

1. To prevent food impaction.
2. To conserve healthy gingival tissue.
3. To make the areas self cleansable.
4. To help ensure permanence of proximal restorations.
5. To maintain normal mesio-distal relationship of the teeth in the dental arch.
6. To improve esthetic appearance, especially on anterior teeth.

PURPOSE OF BREAKING CONTACT POINT

1. To make the areas self cleansable (after restoration)
2. To eliminate caries
3. To place matrix band

EMBRASURES (SPILLWAYS)

- When two teeth in the same arch are in contact, their curvatures adjacent to the contact areas form spillway spaces called *embrasures*.

- The spaces that widen out from the area of contact labially or buccally and lingually are called *labial or buccal and lingual inter proximal embrasures* respectively.

- Above the contact areas incisally and occlusally, the spaces which are bounded by the marginal ridges as they join the cusps and incisal ridges, are called the *incisal or occlusal embrasures.*

- The *gingival embrasure or interproximal* space is a triangular space formed by the contact areas of two teeth and the supporting bone. The base of the triangle is located on the bone.

Purpose

1. It makes a spill way for the escape of food during mastication.

2. It prevents food from being forced through the contact area.

3. Reduce the load of occlusal forces.

4. Permit a slight amount of stimulation to the gingiva.

HEIGHT OF CONTOUR

- The area of greatest circumference on the facial and lingual surfaces of the tooth is called the *height of contour.*

- It protects the gingival tissues by preventing food impaction of the facial and lingual gingiva.

- On the posterior teeth the contour is located in the gingival third of the facial surface and in the middle one-third of the lingual surface.

- These contours divert food over the free gingival margin and they should be placed in the restoration for protection of the periodontium.

MARGINAL RIDGES

- Are those rounded borders of the enamel that form the mesial and distal margins of the occlusal surfaces of premolars and molars and the mesial and distal margins of the lingual surfaces of the incisors and canines.

MAMELON

- It is any one of the three rounded protruberances found on the incisal ridges of newly erupted incisor teeth.

- Each mamelon represents a lobe or the primary section of the formation in the development of crown to which it belongs to.

- They are worn out with usage or they may be missing by birth (as incase of Syphilis, where the central lobe or mamelon will be missing congenitally).

OVERHANG

- The projection of a restoration beyond the cavosurface angle, particularly that which overlays the tooth surface; also the projection of a restoration outward from the normal tooth surface.

CONSEQUENCES OF FAULTY REPRODUCTION OF CONTACTS AND CONTOURS

1. Contact Size

- A contact that is too broad buccolingually or occluso gingivally changes the anatomy of the interdental col, which results in the development of periodontal disease, the areas less able to clean.

- A contact that is too narrow buccolingually or occluso gingivally changes the anatomy of the tooth, which results in food impaction and periodontal disease.

- A contact area placed too occlusally results in a flattened marginal ridge at the occlusal embrasures.

- A contact area placed too buccally or lingually results in a flattened restoration at buccal or lingual embrasures.

- A contact area placed too gingivally results in increased depth of occlusal embrasures and impingement on the interdental col.

- An open (loose) contact results in the continuity of the embrasures with each other and with the interdental papilla.

2. Contact Configuration

- A flat contact area results in a contact area that is too broad buccally, lingually, occlusally, and / or gingivally.

- A contact area with excessive convexity results in diminishing of the extent of the contact area.

3. Contour

i. *Facial and lingual convexities*

- Over convex curvatures result in accumulation of cariogenic and plaque ingredients and depriving of the free and attached gingiva from the massaging, stimulating, keratinizing effect of the food.

ii. *Facial and lingual concavities*

- Deficiency in concavities occlusal to the height of contour results in premature contacts during mandibular movements and excessive concavities result in extrusion, rotation and tilting of cuspal elements.

- Deficiency in concavities apical to the height of contour results in restoration overhangs and excessive concavities result in areas which are difficult to clean.

iii. Areas of proximal contour

- Faulty reproduction of these areas result in restoration overhangs, underhangs, food impaction and impingment on the adjacent periodontal structures.

4. Marginal Ridges

- Improper restoration of the marginal ridges results in.
- Forces direct toward the proximal surface of the adjacent teeth.
- Forces tend to drive the two teeth away from each other.
- Food impaction.

SEPARATION OF THE TEETH

SEPARATORS: These are instruments used to partly displace two neighbouring teeth in opposite directions to create a space in between.

PURPOSE OF SEPARATION

1. To examine the proximal surfaces in the detection of caries.
2. To restore to original positions those teeth which have drifted.
3. To gain access for cavity preparations on anterior teeth.
4. For proper restoration of anatomic proximal contours.
5. For polishing the interproximal restorations.
6. To create a sufficient space for the placement of matrix band interproximally.

METHODS OF SEPARATION

1. Slow or delayed or previous separation.
2. Rapid or immediate separation.

1. SLOW SEPARATION

- Separation should not exceed more than 0.5 mm.

Advantages

1. Comparative absence of soreness of teeth.
2. Less danger to the periodontium.

3. Ability to force away temporarily with gutta-percha, swollen tissue from the gingival margins of cavities.

Disadvantages

1. Time consuming.
2. Repeated application of separating material.

Methods

1. Separating wires.
2. Oversized resin temporaries.
3. Orthodontic appliances.
4. Gutta-percha.
5. Use of wood or rubber.

2. RAPID SEPARATION

- This is a mechanical type of separation which creates either proximal separation at the point of the separator's introduction and / or improved closeness of the proximal surface opposite the point of the separator's introduction.
- It can be used as preparatory to slow tooth movement or to maintain a space gained by slow tooth movement.
- Separation should not exceed 0.2–0.5 mm.

Advantages

1. Quickness.
2. Ability to prevent movement of the teeth during the procedure.

Disadvantages

1. Danger of the rupturing of the periodontal ligament.
2. Pain of too rapid separation.

Methods

A. Wedge Method

- Separation is accomplished by the insertion of a pointed wedge shaped device between the teeth.
- The more the wedge moves facially or lingually, the greater will be the separation.

Example

1. Elliot separator (Fig. 4.1)

Application

- Adjust the two opposing wedges of the separator interproximally so that they are positioned gingival to the contact area.
- Move the knob clockwise so that wedges move towards each other establishing desired separation.

2. Wood or plastic wedges.

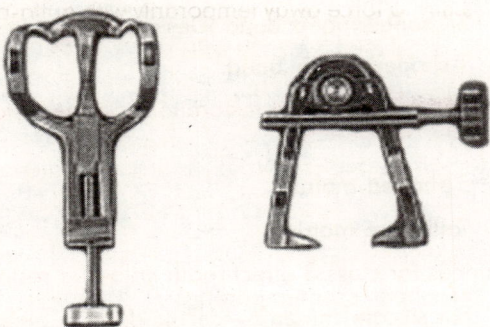

Fig. 4.1

B. Traction Method

- This uses mechanical devices which engage the proximal surfaces of the teeth to be separated by means of holding arms.

Example

1. Non-interfering true separator

- Indicated when continuous stabilized separation is required.
- Advantages are: 1. separation can be increased or decreased after stabilization and 2. is non-interfering.

2. Ferrier double bow separator

- With this device, the separation is stabilized throughout the operation.
- Advantage is that the separation is shared by the contact teeth and not at the expense of one tooth as with the previous type of instrument.

Advantages of mechanical separators

1. For examination of interproximal spaces.
2. For use as preparatory to slow separation.
3. For preparation of cavities.
4. For removal of foreign bodies.
5. To maintain the space gained by slow separation.
6. For insertion and polishing of restorations.

MATRICES

- A dental matrix may be defined as *a properly shaped piece of metal, or other material, used to support and give form to the restoration during its introduction and hardening.*
- Matrix is formed of two parts, i.e. the *band*, which is a piece of metal or polymeric material used to support

and give form to the restorative material during its introduction and hardening and the *retainer*, which is a device by which the band can be retained in its designated position and shape.

- The retainer could be a mechanical device, a wire, dental floss and or compound.

SPECIFICATIONS OF A MATRIX

- It should,
  1. be easy for application.
  2. be easy to remove.
  3. be rigid.
  4. confine the restorative material within the cavity preparation.
  5. be biocompatible.
  6. be economic.

FUNCTIONS

1. Acts as a temporary wall of resistance during the restoration.
2. Gives shape to the restoration.
3. Maintains the form of the restoration during hardening or setting.
4. Assists in holding back the gingiva and rubberdam during restoration.

MATRIX BAND MATERIALS

- Matrix bands are made of stainless steel, copper and celluloid.

MATRIX BAND THICKNESS

- Ranges from to 0.0015" to 0.002".

HEIGHT OF THE MATRIX BAND

- Occlusally should be 1-2 mm above the marginal ridge (Fig. 4.2).

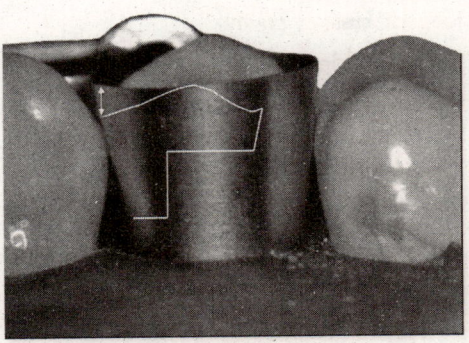

Fig. 4.2

– Gingivally 1 mm below the gingival margin (Fig. 4.3).

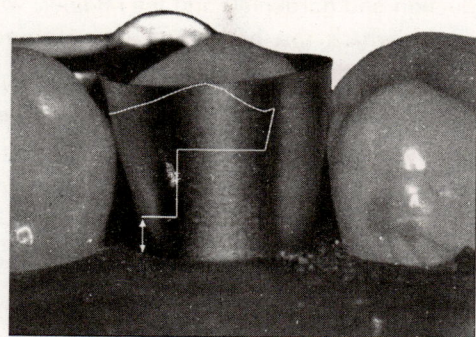

Fig. 4.3

CLASSIFICATION

I.   **Based on the material**

1.   *Metallic matrix:* Made up of stainless steel. Ex: Ivory No: 1 and 8.

2.   *Non-metallic matrix:* Made up of plastic like material. Ex: Myeloid strip.

II. **Based on the retainer**

1.   *With retainer (mechanical):* Needs retainer to keep the matrix in its place. Ex: Ivory No. 1 and 8.

2.   *Without retainer (anatomical):* Do not need retainer. Ex: Automatrix, T-band, Soldered band, compound supported matrix.

III. **Matrices are also classified as**

1.   Circumferential: Ex: Tofflemaire, Ivory No. 8.

2.   Unilateral: Ex: Ivory No. 1, Automatrix.

3.   Mechanical retainer supported.

4.   Compound supported/wedge supported.

5.   Precontoured band.

6.   Uncontoured band.

MATRICES FOR INDIVIDUAL CAVITY PREPARATIONS

I.   **Matrices for class 1 cavity, designs 4, 5, 6, 7 and 8 preparations**

–   Double banded tofflemire matrix.

II. **Matrices for class 2 cavity**

1.   Single-banded tofflemire matrix (Designs 1, 2, 3, 6, 7 and 8).

2.   Ivory matrix No: 1 (unilateral class 2)

3.   Ivory matrix No: 8 (Designs 1, 2 and 3)

4.   Black's matrices (Designs 1, 2 and 3)

5.   Soldered band or seamless copper band matrix (Designs 6, 7 and 8)

6.   The anatomical matrix (Designs 1, 2, 3, 6, 7, and 8)

7.   Roll-in band matrix (auto-matrix)

8.   S-shaped matrix band (Designs 4, 5, and 7)

9.   T-shaped matrix band.

III. **Matrices for amalgam restorations on the distal of the cuspid**

1.   S-shaped matrix.

2.   Tofflemire matrix

IV. **Matrices for class 3 direct tooth coloured restorations**

1.   For silicate cements—celluloid strips, mylar strips.

2.   For resins—cellophane strips, mylar strips.

3.   T-shaped matrix band.

V.   **Matrices for class - 4 direct tooth coloured restorations**

1.   Plastic strip for inciso-proximal cavities.

2.   Aluminium foil incisal corner matrix.

3.   Transparent crown form matrices.

4.   Anatomic matrix.

5.   Modified S-shaped band.

VI. **Matrices for class 5 amalgam restorations**

1.   Window matrix.

2.   S - shaped matrix.

VII. **Matrices for class 5 direct tooth coloured restorations**

1.   Anatomic matrix for non-light cured materials.

2.   Aluminium or copper collars for non-light cured materials.

3.   Anatomic matrix for light and non-light cured materials.

1.   **UNIVERSAL / TOFFLEMIRE MATRIX**

–   It is a circumferential matrix.

–   Available as straight and contrangled (both facially and lingually).

–   Ideally used for MOD cavity and can also be used for class 2 cavity preparation.

Advantages

1.   Can be placed facially or lingually.

2.   Stable band and retainer.

3.   Bands of variable occlusal, gingival heights are available.

4.   Small bands are available for primary dentition.

5.   Provides superior contact and contour.

6.   Helps in holding the cotton rolls in place.

7.   Permits easy removal.

Disadvantage

– Unnecessary space creating on the other side if used in unilateral class 2 preparation.

Tofflemire retainer parts (Fig. 4.4)

1. Set screw
2. Spindle
3. Slide
4. Head
5. Band

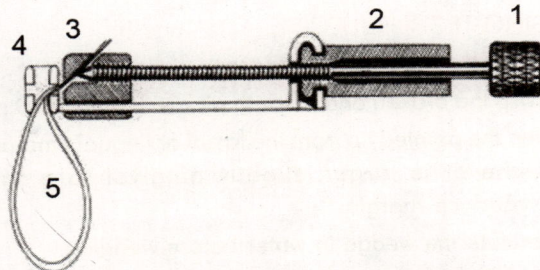

Fig. 4.4

2. IVORY NO. 1

– It is a unilateral matrix (Fig. 4.5).
– Available for premolars and molars.
– The jaws of the retainer should engage the gingival embrasure area.
– Gingival edge has shorter length that allows the retainer to draw the band tight at the gingival margin.

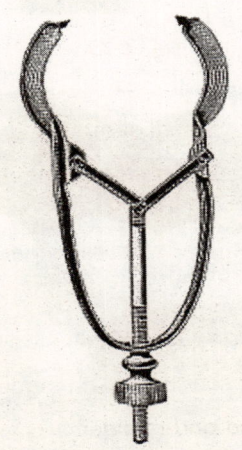

Fig. 4.5

3. IVORY NO. 8

– Indicated in class 2 with buccal or palatal extension; class 2 with no adjacent tooth; MOD and complex cavities.
– Tofflemire is preferred over ivory no. 8.

4. BLACK'S MATRICES

– Of all the different designs for matrices presented by black, only two are mainly used.
– The first is the simplest form and which is recommended for the majority of the small and medium-sized cavities.
– The second form is used for grossly destructed teeth.

5. AUTOMATRIX (Roll-in-band matrix)

– It is a retainerless matrix system with four types of bands that are designed to fit all teeth regardless of circumference.
– **Height:** 4.7- 7.9 mm.
– **Indication:** For extensive class 2 preparation and cuspal restoration.

Advantages

1. Convenience.
2. Improved visibility (retainer is not present).
3. Auto lock loop can be positioned facially or lingually.
4. Decreased time of application.

Disadvantages

1. Cannot be precontoured.
2. Difficult to develop physiological proximal contour.

6. COMPOUND SUPPORTED MATRIX

– Particularly valuable when the amalgam is condensed by mallet force, for example, in the use of the Hollenback pneumatic condenser.
– *Application :* A piece of 0.003 inch stainless steel is placed between the teeth. A wedge is placed at the gingival area both buccally and lingually. After wedging, modelling compound is placed both sides around the exposed portion of the wedge.
– Used in two surface proximal restorations.

7. SOLDERED BAND

– Also called as seamless copper band matrix.
– Indicated in badly broken down teeth, especially for pin-retained amalgam restorations with large buccal and lingual extensions.
– This band is made by taking a measurement of the neck of the tooth and soldering a band of metal to fit.

8. T-SHAPED MATRIX BAND

– These are premade T-shaped stainless steel matrix bands.

– The long arm of the T is bent or curled to encompass the tooth circumferentially and to overlap the short horizontal arm of T. This section is then bent over the long arm, loosely holding it in place.

9. WINDOW MATRIX

– It can be formed using either a Tofflemire matrix or copper band matrix.

– A band is selected and a window is cut in the band slightly smaller than the outside of the cavity. Wedges are placed mesially and distally to stabilize the band.

WEDGES

– Wedge *is a wooden or plastic device placed interproximally which approximates the band on to the tooth and prevents gingival overhang of restoration* (Fig. 4.6).

– In cross-section, the base of the triangle will be in contact with the interdental papillae, gingival to the gingival margin of the proximal cavity.

– The two sides of the triangle should coincide with the corresponding two sides (i.e. mesial and distal) of the gingival embrasure.

– The apex of the triangle should coincide with the gingival start of the contact area.

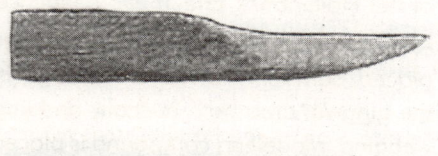

Fig. 4.6

FUNCTIONS

1. To prevent the gingival overhanging of the restorative material.
2. To adapt closely the matrix band to the tooth.
3. To protect gingival interdental papilla.
4. To protect proximal periodontal tissues.
5. To create some separation to compensate for the thickness of the matrix band and minor drifting of the teeth.
6. To establish atraumatic retraction of the rubberdam.
7. To immobilize the matrix band.

TYPES OF WEDGES

1. Wooden
2. Resin (plastic)

Advantages of Wooden Wedge

1. Can be easily cut and trimmed.
2. Absorb water intraorally and swells thus improves interproximal retention.

Advantages of Plastic Wedges

– Can be moulded and bent according to the shape of the interdental papilla.

WEDGING TECHNIQUE (Fig. 4.7 A and B)

– Break off 1–2 cm of round tooth pick.
– Grasp the broken end of tooth pick with a no. 110 plier.
– Insert the pointed tip from the facial or lingual embrasure whichever is larger, slightly gingival to gingival cavosurface margin.
– Lubricate the wedge in water before wedging.

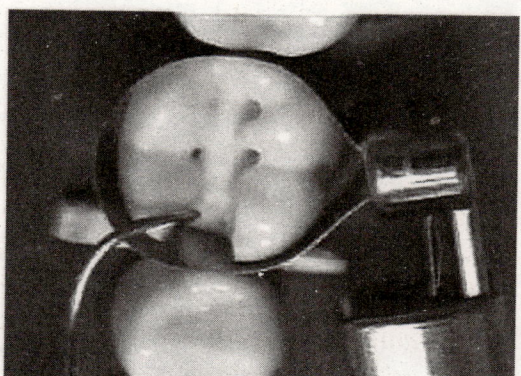

Fig. 4.7 A

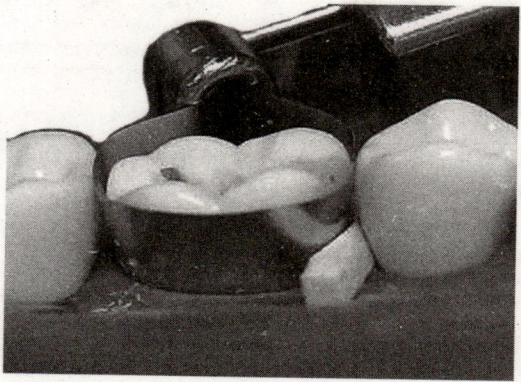

Fig. 4.7 B

CLASSIFICATION OF WEDGES

I. Based on the material,
 1. Plastic
 2. Wooden

II. Based on the shape,

1. Round
2. Triangular (anatomical wedge)

III. Based on either modified or unmodified wedges,

1. Modified wedge: Prevents the distortion of matrix contour, used for very wide spacing between teeth. Ex: A custom made tungblade wedge.

2. Unmodified wedge: Usually inserted into the interdental space from the lingual side because the lingual embrasures are larger.

   – Triangular wedge is indicated for class 2 with deep gingival margin because it has its greatest width at its base.

   – Round wedge is indicated for class 2 with shallow gingival margin because its wedging action is nearer to the gingival margin.

WEDGING TECHNIQUES: (OR TYPES OF WEDGING)

1. Piggy back wedging
2. Double wedging
3. Wedge wedging

1. Piggy back wedging

   – Indication: In cases where there is recession of the interproximal gingiva and gingival recession.

   – Technique: If the first wedge is placed significantly apical to the gingival margin, a second wedge usually smaller than the first one may be piggy back on the first wedge to adequately wedge the matrix band against tooth margins.

2. Double wedging

   – Indication: Occasionally permitted if proximal box is wide faciolingually.

   – Technique: Insert two wedges one from facial embrasure and other one from lingual embrasure.

3. Wedge wedging

   – Used if the concavity on the proximal surface is gingival to the contact area extending into the root.

   – Also used to wedge the matrix band tight against such a margin, a second pointed wedge is inserted between the first wedge and the band.

CHAPTER 05

DENTAL CARIES

Dental caries is an infectious bacterial disease that has afflicted humans since the beginning of recorded history. Since the late 19th century, dentists have been fighting tooth decay by drilling out the decayed tooth structure and filling the tooth with a restorative material. Today, the emphasis in fighting dental caries is shifting from the traditional approach of filling teeth to the new strategies of reducing dental caries. Advances in science and new technologies have placed the emphasis on prevention and early intervention. This chapter discusses the causes, process of tooth decay, types of decay, its diagnosis, management and prevention.

KEY TERMS

1. *Caries:* Tooth decay.
2. *Cavitation:* Formation of a cavity or hole.
3. *Demineralization:* Loss of minerals from the tooth.
4. *Pellicle:* Thin film like coating of salivary materials deposited on tooth surfaces.
5. *Plaque:* Soft deposits on teeth that contain bacteria and their byproducts.
6. *Remineralization:* Replacement of minerals in the tooth.
7. *Xerostomia:* Dryness of the mouth caused by reduction of saliva production.
8. *Fermentable carbohydrates:* Simple carbohydrates such as sucrose, fructose, lactose and glucose.

DEFINITION OF *DENTAL CARIES*

– Dental caries is defined as a progressive irreversible, microbial disease affecting the hard parts of the tooth exposed to the oral environment, resulting in demineralization of the inorganic constituents and dissolution of the organic constituents, thereby leading to a cavity formation.

CLASSIFICATION OF DENTAL CARIES

I. *Based on the severity and progression of the lesion*

1. *Incipient or initial or primary carious lesion*

 – Describes the first attack on the tooth surface and is initial or original carious lesion of the tooth.

 – Are white spot lesions.

 – Reversible lesions.

 – Enamel is intact but demineralised.

 – They can be remineralised.

 – Shape and progression of the lesion depends upon the location, i.e. pit and fissures, enamel smooth suface and root surfaces.

2. *Recurrent or secondary lesion*
   - Is the one which is observed under or around the margins or surrounding walls of an existing restoration.
   - Common sites of recurrent decay are inter proximal margins of a proximal restoration not involving all of the contact area incompletely involved pits and fissures and the areas near fractured sites.

   Causes
   1. Improper cavity preparation (unable to remove all of the decay).
   2. Inadequate cavity restoration (open margins).
   3. Old restorations (microleakage).

3. *Acute or rampant caries*
   - Are rapidly progressing caries that usually involves several teeth.
   - Lesions are multiple, light coloured.
   - Frequently accompanied by severe pulp reactions.
   - Demineralisation exceeds remineralisation.

4. *Chronic caries*
   - Are of variable depth, long standing and are fewer in number.
   - More localized.
   - Lesions are hard in consistency and dark in colour.
   - Remineralisation exceeds demineralisation.

5. *Arrested caries*
   - Arrested caries is the stage where the progress of the decay has stopped and is inactive.
   - The softened dentin has been lost or worn away so that the discoloured (either yellow, brown or black), sound, hard dentin remains. The remaining dentin has a polished look. This is referred to as 'eburnation of dentin'.
   - Arrested carious lesions are found most commonly on lingual and labial aspects of teeth and less common in interproximal areas.

   Formation of arrested caries
   - There are a number of stages are involved in the formation of arrested caries, i.e.

   1. **First stage:** The acids produced by advancing bacteria dissolve the mineral in the surrounding intertubular dentin. The tubule fluid becomes saturated with calcium, magnesium and phosphate ions. The lesion progresses unless the level of metabolic activity of the bacteria is reduced. If less acid is produced then the second stage can occur.

   2. **Second stage:** If bacterial acid production is reduced and the pH increases, the salts precipitate into large crystals of tricalcium phosphate which temporarily block the tubule.

   3. **Third stage:** If further bacterial activity is suppressed, the odontoblast secretes collagen and calcium salts. Small plate like crystals of hydroxyapatite then form and block the tubule more effectively.

6. *Active caries*
   - It is the progressive carious lesion of the tooth where the demineralisation exceeds the remineralisation.

7. *Residual caries*
   - It is the type of caries which is not removed during the tooth preparation either by accident, intention or neglect (Fig. 5.1).
   - When these caries are near the pulp, it may be covered with a pulp capping material to promote reparative dentin deposition.
   - This carious dentin can be excavated at later stage.

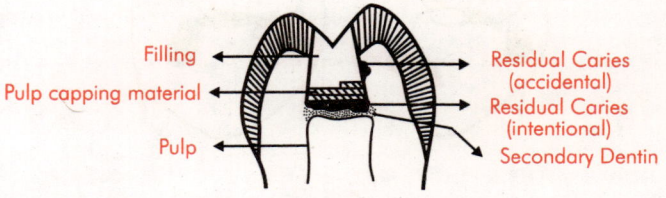

Filling — Residual Caries (accidental)
Pulp capping material — Residual Caries (intentional)
Pulp — Secondary Dentin

Fig. 5.1

II. *Based on the pathway of caries*
   1. *Forward caries (Pit decay)*
      - In this, decay starts in enamel and then it involves the dentin.
      - Extent of caries is greater in enamel than in dentin.

   2. *Backward caries (Smooth surface lesion)*
      - In this, decay attack the enamel from its dentinal side.
      - Extent of caries is greater at DEJ than in enamel.

III. *Based on the number of surfaces involved*
   1. *Simple*
      - That involves only one surface of a tooth (Fig. 5.2).

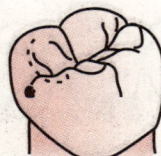

Fig. 5.2

2. Compound

– That involves two surfaces of a tooth (Fig. 5.3).

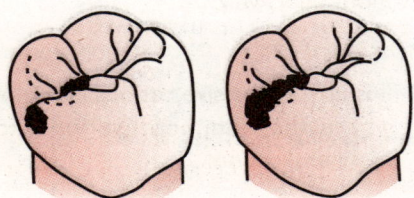

Fig. 5.3

3. Complex

– That involves three or more surfaces of a tooth (Fig. 5.4).

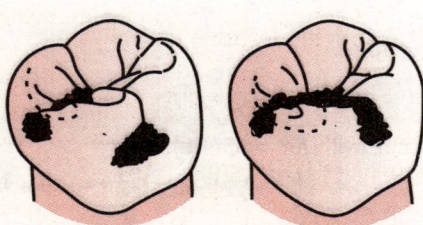

Fig. 5.4

IV. Based on the location on the tooth surface

1. Pit and fissure caries

– The caries originating in the pits and fissures found on the lingual surfaces of maxillary anterior teeth, and on the buccal, lingual and occlusal surfaces of posterior teeth.

– Early lesion difficult to detect clinically.

– Appears as two cones with bases approximating each other.

– Little lateral spread occurs until DEJ is reached.

– *Occurence:* May be due to defective formation or incomplete coalescence of enamel by developmental enamel lobes or complete coalescence enamel where shallow grooves and fossa become carious due to neglect.

2. Smooth surface caries

– The caries originating in all surfaces without pits, fissures or grooves.

Locations

1. Proximal surfaces cervical to the contact area.

2. Facial or lingual surfaces cervical to the height of contour.

– Caries occurs due to lack of adequate plaque removal.

– Shape is two triangles / cones.

– Base of enamel triangle is at the enamel surface.

– Apex of enamel cone contacts the base of dentin cone caries due to lateral spread at DEJ.

3. Senile (root) caries

– Located exclusively on the cementum and dentin of the root surfaces of the teeth.

– Progresses more rapidly than enamel caries.

– Sometimes associated with partial denture clasps.

– Associated with aging process.

V. G.V. blacks classification

– It is a therapeutic classification.

– It is based on the treatment and restoration design.

Class I: Pit and fissure cavities that occur in the occlusal surfaces of bicuspids and molars; the occlusal two-thirds of the buccal and lingual surfaces of the molars and the lingual surfaces of incisors. Cavities beginning in structural defects that occasionally occur on the occlusal or incisal two thirds of all teeth (Fig. 5.5).

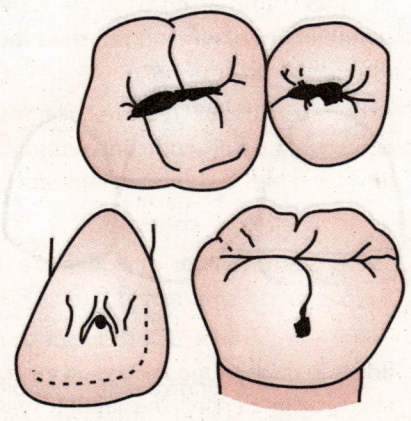

Fig. 5.5

Class II: Cavities in the single proximal surfaces of bicuspids and molars (Fig. 5.6).

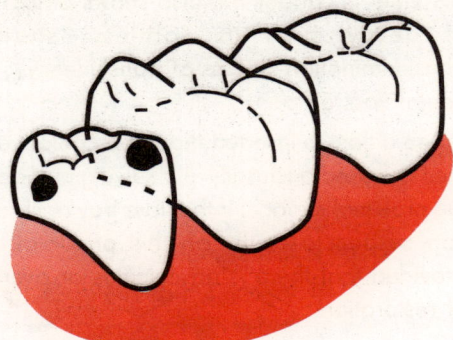

Fig. 5.6

Class III: Cavities in the proximal surfaces of incisors and cuspids not involving the incisal angle (Fig. 5.7).

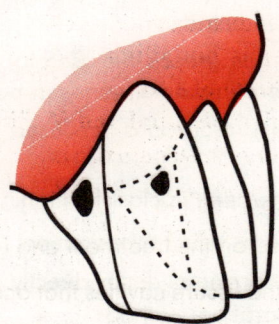

Fig. 5.7

Class IV: Cavities in the proximal surfaces of incisors and cuspids involving the incisal angle (Fig. 5.8).

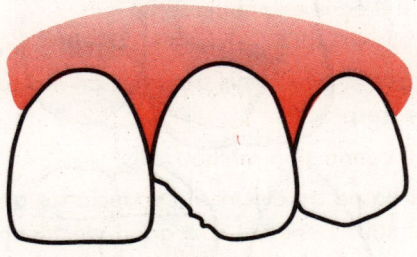

Fig. 5.8

Class V: Cavities in the gingival third, not pit and fissure cavities, of the labial, buccal and lingual surfaces of all teeth (Fig. 5.9).

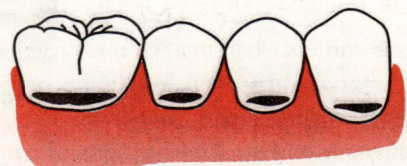

Fig. 5.9

Class VI: Cavities on both mesial and distal proximal surfaces of bicuspids and molars that when restored will share a common occlusal isthmus or cavities on the incisal edges of anterior or cusp tips of posterior teeth (Fig. 5.10).

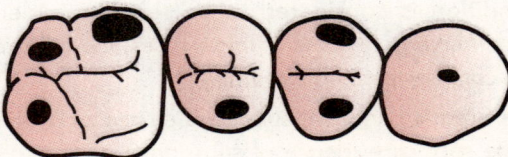

Fig. 5.10

DEVELOPMENT OF CARIES

– Dental caries is a disease caused by multiple factors.

– For caries to develop, the following three factors must present at the same time,

1. A susceptible tooth

2. Diet rich in fermentable carbohydrates

3. Specific bacteria (*Streptococcus mutans*, Lacto-bacillus; regardless of other factors, caries cannot occur without bacteria).

– The bacteria in dental plaque feed on the fermentable carbohydrates that found in the regular diet. Just as wastes are a byproduct of eating, the bacteria produce acids as a byproduct of their metabolism. Acid from the plaque travels into the tooth and dissolves the minerals of the enamel or dentin. If this process progresses, decay develops.

Stages of caries development

– It can take months or even years for a carious lesion to develop.

– Carious lesions occur when more minerals are lost from the enamel than are deposited.

– Caries develop in two stages, i.e.,

1. **First stage,** the *incipient caries* or *incipient lesions*:

   – Occurs when caries begin to demineralize the enamel.

2. **Second stage,** the *overt lesion* or *frank lesion*:

   – Characterized by the development of cavity.

CRITERIA FOR THE DIAGNOSIS OF DENTAL CARIES

1. The area is carious when the explorer 'catches' or resist removal after the insertion into a pit or fissure with moderate to firm pressure and when this is accompanied by one or more of the following signs of caries:
   i. A softness at the base of the area.
   ii. Opacity adjacent to the pit or fissure as evidence of undermining or demineralisation.
   iii. Softened enamel adjacent to the pit or fissure which may be scraped away with the explorer.

2. The area is carious of there is loss of the normal translucency of the enamel, adjacent to a pit, which is in contrast to the surrounding tooth structure. This condition is considered to be reliable evidence of undermining. In some of these cases, the explorer may not catch or penetrate the pit.

3. The area is carious if surface is etched or if there is a white spot as evidence of subsurface demineralisation and if the area is found to be soft by,
   i. Penetration with explorer.
   ii. Scraping away enamel with explorer.

4. The area is sound when there is apparent evidence of demineralisation (etching or white spots) but no evidence of softness.

DIAGNOSIS OF DENTAL CARIES

1. Visual examination
   - The tooth must be clean, dry and well illuminated when carrying out a visual examination.
   - Discoloration gives the suspicion of decay.
   - Observing a grey hue in a marginal ridge can be a suspicion of a proximal cavity under that ridge.

2. Enhanced visual examination
   #### 1. Transillumination
   - It uses an intense beam of visible light, usually directed on the lateral surface of the tooth to transilluminate it.
   - This technique is most useful in the diagnosis of anterior approximal caries and cracked teeth.

   #### 2. Fibre-optic transillumination
   - It uses a fibre-optic light source which is placed palatal/lingual to anterior teeth and are viewed from the facial surface to diagnose the anterior approximal caries.

   #### 3. Magnification
   - It is used most commonly in the form of magnification loupes in adjacent to clinical examination and radiographic evaluation.

3. Tactile examination
   #### 1. Explorer
   - Any discontinuity of the enamel in which an explorer will enter is carious if it also shows other evidence of decay such as softness, shadow by transillumination or loss of translucency.

   #### 2. Dental floss or tape
   - When a floss is inserted though a contact area and then dragged occlusally in a sawing motion against the proximal surface, if the floss fray or shread, one can suspect a cavity on this proximal surface, provided that there is no calculus or overhanging of restoration.

4. Patient complaint
   - When the patient consumes hot or cold items that change osmotic pressure in the dentin, cause subjective compliants, which can be suspicion of dentinal involvement of caries.

5. Radiographic examination
   - Radiographs are used to confirm a clinical suspicion of caries, to detect early lesions and for monitoring the disease activity.
   - Bitewing radiographs are used for the diagnosis of occlusal and proximal caries in posterior teeth.
   - Periapical radiographs are used for the anterior teeth.

6. Tooth separation method
   - It is a type of visual examination.
   - To see the proximal decay directly, one can use the tooth separation method.

7. Dyes
   - A variety of different dyes that stain caries are currently available, which make the visualisation of caries earlier.

8. Laser fluorescence
   - Lasers are used for the detection of caries especially for the early enamel lesions.
   - Caries illuminated by a laser will fluoresce, the degree to which this occurs is an indicator of the disease process.

9. Electrical conduction method
   - It is based on electrical conductance and the fact that sound enamel is a good electrical insulator; however, carious teeth allows the passage of an electrical current more readily, which results in a drop in the electrical resistance.
   - The degree to which the resistance drops is an indicator of the extent of caries.

IDENTIFICATION OF OCCLUSAL CARIES

1. Chalkiness of enamel on the walls and the base of the pit or fissure.

2. Softened base at the pit or fissure.

3. Brownish grey discoloration under the enamel adjacent to the pit or fissure.

4. Presence of radiolucency below the occlusal enamel.

IDENTIFICATION OF PROXIMAL CARIES

1. Broken surface, which can be detectable visual or tactile methods.

2. Discoloured marginal ridge.

3. Opaque area in dentin on transillumination of the tooth.

4. Presence of radiolucency, i.e. bitewing radiographs.

DANGER AREAS FOR CARIES

- G. V. black recognised the tooth surfaces on which dental plaque easily accumulates as the areas most prone to caries attack. These surfaces which he regarded as "danger areas".

- They are,

  1. **Pits and Fissures:** Are found on occlusal surfaces of molars and premolars and also near the cingular of maxillary incisors and canines (lingual pits).

  2. **Approximal surfaces of all teeth.**

  3. **Gingival thirds of all teeth,** both on facial and lingual surfaces.

INFECTED DENTIN

- It is highly demineralised.

- It is unremineralisable.

- It is superficial layer.

- It lacks sensation.

- It can be stained by,

  - 0.5% basic fuschisin

  - 10% acid red solution

  - 0.2% propylene glycol

- Intertubular dentin is greatly demineralised with irregularly scattered crystals.

- The collagen fibres are broken down and only indistinct cross bands and no inter bands are observed.

- This infected dentin should be excavated.

AFFECTED DENTIN

- Intermedially demineralised.

- It is remineralisable.

- It is deeper layer.

- It is sensitive.

- It does not stain with any solution.

- Intertubular dentin is partly demineralised with distinct cross bands and inter bands.

- It should be left to remineralise.

DIRECT PULP EXPOSURE

Causes

1. Iatrogenic

2. Trauma

Type of exposure	Indication	Rx
A pin-point exposure with sound dentin at the periphery of the exposure with haemorrhage.	No inflammation or mild inflammation restricted to the exposure site.	Can be successfully repaired.
Pin-point exposure with sound dentin at the periphery with a drop of blood that coagulates immediately on the cavity floor in the form of a button.	Mild pulpul inflammation restricted to exposure site.	Can be successfully repaired.
Exposure with infected carious dentin at the periphery.	Inflammation beyond the exposure site	Doubtful repair.
Exposure with profuse haemorrhage.	Inflammation involving pulpal and root canals	Usually beyond repair.
Exposure with pus or inflammatory fluids.	Extensive inflammation and destruction of the pulpal and root canal.	Definitely beyond repair.

DIRECT PULP CAPPING

Definition

- Involves the placement of a bio-compatible agent on healthy pulp tissue that has been inadvertently exposed from caries excavation or traumatic injury.

Objective

- To seal the pulp against bacterial leakage, to encourage the formation of reparative dentin and to maintain the vitality of the underlying pulp tissue.

Indications

- Following traumatic injuries.
- Mechanical exposure less than 1mm² in a asymptomatic vital young permanent tooth.

Contraindications

1. Spontaneous and nocturnal toothache.
2. Excessive tooth mobility.
3. Thickened periodontal ligament.
4. Radiographic evidence of furcal or periradicular degeneration.
5. Uncontrollable bleeding at the time of haemorrhage.
6. Purulent exudate from the site of exposure.

Materials Used

1. Calcium hydroxide.
2. Unmodified zinc oxide eugenol.

Procedure

- All undesirable and / or undermined enamel and unsound dentin should be removed.
- The cavity floor and exposure site should be gently washed and irrigated with sterile water.
- Dry with cotton pellets.
- Either calcium hydroxide or unmodified zinc oxide eugenol can be used as a capping material.
- When ZOE is used, sound dentin shavings are cut from surrounding walls and deposited at the exposure site and then covered with a creamy mix of unmodified ZOE.
- When using calcium hydroxide, a creamy mix is prepared and placed directly on the exposure site.
- The permanent restoration should be placed.
- The patient should be informed of the signs and symptoms of pulpal degeneration.
- Patient is recalled after 6-8 weeks if calcium hydroxide is placed or 8-9 weeks if the unmodified ZOE is placed.
- Radiograph is taken to evaluate the status of the tooth.

INDIRECT PULP CAPPING

Definition

- The application of a medicament over a thin layer of remaining carious dentin, after deep excavation with no exposure of the pulp.

Indications

1. *History*
   i. Mild discomfort from chemical and thermal stimuli.
   ii. Absence of spontaneous pain.
2. *Clinical examination*
   i. Large carious lesion.
   ii. Absence of lymphoadenopathy.
   iii. Normal appearance of adjacent gingiva.
   iv. Normal colour of tooth.
3. *Radiographic examination*
   i. Deep carious lesion in close proximity to the pulp.
   ii. Normal lamina dura.
   iii. Normal periodontal ligament space.
   iv. No inter radicular or periapical radiolucency.

Contraindications

1. *History*
   i. Sharp, penetrating pain that persists after withdrawal of symptoms.
   ii. Prolonged spontaneous and nocturnal toothache.
2. *Clinical examination*
   i. Excessive tooth mobility.
   ii. Tooth discoloration.
   iii. Non-responsiveness to pulp tests.
3. *Radiographic examination*
   i. Large carious lesion with apparent pulp exposure.
   ii. Interrupted or broken lamina dura.
   iii. Widened periodontal ligament space.
   iv. Periapical radiolucency.

Materials used

1. Calcium hydroxide.
2. Zinc oxide eugenol.

Procedure

- 3 techniques are commonly used.

Technique 1 : A thin layer of calcium hydroxide paste is placed over the site of near exposure. A thick layer of zinc oxide eugenol is then applied. Patient is recalled after 6-9 weeks; the tooth is reopened and the remaining carious material removed. A sound layer of dentin should be present. Calcium hydroxide is placed as dressing and the tooth is restored by routine procedures.

Technique 2 : A thin layer of zinc oxide eugenol paste is placed over the area of near exposure. A thick layer of zinc oxide eugenol is then applied. The tooth is reopened after 6-8 weeks and the remaining carious material is removed. A sound layer of dentin should be present. Calcium hydroxide is placed as dressing and the tooth is restored by routine procedures.

Technique 3 : Routine cavity preparation is completed. Remove the gross caries. A dressing of calcium hydroxide paste with or without zinc oxide eugenol is placed over the residual caries. An amalgam restoration is placed over the dressing. Complete removal of caries is delayed for 6-8 weeks. Do not re-enter the tooth if it appears clinically and radiographically healthy.

METHODS OF CARIES INTERVENTION (PREVENTION)

– Even though the dentist restores the carious tooth, there is still the risk for further decay. This is because, restoring teeth has no effect on the bacteria still living in mouth.

– The caries process can be interrupted or prevented in the following ways,

1. Proper general health
2. Fluoride exposure
3. Immunization
4. Proper salivary functioning
5. Antimicrobial agents
6. Balanced diet
7. Proper oral hygiene
8. Xylitol gums
9. Pit and fissure sealants
10. Restorations

PIT AND FISSURE SEALANTS

– Dental caries are highly prevalent in cases of deep pit and fissures.

– Buonocore introduced the filling of filler resin with bonded resin.

– Bodecker introduced fissure eradication technique in order to transform the retentive fissures into cleansable areas.

Classification

I. Based on Polymerization Methods

1. Self activation
2. Light activation
    i. First generation sealant. UV light (365 nm) Ex: Nuvaseal.
    ii. Second generation sealant. Self cure (chemical cure) Ex : Delton.
    iii. Third generation sealant. Visible light cure (430-460 nm) Ex: Fissurit.
    iv. Fourth generation sealant contain fluoride releasing agents incorporated in resins.

II. Based on Resin Systems

1. BISGMA
2. Urethaneacrylate

III. Filled and unfilled resins

IV. Clear and tinted resins

Recommended age groups for sealant application

– 3-4 years for primary molars.
– 6-7 years for first permanent molars.
– 11-13 years for second permanent molars.

Indications

– Newly erupted both primary molars and permanent bicuspids and molars with open or sticky grooves.
– Tooth should have erupted less than 4 years ago.

Procedure

1. Isolation of tooth.
2. Polishing is not recommended as the polish slurry would interfere with normal acid etching procedure.
3. Tooth is dried.
4. 30-50% orthophosphoric acid is applied over recommended area using an applicator tip.
5. After a period of 60 sec tooth is washed and dried. Following studies, it has been established that waiting period of 15 sec is enough following acid etching during which time retentive property of etched surface is enhanced.
6. Then etched surface is washed and dried.
7. A characteristic chalky white and or froasty appearance is observed.
8. The sealant is applied over the etched area following which it is cured.

Test for retention

– An explorer is run along margin of treated tooth and any catch would indicate the presence of an air void in which case procedure should be repeated.

ENAMELOPLASTY

– Also called as *Dimpling*.
– It was proposed by Dr. Miles Markley.

– It is the removal of a shallow enamel developmental fissure or pit to create a smooth, saucer shaped surface that is self-cleansing or easily cleaned.

– Maximum removal of one-third of enamel thickness is allowed.

– Restoration cavosurface angle should not be less than 80 degrees.

PROPHYLACTIC ODONTOTOMY

– Proposed by Hyatt in 1923.

– It is characterized by minimally preparing and filling with amalgam on developmental, structural imperfections of the enamel, such as pits and fissures, to prevent caries originating in these sites.

– It is an outdated concept and hence no longer advocated as a preventive measure.

Technique

– When the tooth is erupted into oral cavity the occlusal surface was restored with amalgam or oxyphosphate cement. Later when the tooth achieves occlusion the tooth is restored with amalgam after a shallow cavity preparation.

CHAPTER 06

FUNDAMENTALS OF CAVITY PREPARATION AND RESTORATIONS

1. **Angle:** The union of two surfaces.
2. **Line angle:** The union of two surfaces along a definite line.
3. **Point angle:** The union of two surfaces along of three surfaces at a point.
4. **Axial line angle:** A line angle running parallel with the long axis of the tooth.
5. **Pulpal line angle:** A line angle running horizontally to the long axis of the tooth.
6. **Cavo surface angle:** The angle formed by the junction of the walls of the cavity with the surface of the tooth.
7. **Margin:** The junction of the walls of a cavity with the surface of a tooth.
8. **Marginal out line:** The shape of the cavity along its margins.
9. **Cavo surface margin:** The surface periphery of the cavity preparation, which is the junction between the cavity wall (floor) and the adjacent tooth surface.
10. **Floor:** Refers to those portions of the preparation which are almost at right angles to the surrounding walls. Floors are usually composed of dentin only (pulpal floor), but they can be formed of enamel and dentin (gingival floor).
11. **Seat:** The bottom or floor in simple cavities, either the axial or pulpal wall; in proximo incisal and proximo occlusal cavities, the gingival wall.
12. **Step:** The auxillary portion of the compound mortise form, consisting of the axial and pulpal walls in complex cavities.
13. **Wall:** One of the internal boundaries of a cavity.
14. **Enamel wall:** That part of a cavity wall composed of enamel.
15. **Dentin wall:** That part of a cavity wall consisting of dentin.
16. **Subpulpal wall:** When the pulp is removed the pulpal wall disappears and the base of the pulp chamber becomes the subpulpal wall.

WALLS OF THE CAVITY PREPARATION

– Extracoronal cavity walls carry the name of the surface that is reduced and the intracoronal walls of the preparation also take the name of the surface from which they are derived.

1. **For Occlusal Class I preparation:** It has 4 surrounding walls, i.e. Distal, Mesial, Facial and Lingual (Fig. 6.1).

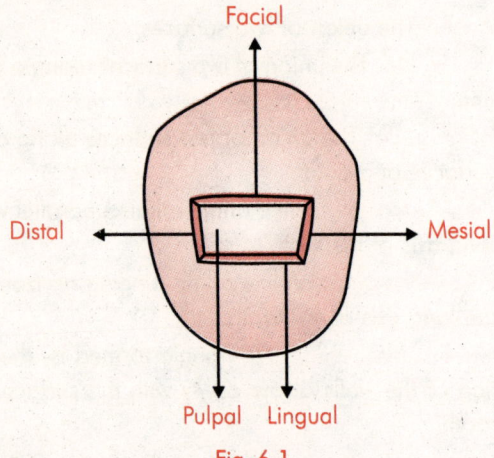

Fig. 6.1

2. **For Class II (MO) preparation:** It has 6 walls, i.e. Distal, Lingual, Facial, Pulpal, Axial and Gingival (Fig. 6.2).

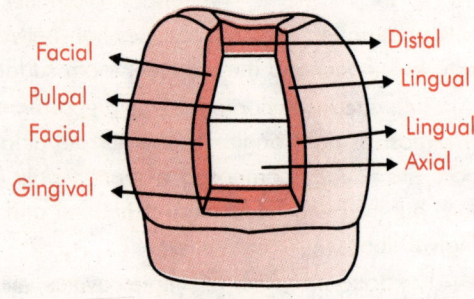

Fig. 6.2

3. **For Class III preparation:** It has 4 walls, i.e. Facial, Lingual, Gingival and Incisal wall (only occasionally) (Fig. 6.3).

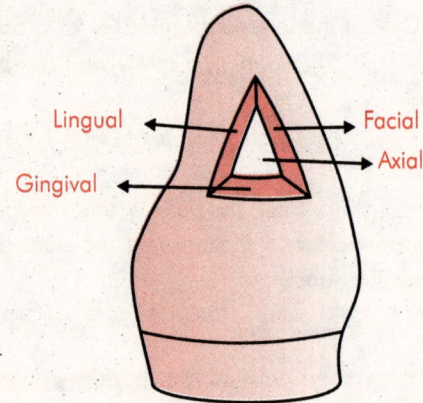

Fig. 6.3

4. **For Class IV preparation:** It has 6 walls, i.e. Mesial, Facial, Axial, Lingual, Pulpal and Gingival (Fig. 6.4).

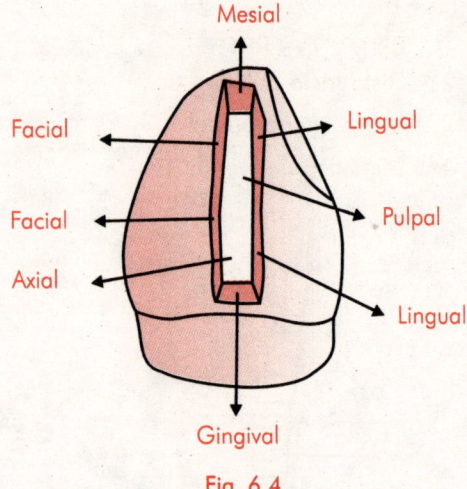

Fig. 6.4

5. **For Class V preparation:** It has 5 walls, i.e. Incisal, Mesial, Axial, Gingival and Distal (Fig. 6.5).

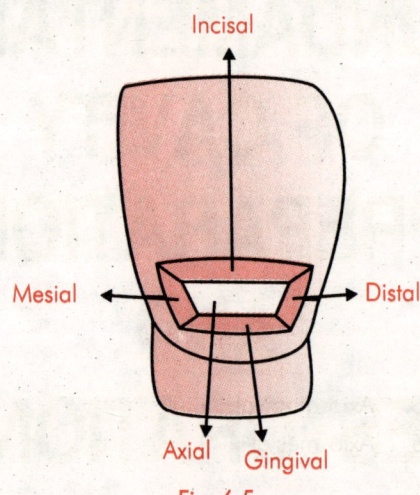

Fig. 6.5

6. **For Class VI preparation:** Same as an occlusal class I preparation.

ANGLES OF THE CAVITY PREPARATION

1. **For Occlusal Cavity: (Class I)** (Fig. 6.6)
   A. **Line angles : (8)**
      1. Mesio facial
      2. Mesio lingual
      3. Disto facial
      4. Disto lingual
      5. Facio pulpal
      6. Linguo pulpal
      7. Mesio pulpal
      8. Disto pulpal

B. Point angles: (4)
1. Mesio facio pulpal
2. Disto facio pulpal
3. Mesio linguo pulpal
4. Disto linguo pulpal

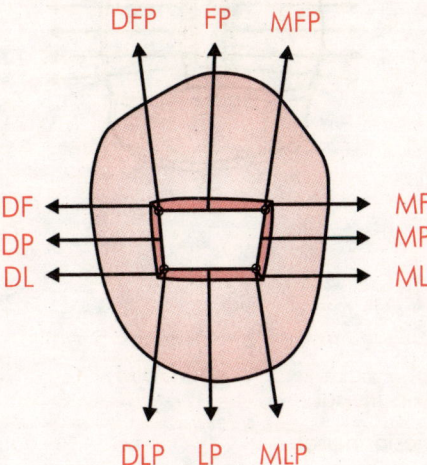

Fig. 6.6

2. For Buccal or Lingual cavities on Posterior teeth

A. Line angles: (8)
1. Mesio gingival
2. Disto gingival
3. Mesio occlusal
4. Disto occlusal
5. Axio gingival
6. Axio mesial
7. Axio occlusal
8. Axio distal

B. Point angles: (4)
1. Axio mesio gingival
2. Axio mesio occlusal
3. Axio disto gingival
4. Axio disto occlusal

3. For Proximo Occlusal cavity:(Class II) (Fig. 6.7)
There are 11 line angles and 6 point angles, i.e.

(i) In the mesial or distal portion: (5 line and 2 point angles)

A. Line angles
1. Bucco gingival
2. Linguo gingival
3. Bucco axial
4. Linguo axial
5. Gingivo axial

B. Point angles
1. Gingivo bucco axial
2. Gingivo linguo axial

(ii) In the step portion: (5 line and 2 point angles)

A. Line angles
1. Bucco distal (or mesial)
2. Linguo distal (or mesial)
3. Disto (or mesial) pulpal
4. Linguo pulpal
5. Bucco pulpal

B. Point angles
1. Disto (or mesio) bucco pulpal
2. Disto (or mesio) linguo pulpal

– Also an *axio pulpal line angle* and *pulpo linguo axial* and *pulpo bucco axial point angles* may be named.

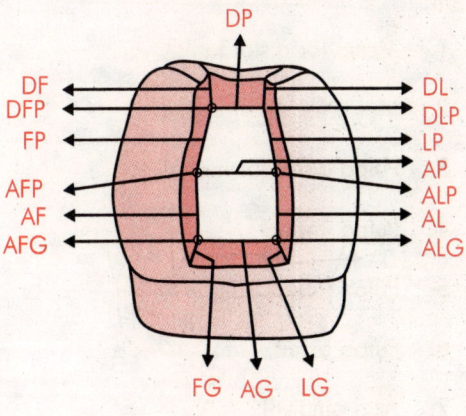

Fig. 6.7

4. For Mesial and Distal cavities on Anterior teeth (Class III) (Fig. 6.8)

A. Line angles: (6)
1. Labio (facio) gingival
2. Linguo gingival
3. Axio incisal
4. Axio labial (facial)
5. Axio lingual
6. Axio gingival

B. Point angles: (3)
1. Axio labio gingival
2. Axio linguo gingival
3. Axio incisal

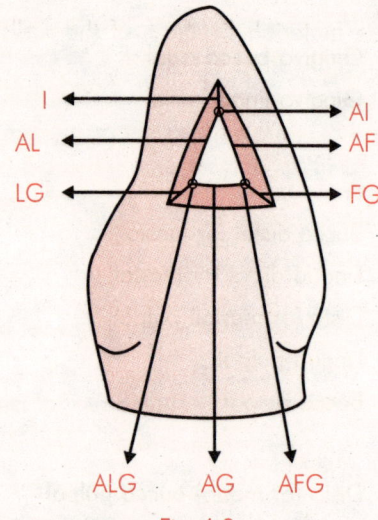

Fig. 6.8

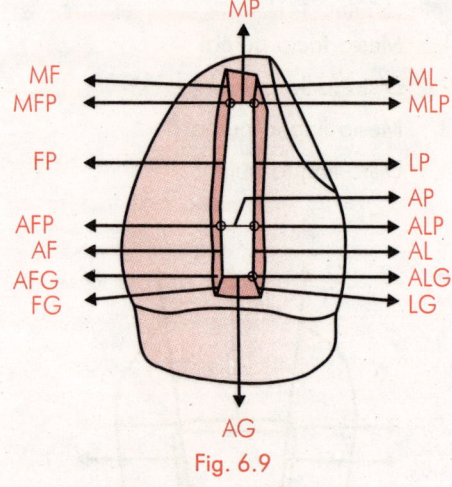

Fig. 6.9

5. For Proximo Incisal cavity: (Class IV) (Fig. 6.9)

A. Line angles: (11)

1. Mesio (or disto) labial

2. Mesio (or disto) lingual

3. Pulpo distal (or mesial)

4. Pulpo lingual

5. Pulpo labial

6. Pulpo axial

7. Axio gingival

8. Facio gingival

9. Linguo gingival

10. Axio facial

11. Axio pulpal

B. Point angles: (6)

1. Mesio (or disto) pulpolabial

2. Mesio (or disto) pulpo lingual

3. Axio facio gingival

4. Axio linguo gingival

5. Axio facio pulpal

6. Axio linguo pulpal

6. For a Class-V cavity (Fig. 6.10)

A. Line angles : (8)

1. Axio incisal

2. Mesio incisal

3. Axio mesial

4. Mesio gingival

5. Axio gingival

6. Disto gingival

7. Disto incisal

8. Axio distal

B. Point angles : (4)

1. Axio disto incisal

2. Axio mesio incisal

3. Axio mesio gingival

4. Axio disto gingival

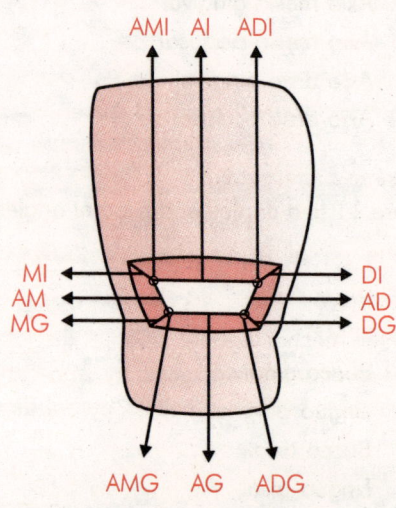

Fig. 6.10

PRINCIPLES OF THE CAVITY PREPARATION

CAVITY: Refers to *a defect in enamel or in enamel and dentin, resulting from the pathologic process of dental caries.*

CAVITY PREPARATION

Defined as *"the mechanical alteration of defective, injured or diseased tooth in order to best receive restorative materials which will re establish the form, function and esthetics".* Or also defined as *"the orderly operating procedure required to establish in a tooth the biomechanically acceptable form necessary to receive and retain a restoration".*

Cavities are prepared with rotary and hand cutting instruments, by a sequential follow-up of a series of steps.

OBJECTIVES OF CAVITY PREPARATION

1. To remove all the defects and to give necessary protection to the pulp.
2. To locate the margins of the restoration in a consecutive manner.
3. To form the cavity, that will not allow the fracture of the tooth or restoration and the displacement of the restoration.
4. To allow for the esthetic and functional placement of a restoration.

FACTORS AFFECTING CAVITY PREPARATION

1. **Diagnosis**
   - Caries, fractured teeth, esthetics.
   - Occlusal relationships.
   - Risk potential.
2. **Knowledge of dental anatomy**
3. **Patients factors**
   - Age, economic status.

STAGES OF CAVITY PREPARATION

1. **1st Stage: Initial cavity preparation**

   Includes the mechanical alteration of the tooth which is extended to enamel, supported by, non-carious dentin in all directions but into a limited pulpal depth.

2. **2nd Stage: Final cavity preparation**

   Includes the completion of the cavity, i.e. excavation of remaining infected carious dentin, removal of the old restorative material, finishing of the walls, cleaning, inspection and varnishing of the cavity.

STEPS IN CAVITY PREPARATION: (G.V. Black)

I. **Initial cavity preparation stage**
   1. Obtaining outline form and initial depth.
   2. Obtaining primary resistance form.
   3. Obtaining primary retention form.
   4. Obtaining convenience form.

II. **Final cavity preparation stage**
   1. Removal of carious tooth portion and old restoration if any.
   2. Secondary resistance and retention form.
   3. Finishing of external walls.
   4. Debridement of the preparation.

1. *OUTLINE FORM AND INITIAL DEPTH*

- Outline form is *the shape of the area of the tooth surface included within the cavo surface margins of the prepared cavity.*
- Outline form usually varies according to the type of restorative material and to the class of preparation.
- Initial depth varies from 0.2–0.8 mm pulpally of the DEJ.

Principles of establishing outline form are,

1. All weakened enamel should be removed.
2. All faults should be included.
3. All margins should be placed in esthetically pleasing position.

Factors determining the outline form are,

1. Extent of caries, defect or faulty or old restoration.
2. Occlusal condition.
3. Cavo surface marginal configuration.
4. Adjacent tooth contour.
5. Esthetic consideration.

Significance of outline form

Provides sufficient access for the proper cavity preparation and for the placement and finishing of the restoration.

2. *PRIMARY RESISTANCE FORM*

- Defined as *the shape given to the preparation that enables the restoration and remaining tooth structure to withstand masticatory stresses without fracture.*

- This property is chiefly obtained by the bulk of the cavity form in an axio pulpal direction; the bulk in turn produces thickness for the restoration and the optimum compressive and tensile strengths.

- Primary resistance is obtained by the following features during cavity preparation, i.e.

  1. Flat pulpal and gingival wall.
  2. Box shaped cavity.
  3. Inclusion of weakened tooth structure.
  4. Restricting the extension of external walls.
  5. Preservation of cusps and marginal ridges.
  6. Rounding internal line angles.
  7. Providing adequate thickness of restorative material.
  8. Reduction of cusps for capping when indicated.
  9. Parallelism of the walls.

3. PRIMARY RETENTION FORM

- Defined as *the shape given to the preparation that resists displacement or removal of the restoration from the tipping or lifting forces.*

- Retention means are divided into principal and auxillary types according to their efficiency in retaining the restoration.

A. Principal means of retention

i. Frictional retention

It can be obtained (i) by increasing the surface area of contact between tooth structure and restorative material (ii) by creation of opposing walls or surfaces, (iii) by producing parallelism between opposing walls, (iv) by bringing the restorative material closer to tooth structure during insertion.

ii. Elastic deformation of dentin

It can be done by changing the position of dentinal walls and floors microscopically by using condensation energy within the dentin's proportional limit.

It creates more gripping action by the tooth on the restorative material.

iii. Undercuts or inverted truncated cones

Usually placed in the point angles of the cavity.

iv. Dove-tail retention

Dove-tail is *a widened or fanned-out portion of the prepared cavity, usually established to increase the retention and resistance form.*

B. Auxillary means of retention

i. Grooves cut in dentin without undermining the adjacent enamel whenever bulk allows.

ii. Internal boxes have definite walls and floors.

iii. Posts are made from wrought or cast metal and placed in the root canals.

iv. Pins are made from cast or wrought metal. They may be parallel or non-parallel, vertical or horizontal, threaded or cemented.

v. Triangular areas: are placed within the dentin and are located laterally without undermining overlying enamel plates.

vi. Acid conditioning or etching of enamel creates mechanical locks and increases surface areas of contact between tooth structure and the restorative material. Sometimes, it is considered as a principal retention mode.

vii. Cements or Luting agents: Least effective auxillary means of retention.

4. CONVENIENCE FORM

Defined as, *the shape given to a tooth preparation or modification added to the basic preparation, to facilitate proper instrumentation for the preparation of the cavity or insertion of the restorative material.*

i. Modifications in tooth preparation: Include flaring of some walls more than otherwise necessary for resistance or retention to decrease distortion errors during the fabrication of intermediate materials (castings); decreasing the roundness of some walls more than normally needed; extension of margins more than otherwise necessary.

ii. Instrument modification: Includes contra-angling, bayonetting or the addition of several angles to the shank of an instrument.

iii. Separation: Includes the use of wedges interproximally during proximal surface instrumentation.

5. REMOVAL OF CARIOUS TOOTH PORTION AND OLD RESTORATION IF ANY

- Removal of caries is the mechanical elimination of carious dentin and debris from the cavity preparation.

- If the decay is soft, removal should be done with the broadest discoid or spoon excavator, directing it with scooping actions from the cavity peripheries to the center.

– If the decay is hard, a large round bur is used in addition to excavator. Bur should be in slow revolving motion, used with brushing strokes from the peripheries of the cavity preparation to the center, with a lot of water coolant.

6. SECONDARY RESISTANCE AND RETENTION FORM

– After the removal of infected dentin and/or old restorative material, pulpal protection is provided.

– Now, resistance and retention features are necessary for the preparation.

– The secondary resistance and retention forms are of 2 types:
  A. Mechanical preparation features.
  B. Treatments of the preparation walls with etching, priming and adhesive materials.

A. Mechanical Features

I. Retention Locks, Grooves and Coves

1. Retention locks

Proximal retention locks in the axiofacial and axiolingual line angles significantly *strengthen the isthmus of a class II restoration* and are superior to axiogingival grooves in *increasing the restoration's fracture strength*, and *prevents the proximal displacement of the restoration.*

Characteristics

There are 4 characteristics or determinants of proximal locks, i.e.
1. Position
2. Translation
3. Depth and
4. Occlusogingival orientation

Position refers to the axiofacial and axiolingual line angles of initial tooth preparation (0.2 mm axial to DEJ). *Retention locks should be placed 0.2 mm inside the DEJ, regardless of the depth of the axial walls and axial line angles.*

Translation refers to the direction of movement of the axis of the bur.

Depth refers to the extent of translation (i.e 0.5 mm at gingival floor level).

Occlusogingival orientation refers to the tilt of the No. 169 L bur which dictates the occulusal height of the lock, given a constant depth.

Preparation

– To prepare a retention lock, use a no.169 L bur with air coolant (to improve vision) and reduced speed (to improve tactile 'feel' and control).

– The bur is placed in the properly positioned axiolingual line angle and directed to bisect the angle approximately parallel to the DEJ. This positions the retention lock 0.2 mm inside the DEJ, thus maintianing the enamel support.

– The bur is titled to allow cutting to the depth of the diameter of the end of the bur at the point angle and permit the lock to diminish in depth occlusally, terminating at the axiolinguopulpal point angle.

– In a similar manner facial lock is prepared in the axiofacial line angle.

– If the axial line angle is too shallow, the lock may undermine the enamel of dentinal support.

– If the line angle is too deep, preparation of the lock may result in exposure of the pulp.

2. Retention grooves

– Grooves are for cast metal restorations and also root surface tooth preparation in composites.

– Grooves are horizontally oriented.

– Are prepared in most class III and V preparations for amalgam and in some root surface tooth preparations for composite.

1. In Class II Amalgam

– Prepare the retention grooves with a no. ¼ bur into the occlusoaxial and gingivoaxial line angles, 0.2 mm inside the DEJ or 0.3 to 0.5 mm inside the cemental cavosurface margin.

– The depth of these grooves is one half the diameter of the bur head (i.e 0.25 mm).

– The bur is directed to bisect the angle formed by the junction of occlusal (or gingival) and axial walls.

– Ideally, the direction of the occlusal groove is slightly more occlusal than axial, and the direction of a gingival groove would be slightly more gingival than axial.

2. In Class III Amalgam

– Prepare the gingival retention groove by placing a no. ¼ bur in the axio faciogingival point angle.

– It is positioned in the dentin to maintain 0.2 mm of dentin between the groove and the DEJ.

– Move the bur lingually along the axiogingival line angle with the angle of cutting generally bisecting the angle between the gingival and axial walls.

3. **In Class V Amalgam**

- Use a no. ¼ bur to prepare two retention grooves, one along the incisoaxial line angle and the other along the gingivoaxial line angle.
- The handpiece is positioned so that the no. ¼ bur is directed generally to bisect the angle formed at the junction of the axial wall and the incisal (or occlusal) wall.
- The depth of the grooves should be approximately 0.25 mm which is half the diameter of the bur.

4. **In Class III composite**

- Groove retention may be necessary in root surface preparations.
- The retention groove created helps in (1). Minimizing the negative effects of polymerization shrinkage, (2) enhance the marginal seal by resisting flexural forces placed on the cervical portion of the restoration.
- A continuous retention groove can be prepared in the internal portion of the external walls using a no. ¼ round bur.
- The groove is located 0.25 mm from the root surface and is prepared to a depth of 0.25 mm.
- This groove is directed as the bisector of the angle formed by the junction of the axial wall and the external wall. For its entire length, the groove should be parallel to the root surface.

5. **In Class IV Composite**

- A gingival retention groove can be prepared using a no. ¼ round bur.
- It is prepared 0.2 mm inside the DEJ at a depth of 0.25 mm and at an angle bisecting the junction of the axial wall and gingival wall.
- The groove should extend the length of the gingival floor and slightly up the facioaxial and linguoaxial line angles.

6. **In Class V Composite**

- Retention grooves are prepared with a no. ¼ bur along the full length of the gingivoaxial and inciso axial (occlusoaxial) line angles.
- These grooves are prepared 0.25 mm in depth into the external walls and next to the axial wall at an angle that bisects the junction between the axial wall and the gingival or occlusal (or incisal) wall.

3. **Retention coves**

Retention coves are appropriately placed undercuts for the incisal retention of class III amalgams, occlusal portion of some amalgam restorations, some class V amalgams and occasionally for facilitating the start of insertion of certain gold foil restorations.

1. **In Class - III Amalgam**

- If less retention form is needed, two gingival coves may be used, as opposed to a continuous groove.
- One each may be placed in the axiogingivo facial and axiogingivo lingual point angles.
- The diameter of the bur is 0.5 mm and the depth of the groove should be half this diameter or 0.25 mm.
- Prepare an incisal retention cove at the axiofacio incisal point angle with a no. ¼ bur in dentin, being careful not to undermine the enamel.
- It is directed similarly into the incisal point angle and prepared to one half the diameter of the bur.
- Undermining the incisal enamel (or incisal canopy) should be avoided.

2. **In Class - I Amalgam**

- No. 33 ½ bur may be used to prepare a retention cove in the faciopulpal line angle.
- The tip of the No. 245 bur held parallel to the long axis of the tooth crown also might be used to prepare this cove.
- This retention cove is recommended only if occlusal convergence of the mesial and distal walls of the occlusal portion is absent or inadequate.

3. **In Class V Amalgam**

- Four retention coves may be prepared, one in each of the four axial point angles of the preparation.
- Using four coves instead of two full length grooves conserves dentin near the pulp.

II. **Groove extensions**

- These are obtained by extending the preparation for molars onto the facial or lingual surface to include the facial or lingual groove.
- These extensions are given for cast metal restorations.
- This feature enchances resistance for the remaining tooth.

III. **Skirts**

- Skirts are preparation features that extend the preparation around the line angles of the tooth.
- Skirts increase the resistance form by enveloping the tooth.
- Used in cast gold restorations.

IV. Beveled enamel margins

- These are primarily used to provide a better junctional relationship between the metal and the tooth.
- Bevel provides increased surface area for etchable enamel in composite restorations.
- Used in cast gold/metal restorations.

V. Pins, slots, steps and amalgapins

- These are indicated when there is unusually great need for increased retention form.
- Mostly for amalgam restorations.

B. Placement of Etchant, Primer or Adhesive on prepared walls

Along with mechanical alterations, certain etchants and primers are used for increased retention and resistance.

1. Enamel wall etching

- Etching results in microscopically roughened surface to which the bonding material is mechanically bound.
- Enamel walls are etched for porcelain, composite and amalgam materials.

2. Dentin treatment

- Dentin surface require etching and priming for bonded porcelain, composite or amalgam restorations.

7. FINISHING OF EXTERNAL WALLS

Objectives

1. To create best marginal seal between restorative material and tooth structure.
2. To afford a smooth marginal structure.
3. To provide maximum strength to the tooth and the restorative material near the margin.

For an ideal enamel wall, *Noy* formulated certain structural requirements. They are,

1. The enamel wall must rest upon sound dentin.
2. The enamel rods which form the cavosurface angle must have their inner ends resting on sound dentin.
3. The enamel rods which form the cavosurface angle must be supported, or be resting on sound dentin and their outer ends must be covered by the restorative material.
4. The cavosurface angle must be trimmed or beveled so that the margins will not be exposed to injury in condensing the restorative material against it.

8. DEBRIDEMENT (TOILET) OF THE PREPARATION

- Defined as *the act of freeing the preparation walls and margins from objects that may interfere with the proper adaptability and behaviour of the restorative material.*

- It includes the freeing of all preparation walls, floors and margins from enamel and dentin chips resulting from excavation and grinding; drying the preparation walls, floors and margins from any introduced moisture; sterilization of preparation of walls and floors.

Methods

1. Water, air or combinations of air-water jets, using the water-air syringe is very efficient in removing.
2. Dry cotton pellets is a safer way to dry the cavity.
3. Cavity cleaners which are solutions of very low concentration of citric, ascorbic and acetic acids are sometimes used to remove the debris. They should be used in shallow cavities and should be followed by long period of water jet rinsing.
4. A dilute solution of hydrogen peroxide is a very efficient debris removing agent.
5. Scrapping preparation walls, floors and margins with sharp hand instruments especially chisels is most effective way of freeing the lodged debris.
6. Smear layer of the preparation can be removed by a solution of 10% EDTA.

EMPHASIS ON CONSERVATIVE CAVITY PREPARATION

- Inspite of tremendous improvements in dental biomaterials, we still do not have an ideal restorative material.
- Every restorative material has its own disadvantages and hence, it is not equal to normal healthy tooth structure.
- So, during cavity preparation, we should emphasize on complete removal of the diseased tooth structure and minimal necessary removal of normal tooth structure for better resistance and retention purposes.

RESTORATIONS

- Restoration is defined as *filling material or prosthesis used to restore or replace a tooth, a portion of a tooth, multiple teeth or other oral tissues.*

Classification

I. Based on fabrication

1. Direct restoration
2. Indirect restoration

II. Based on longevity

1. Intermediate/temporary
2. Permanent

1. Direct Restoration

Defined as a *cement, metal or resin-based composite that is placed and formed intra orally to restore teeth or enhance esthetics.*

Ex: Amalgam, GIC, Composite, DFG, etc.

2. Indirect Restoration

Defined as a *ceramic, metal, metal-ceramic, or resin-based composite used extraorally to produce prosthesis, which replace missing teeth, enhance esthetics and/or restore damaged teeth.*

3. Intermediate / Temporary Restoration

Defined as a *tooth filling or prosthesis that is placed for a limited period, from several days to months, and is designed to seal teeth and maintain their position until a long-term restoration is placed.*

4. Permanent Restoration

Defined as a *long-lasting replacement or restoration for missing damaged or discoloured teeth.*

Indications for Restorations

1. Caries
2. Replacement or repair of old restorations
3. Fractured teeth
4. To restore form and function
5. Esthetic desire
6. To fulfil other restorative needs

Factors affecting the placement of the restoration

1. Extent of caries.
2. Strength of remaining tooth structure.
3. Patient's oral hygiene and dental caries history.
4. Economic status.
5. Ability of the dentist to perform the procedure.
6. Preferences of the dentist and the prevailing standard of care.
7. Patient's acceptance.

CHAPTER 07

DENTAL AMALGAM RESTORATIONS

A. INITIAL TOOTH PREPARATION

1. Outline form

- The class I amalgam tooth preparation should include only the faulty, defective occulsal pits and fissures.

- Cavity margins occulsally should be located on smooth surfaces, inclined planes of cusps, marginal ridges and crossing ridges.

- Begin, the tooth preparation by entering the deepest faulty pit with a `punch cut' using a no. 245, round carbide bur.

- Bur should be positioned parallel to the long axis of the tooth.

- Entering the distal pit first provides increased visibility for mesial extension.

- For a class I preparation, a faciolingual width of not more than 1 to 1.5 mm or one-fourth of intercuspal distance and a depth of 1.5 to 2mm is ideal, and the depth measured at the central fissure.

- Extension of the cavity is made using a plain straight fissure carbide bur.

- Cavity is extended along the central fissure toward the mesial pit following the DEJ creating a flat pulpal floor.

2. Primary Resistance form

- Flat pulpal floor in sound tooth structure to resist forces directed in long axis of the tooth.

- Occlusal buccopulpal and linguopulpal line angles are rounded.

- Minimal extension of external wall.

- Strong, ideal enamel margins.

- Adequate depth.

3. Primary Retention form

- Parallelism or right occlusal converge of two or more opposing external walls.

4. Convenience form

- Shape and form of the cavity gives the accessibility during the restoration.

B. FINAL TOOTH PREPARATION

- Removal of the remaining enamel pit-and-fissure in the pulpal floor.

- The floor of the cavity is deepened to eliminate the fault and to remove the caries.

- Infected dentin is best removed by discoid type spoon excavator or a slow revolving round carbide bur.

- When removing the infected dentin, stop the excavation when the tooth structure feels hard or firm.

- External walls are finished, providing an approximate of 90 to 100 degree cavosurface angle.

- Prepared tooth is inspected and cleaned before restoration.

- Tooth is rinsed with air water syringe.

DESIGNS OF CLASS I CAVITY PREPARATION

1. Class I, Design 1 (Fig. 7.1)

- *Involves occlusal surfaces of molars and premolars.*

- *Indications*

1. Penetration of caries does not exceeding 0.5 mm to 1mm into dentin.

2. Decay not involving more than one-fourth of the intercuspal distance.

3. Patients with good oral hygiene and low caries index.

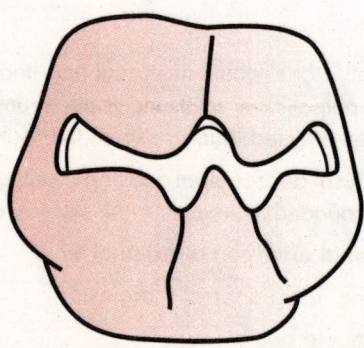

Fig. 7.1

2. Class I, Design 2 (Fig. 7.2)

- *Involves occlusal surfaces of molars and premolars.*

- *Indications.*

1. Penetration of caries exceeding 1mm into dentin.

2. Decay involving more than one-fourth of the intercuspal distance.

3. Patients with high plaque and caries indices.

4. Teeth with intact cusps.

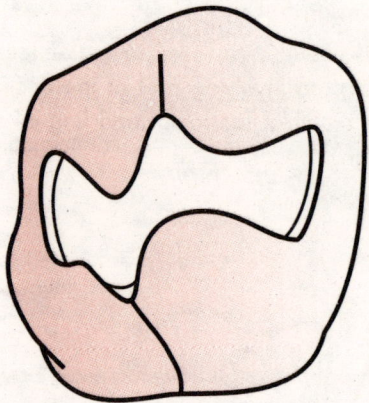

Fig. 7.2

3. Class I, Design 3 (Fig. 7.3)

- Involves the occlusal one- to two-third of the facial and lingual surfaces of molars and on the lingual surfaces of upper anterior teeth (usually the lateral incisors).

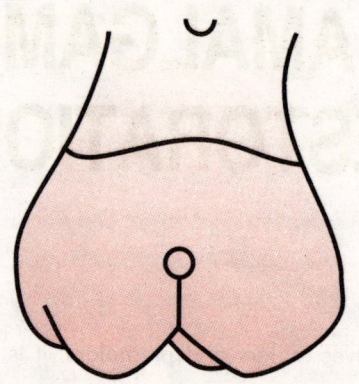

Fig. 7.3

4. Class I, Design 4 (Fig. 7.4)

- Involves molars in addition to involvement of occlusal surfaces, the grooves of facial and or lingual surfaces are also involved.

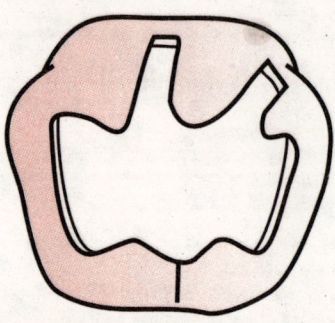

Fig. 7.4

5. Class I, Design 5 (Fig. 7.5)

   – Involvement is confined to molar teeth, where in addition to involving part of the occlusal surface, most or all of the facial and lingual surfaces are also involved.

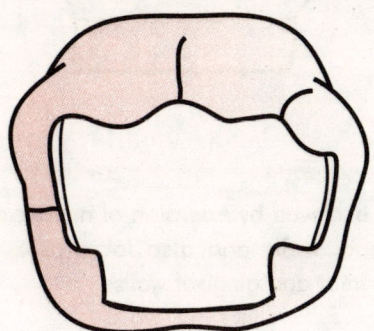

Fig. 7.5

6. Class I, Design 6

   – Involves a part of the occlusal surfaces of molars or premolars and a portion of the facial, proximal or lingual surface in the form of a table of an entire cusp (marginal ridge) or a section of a cusp (marginal ridge).

7. Class I, Design 7

   – Involves the occlusal, facial and / or lingual surfaces of molars and premolars.

8. Class I, Design 8

   – Involves molars and premolars, it is used on the occlusal and sometimes on the occlusal and / or facial lingual surfaces. Also used on the lingual surfaces of anterior teeth.

CLASS II CAVITY PREPARATION

Factors affecting the success of Class II Amalgam Restoration

1. Tooth preparation.
2. Proper matrix selection and adaptation of matrix.
3. Isolation of the operating field.
4. Proper manipulation of restorative material.

A. Initial tooth preparation

1. Occlusal outline form (Fig. 7.6)

   – Occlusal outline is similar to that of class I amalgam tooth preparation.

   – Begin the tooth preparation by entering into the pit nearest involved proximal surface punch cut using no. 245 bur.

   – Bur should be positioned parallel to the long axis of the tooth, create facial, lingual and distal walls with slight occlusal convergence.

   – Initial depth is 1.5–2mm or 1/2 to 2/3 of the cutting length of no. 245 bur. Depth is measured from central fissure.

   – Dovetail is created at the opposite end of the proximal involvement.

   – Width of the cavity is 1/4th of the intercuspal distance.

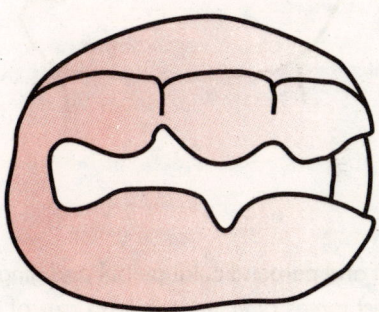

Fig. 7.6

2. Proximal outline from (Fig. 7.7)

   – Visualize and locate the facial and lingual walls of the proximal box relatively to the contact area.

Objectives of extension of proximal margins

   – to include all caries.

   – to create 90° cavosurface margin.

   – to establish 0.5 mm clearance with the adjacent proximal surface facially, lingually and gingivally.

Proximal ditch cut

   – Position the bur over the pulpal floor next to the remaining marginal ridge, cut the ditch gingivally along the exposed DEJ.

   – 2/3rd of the expense of the dentin (0.5 to 0.6 mm)

   – 1/3rd at the expense of the enamel (0.2 to 0.3 mm)

   – Pressure is directed gingivally and the bur move facially and lingually.

   – *Gingival seat is located 1–2 mm below the contact area.*

– *Axial depth of gingival seat is about 0.6 to 0.8 mm in dentin.*

– Proximal ditch cut may be diverged gingivally to make the facial lingual extension gingivally greater than occlusal and this is done by using no. 245 inverted cone bur.

– Removing the remaining undermined enamel with enamel hatchet in a scrapping motion on facioproximal, linguoproximal and gingival wall.

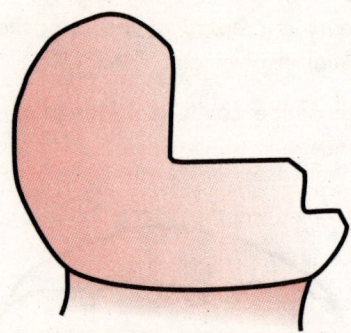

Fig. 7.7

3. Primary Resistance form

– Flat and perpendicular pulpal and gingival walls to resist forces directed with long axis of the tooth.

– Restricting the extension of walls to allow strong cusp ridges to remain with sufficient dentin support.

– Restricting the occlusal step.

– Reverse curve at the junction of occlusal step and proximal box gives strength to amalgam and tooth (Fig. 7.8).

– *Internal line angles are rounded.*

– *Axiopulpal line angle is rounded.*

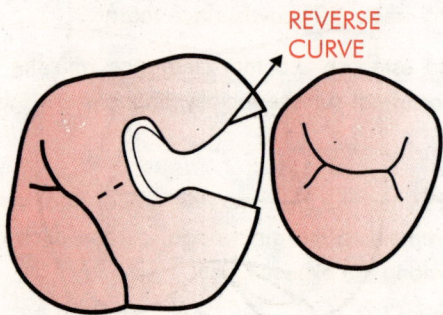

REVERSE
CURVE

Fig. 7.8

4. Primary Retention form (Fig. 7.9)

– Occlusal convergence of facial and lingual proximal wall.

– Dovetail design on the occlusal step.

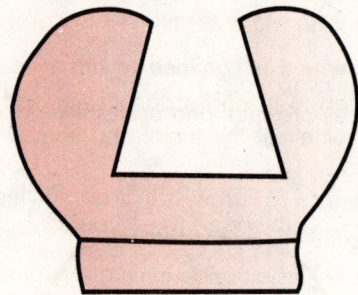

Fig. 7.9

5. Convenience form

– It is achieved by extension of mesial, distal, facial, lingual walls and also facio proximal, linguo proximal and gingival walls.

B. FINAL TOOTH PREPARATION

– Removal of any remaining defective enamel and infected carious dentin.

– Removal of old restoration.

– Infected carious dentin is removed with slow speed round bur or discoid type spoon excavator.

1. Pulp Protection

– Base applied is zinc poly carboxylate or zinc phosphate.

2. Secondary Resistance and Retention form

– Restricting of extension of external walls.

– *Bevelling the axiopulpal line angle.*

– Induction of retentive locks located occlusal to the axiopulpal line angle prove more resistance.

– Proximal retentive locks in the axiofacial and axiolingal line angles.

– Induction of grooves in the proximal box.

– The occlusal convergence of the facial and lingual wall and the dovetail design provide sufficient retention form.

– Introduction of proximal locks by using no. 169L bur.

3. Procedure for finishing external walls

– Preparation walls should be free of unsupported enamel rods and marginal irregularities.

– 90 degree cavosurface angle at the proximal margin.

– Use GMT to establish a slight cavosurface bevel at the gingival margin.

– Prepared tooth is cleaned and inspected before restoration.

– Disinfectants are used for cleaning tooth preparation.

DESIGNS OF CLASS II CAVITY PREPARATION

1. **Class II, Design 1 (Conventional Design) (Fig. 7.10)**

   – *Involves proximal and occlusal surfaces.*

   – Indications.

   1. Moderate to large size proximal lesion with the involvement of occlusal surface.
   2. Proximal lesion undermining an adjacent marginal ridge or not accessible through any other means but involvement of the occlusal surfaces.
   3. A class II in stress bearing areas.
   4. An oral environment where local cariogenic conditions contraindicate a modern design.

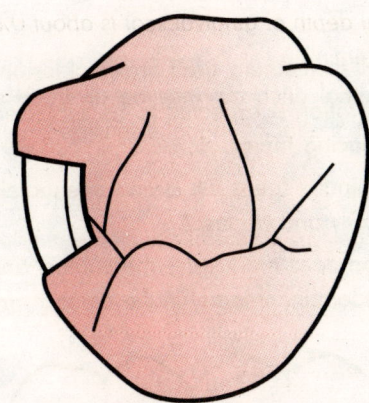

Fig. 7.11

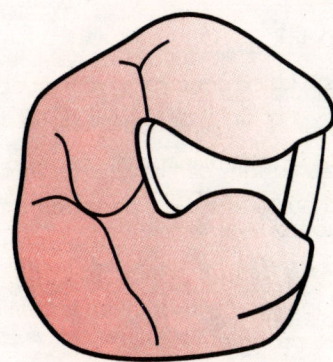

Fig. 7.10

2. **Class II, Design 2 (Modern Design) (Fig. 7.11)**

   – *Involves proximal and occlusal surfaces.*

   – Indications.

   1. A moderate to small sized proximal lesions.
   2. A class II in a stress bearing area.
   3. An occlusal lesion undermining one or both marginal ridges and not exceeding a width of 1/4 of the intercuspal distance.

3. **Class II, Design 3 (Conservative Design)**

   – *Involves primarily the proximal surface and a very limited part of the occlusal surface not extending beyond the adjacent triangular fossa.*

   – Indications.

   1. The decay is restricted to the proximal surface only and the occlusal surface is completely sound.
   2. When the restoration is expected to be subjected to minimal loading.
   3. There are sound pronounced occlusal crossing ridges and the inclined planes of the adjacent cusps are smooth and are devoid of any crossing fissures.

4. **Class II, Design 4 (Simple Design) (Fig. 7.12)**

   – *Involves proximal surfaces only.*

   – Indications.

   1. Decay is restricted to contacting or proximal surfaces without undermining the corresponding marginal ridges.
   2. When there is diastemaor the adjacent tooth is missing and facilitating direct access.
   3. The affected tooth is rotated or inclined so that the contacting surface is not the anatomical proximal one, again facilitating access.
   4. The proximal lesion is located very gingivally at or apical to the CEJ, accompanied by gingival recession.
   5. The proximal lesion occurs on tapered teeth with wide gingival embrasures facilitating facial or lingual access to the lesion.

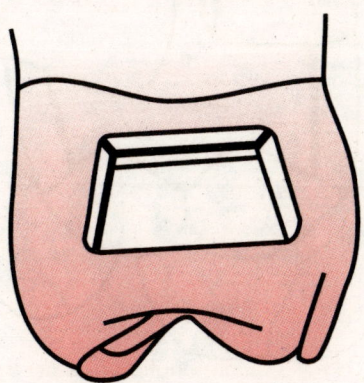

Fig. 7.12

5. **Class II, Design 5 (Fig. 7.13)**

   – *Involves part of the proximal surface with a very limited access area on the facial and lingual areas.*

– Indications.

1. Small to medium sized proximal lesions.

2. Restoration is expected to be subjected to normal displacing forces.

3. Marginal ridge is intact and adequately supported apically and occlusally.

4. Lesion does not involve the contact area nor does it undermine enamel in the contact area.

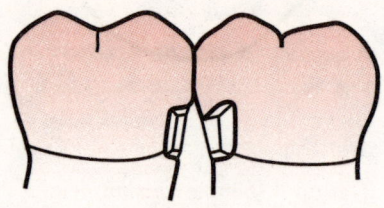

Fig. 7.13

6. **Class II, Design 6** (Fig. 7.14)

   – *Involves the occlusal, proximal and part of the facial and / or lingual surfaces.*

   – Indications.

1. Cusp is completely missing or undermined.

2. The cusp length is double or more its width either throughout or at certain portions of the cusp.

3. When a foundation for cast restoration is required.

4. Teeth with a doubtful prognosis both endodontically and periodontally.

5. A cast restoration is not indicated.

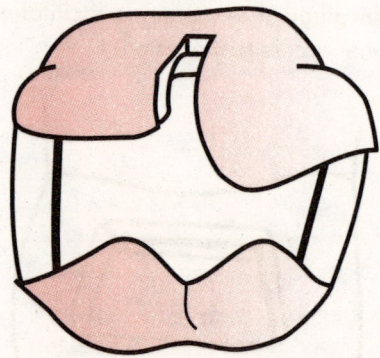

Fig. 7.14

7. **Class II, Design 7 (Combination of Class II with Class V)** (Fig. 7.15)

   Shape A : The junction between the class II and class II via the proximal, crossing the axial angles.

   – *Involves the occlusal, proximal and part or all of the gingival third of the facial and or lingual surfaces with the intervening part of the axial angle.*

– · Indications.

1. A location apical to the contact area, an occluso-proximal lesion joins a senile decay.

2. Class V lesion undermines enamel or directly involves tooth structure of the adjacent axial angles in a tooth having a proximoocclusal lesion.

3. Surface defects or decalfications at the axial angle of the tooth are continuous with a proximo occlusal cavity preparation or lesion apical to the contact area.

Shape B :   The junction between the class II and class V is through the occlusal via the buccal and or lingual grooves.

   – *Involves the proximal, occlusal, facial and or lingual surfaces.*

   – Indications.

1. A class V lesion connecting with an occlusoproximal lesion via a facial or lingual fissured groove.

2. Surface defects or decalcifications on the facial or lingual surface connecting a class V lesion with an occlusoproximal lesion.

3. A class V lesion which is continuous with a class I, design 4 which inturn is continuous with an occluso proximal lesion.

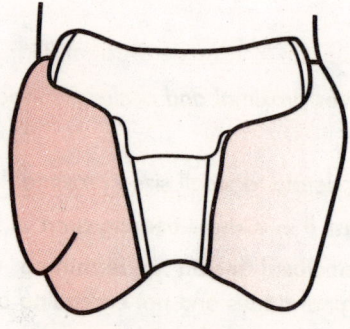

Fig. 7.15

8. **Class II, Design 8**

   – *Involves two or more surfaces of an endodontically treated tooth that does not require post retention.*

   – Indications.

1. The remaining tooth structure, after endodontics can support and retain an amalgam restorations.

2. The tooth has a sufficient pulp chamber to accommodate, retaining, self resisting amalgam bulk, i.e. a minimum 2 mm thickness in three dimensions.

3. The post endodontic pulp chamber has at least two opposing intact walls.

4. The tooth contains sufficiently large root canals to accommodate, retaining, resisting amalgam bulk at its occlusal 1/3rd.

5. A foundation is needed for a reinforcing restoration.

MODIFICATIONS IN TOOTH PREPARATION FOR CLASS II CAVITY

1. Rotated Teeth

- Tooth preparation for rotated teeth follows the same principles as normally aligned teeth.

- The outline form for a tooth preparation on the rotated mandibular second premolar differ from normal, i.e. proximal box is displaced facially as the proximal caries involves the mesiofacial line angle of the tooth crown.

- In case the tooth is rotated to 90 degrees, then the preparation requires an isthmus that includes the cuspal eminence.

- If in case the lesion is small, then slot preparation is required.

2. Unusual Outline Form

- The outline form should conform to the restoration, requirement of the restoration.

Example

1. Usually, a dovetail is not required in the occlusal step of a single proximal surface preparation unless a fissure, emanating from the occlusal step is involved.

2 In an occlusal fissure, i.e. segmented by coalesced enamel, if the preparations are separated by approximately 0.5 mm or more of sound tooth structure then it should be restored with individual amalgam restoration.

3. Adjoining Restorations

- When two restorations adjoin, care must be taken that the outline of the second restoration does not weaken the amalgam margin of the first.

- The preparation requires, that the intersecting margins of the two restoration be at right angles.

4. Abutment Teeth for Removable Partial Denture

- When the tooth is an abutment for a planned removable partial denture, the occlusoproximal outline form adjacent to edentulous area needs additional extension for the rest seat.

- If the rest seat is to be within the amalgam margins then 0.5 mm of amalgam between the rest seat and the margins is recommended.

- If the rest seat involves both amalgam and enamel no modification of the outline form of the tooth preparation is indicated.

5. Tunnelling / Amalgam Tunnel Tooth Restorations

- This preparation joins an occlusal lesion with a proximal lesion by means of a prepared tunnel under the involved marginal ridge.

- Marginal ridge remains essentially intact.

- Developing appropriately formed preparation walls and excavating caries may be compromised by lack of access and visibility.

6. Amalgam Box only Tooth Restorations

- Box only tooth preparations are advocated for posterior teeth in which a proximal surface requires restoration but the occusal surface is not faulty.

- Proximal box is prepared and specific retention form is provided.

- An occlusal step is included.

- These restorations are more conservative as less tooth structure is removed.

REVERSE CURVE

- *The external outline of the occlusal surface where the isthmus joins the buccal proximal flare is often in the form of a convex or a straight line. When the position of the isthmus and the proximal external outline becomes substantially offset buccal-lingually, a reverse curve taking the form of a concave curve is used as a means of conserving sound tooth tissue* (Fig 7.16).

- *Significance :* Preserves the triangular ridge of the affected cusp.

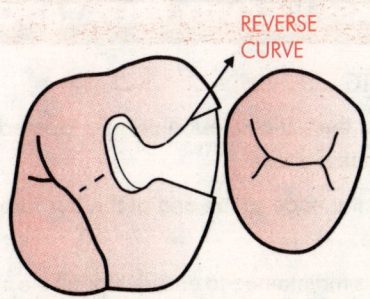

REVERSE CURVE

Fig. 7.16

CLASS III CAVITY PREPARATION

- This is the basic design for the distal aspect of cuspids.

- A lingual access preparation is recommended.

A. INITIAL TOOTH PREPARATION

- Outline form is similar to the conventional class III composite preparation.
- No. 2 bur is used for initial entry on distolingual marginal ridge and bur penetrates the carious lesion beneath contact area.
- Bur is positioned perpendicular to lingual surface of the tooth.
- Initial axial depth is 0.5 to 0.6 mm into the DEJ.
- The cavosurface angle should be 90 degree at all margins.
- Internal line angles are rounded.

B. FINAL TOOTH PREPARATION

- Removal of remaining infected dentin.
- Finishing of external walls.
- Secondary retention form is provided by gingival groove in the axiofacio gingival point angle and it is positioned in the dentin of 0.2 mm between the groove and the DEJ.
- Alternatively retention is obtained by incisal cove and lingual dovetail.
- Axiopupal line angle is bevelled using gingival margin trimmer.
- Remove any unsupported enamel, smoothen the enamel walls and margins and refine cavosurface angles.
- Completed tooth preparation is carefully inspected and cleaned.

CLASS V CAVITY PREPARATION

A. INITIAL TOOTH PREPARATION

- Enter the carious lesion using a tapered surface bur of suitable size.
- Use the edge of the end of the bur to penetrate the area.
- Bur is maintained to ensure that all the external walls are perpendicular to the external tooth surface.
- Initial axial depth is 0.5 mm inside the DEJ.
- And if the root surface is involved, the axial depth, is approximately 0.75 mm.
- For tooth preparation, which is extended inciso gingivally, the axial wall should be more convex.
- Round bur is used to define internal line angles.

B. FINAL TOOTH PREPARATION

- Remove the remaining infected dentin with no. 2 or no.4 round bur.
- Remove the old restoration.
- Use a no. 1/4 bur to prepare two retention grooves, one on incisoaxial line angle and other, on gingivoaxial line angle.
- Or alternatively four retention coves may be prepared, one in each of the four axial point angles.
- Depth of grooves : 0.25 mm.
- In case of inadequate accessibility an angle former chisel can be used to prepare the retention form.
- Clean the preparation.
- Inspect for completeness.

FAILURES OF AMALGAM RESTORATIONS

- The causes are,

1. Wrong selection of cases
   - Amalgam restoration is not suitable for very large caries involving multiple surfaces.

2. Improper cavity preparations
   - It affects the resistance and retention of amalgam restoration leading to fracture or dislodgement of restoration.

3. Delayed expansion
   - Due to moisture contamination the zinc content of amalgam reacts to release hydrogen gas and causes pressure effects and pain.

4. Inadequate cleaning of the cavity

5. Inadequate pulp protection
- Results in microleakage causing secondary caries and pain.

6. Inadequate matrix application
- Causes improper interproximal contours, overhanging restoration which further leads to food impaction and periodontal disease.

7. Improper manipulation of materials
   i. Improper selection of amalgam
   ii. Improper Hg / Alloy Ratio
      - Decreased strength
      - Increased creep
      - Increased expansion of amalgam
      - Decreased corrosion resistance

iii. *Improper trituration*

iv. *Improper condensation*

- High condensation: Amalgam constriction
- Low condensation: Amalgam expansion
- Low condensation pressure :
  - Decreased strength
  - Increased creep rate
  - Decreased corrosion resistance

8. Improper or non-carved amalgam are susceptible to fracture.

9. Failure to polish decreases corrosion resistance.

FINISHING AND POLISHING OF AMALGAM RESTORATIONS

- Finishing of amalgam restoration is necessary to correct a marginal discrepancy or improve the contour.

- Amalgam polishing is done usually after 24 hours of insertion because crystallization is not complete within 24 hours.

1. ### Occlusal Surfaces

   - Any irregularities are removed with green stones. Stones are tapered or inverted cone.

   Initial polishing

   A. Unwebbed rubber cup and soft cup brush with a slurry of silex is used.

   B. Finishing burs of different sizes and shapes.

2. ### Proximal Surfaces

   - Overhangs are eliminated with no. 12 BP blade or gold foil knives or spoon excavators.

   Finishing and polishing

   - Narrow, fine water resistant finishing strips and / or dental tape are placed beneath the contact and passed back and forth

3. ### Buccal and Lingual proximal margins

   - Finished with adequately fixed extra fine water proof disk.

4. ### Final Polishing

   - Of the occlusal surface and accessible area of proximal surface, with a fine grit rubber polishing point or with the rubber cup with flour of pumice followed by a high luster agent such as precipitated chalk.

PIN RETAINED AMALGAM RESTORATIONS

- Pin retained amalgam restorations are defined as any restoration requiring placement of one or more pins for providing adequate retention.

INDICATIONS

1. It is mainly indicated to restore badly broken young permanent teeth where there is insufficient amount of dentin present to get retention form, by means of grooves or slots but sufficient amount of dentin present for placement of pins.

2. It can be used as a transitional restoration prior to endodontic, periodontic, orthodontic treatments.

3. Pin retention is required in foundations for partial or full veneer cast restoration or metalo-ceramic restorations.

4. As an auxiliary or reciprocal retention.

CONTRAINDICATIONS

1. In extremely large pulp chamber (due to insufficient amount of dentin for placement of pins).

2. Subgingivally deep calculus.

ADVANTAGES

1. More conservation of tooth structure.

2. Less time consuming.

3. Economic.

DISADVANTAGES

1. Since pins help only in retention but will does reinforce amalgam, it cannot be used in very high stress bearing area.

2. Difficult to achieve proper contact and contour.

3. Risk of possibility of perforation of pulp, or periodontal ligament space unless skillfully done.

4. Microleakage.

5. Decreased tensile strength of silver.

GUIDELINES FOR THE PLACEMENT OF PINS

- Pin should be located close to the line angles of tooth.

- Pin hole should be at least 0-5 mm from the Dentinoenamel junction.

- The optimum interpin distance is 5 mm.

- Pins should be placed so that their axes are not parallel.

- Pins should be placed 0.5 mm from the vertical wall of the tooth.

- The fewest number of pins which will provide adequate retention should be used.

- The choice of pin size should be made on the basis of the amount of tooth structure remaining and need for retention.
- Increase in diameter increases retention.
- Pin retention increases with increased embedment in dentin.
- The optimum length of a pin is 2 mm.
- The number of pins placed varies with amount of tooth structure lost.
- Ex: For molar 1 pin per missing cusp.
  For premolars 2 pins per missing cusp.

TYPES OF PINS

- Classified on the basis of *retentive mechanism*,
  1. Cemented pins.
  2. Friction lock (Frictional grip pins).
  3. Self threading / self shearing pins.

1. CEMENTED PINS

- In this type, *pin channel is larger in diameter than the pin*.
- Available in two sizes.

Pin channel diameter	Pin diameter
0.027″	0.025″
0.021″	0.020″

Indications

1. Ideal for all pin retained restorations (as it creates least crazing and stresses in the tooth).
2. Only technique to be used for endodontically treated teeth.
3. Only techniques to be used when the pin location is very close to DEJ (0.5–1.0 mm distance is enough).
4. Only technique for using U- and L-shaped pins in Class 4 restorations and foundations.
5. Used when limited bulk of dentin is available for pin placement.
6. Ideal technique for a sclerosed, tertiary, calcified barrier or any other highly mineralized or dehydrated dentin.
7. Only technique for the cross-linking of two parts of the same tooth.

Disadvantages

1. Cementing medium is necessary for its retention.
2. Least retentive.

3. Requires additional step, in technique for the cementation.
   - Pin holes are placed at a depth of 3 to 4 mm.
   - Reinforced ZOE or GIC is used for the cementation of pin.

2. FRICTION LOCK PINS

- *The pin channel is slightly narrower in diameter than the pin.*
- Available in one size,

Pin channel diameter	Pin diameter
0.021″	0.022″

Indications

- Least used of all pin techniques because of the following requirements,
1. Should be used in vital teeth only.
2. At least 4 mm bulk of dentin should be present around the pin (in all three dimensions).
3. Pin should be located at least 2.5 mm from the DEJ.
4. Should be used only in the accessible areas of the mouth (so that the seating force will be parallel to the long axis of the pin).

Disadvantages

1. Maximum stresses are exhibited.
2. Strict indications
   - Pin holes are placed at a depth of 2-3 mm.
   - It is retained by frictional resistance and resiliency of dentin.
   - These are 2-3 times more retentive than cemented pins.

3. SELF THREADED PINS

- *The pin channel diameter is narrower than the pin.*
- Available as,

Pin channel diameter	Pin diameter
0.027″	0.031″
0.021″	0.023″
0.018″	0.020″
0.013″	0.015″

Indications

- It is the most applicable and feasible technique.
1. Used for vital teeth.
2. The dentin to be engaged for the pin (whether it is primary or secondary) should be properly hydrated.
3. Pin location should be at least 1.5 mm from DEJ.
4. When a minimal number of pins are needed.
5. When the maximum retention is needed.

Disadvantages

Dentinal trauma may be caused as the threads cut into the tooth structure.

- Pin holes are placed at a depth of 1.3-2 mm.
- They rely on the mechanical grasp of the threads into dentin.
- They are 2-3 times more retentive than the cemented pins.

PIN-CHANNEL PREPARATION

- Three basic instruments are used for the preparation.

1. The Twist drill

- It is an end cutting, revolving instrument with two blades, bibevelled in longitudinal section.
- It should be used at ultra low speed (300 - 500 RPM).
- Should be used in direct cutting acts and do not use in lateral cuttings as it widens the pin channel and lead to drill fracture.
- Should be finished in one or two thrusts.
- Never use-the drill in enamel as they do not cut enamel and become dull.

2. No.1, 2 or 3 round burs :
Are used to establish a leading hole in the center of which pin channel drilling is started. This avoids the skidding of the twist drill.

3. Measuring probes or depth gauge
are used to verify the depth of the pin channel.

Danger areas for pin placement

1. Mesial surface of upper 1st premolar.
2. Mesiobuccal line angles of upper and lower first molar.

Failure of pin-retained restorations

- Failure may occur,
  1. Within the restoration: restoration fracture.
  2. At the interface between the pin and the restorative material: pin restoration separation.
  3. Within the pin: pin fracture.
  4. At the interface between pin and dentin pin dentin separation.
  5. Within the dentin : dentin fracture.

Failure locations for different types of pins

1. In case of cemented pins, failure usually occurs at the cement dentin interface.
2. In case of friction grip pins, failure always occurs at the pin dentin interface.
3. In case of small threaded pins, failure usually occurs within pin themselves.
4. In case of large threaded (regular) pin, failure usually occurs in the dentin itself.

Pin Hole Perforations

- Whenever a pin hole is placed, the tooth is examined for possible perforations.
- The tooth is dried and an endodontic paper point should be placed in the pin hole.
- If a perforation exists paper point will become moistened.
- If no perforation the paper point should be dry.
- Pulpal perforation is treated by placing a calcium hydroxide intermediary base into the pin hole.
- Periodontal perforations are sealed using amalgam.

Enlarged Pinholes

- If the pin fails to engage itself and the threads do not hold the pin, then the pin hole is too large.
- To overcome this one can,
  - Drill the hole deeper and reinsert a fresh pin.
  - Redrill a larger hole and use a larger pin.
  - Cement the existing pin in place.

MECHANICS OF PIN-RETAINED RESTORATIONS

A. Stressing Capability of Pins

1. Type of pins

- Maximum stresses are associated with friction grip pins.
- Little or no stresses with cemented pins.
- Intermediate stresses with threaded pins when compared to other pins.

2. Diameter of pins

- The greater the diameter of the pin, the greater will be the stress induction.

3. Depth of the pin

- The greater the depth of the pin channel, the greater will be stress induction.

4. *Bulk of dentin*

   – The greater the amount of dentin pulpally or toward the surface from the pin, the lesser will be the stress induction.

5. *Types of dentin*

   – Primary dentin of young teeth is least affected by stress induction due to its high elastic and plastic limit.

   – The greater the mineralization and dehydration of the dentin, the lesser will be the dentinal tolerance to the stresses.

   – *The order of stress tolerance of different types of dentin in the decreasing order is primary dentin, secondary dentin, sclerosed dentin, tertiary dentin and calcific barrier.*

   – Stress tolerance is greatly decreased when the dentin looses its vitality.

   – Accordingly, threaded or frictional grip pins are not used in endodontically treated teeth and in the dentinal areas with dead tract formation. So cemented pins are routinely used in this situation.

   – Friction grip and threaded pins are not used in the areas of tertiary dentin, sclerosed dentin and calcific barrier. Cemented pins are preferred for this.

6. *The inter-pin distance*

   – The lesser the distance between the pins, the greater will be the concentration of stresses.

7. *Number of pins*

   – The lesser the number of pins per tooth, the less will be the stresses.

B. Retention of Pins

1. *Types of pins*

   – Cemented pins are least retentive.

   – Friction grip pins are 2-3 times more retentive than cemented pins.

   – Self-threading pins are 5-6 times more retentive than cemented pins.

2. *Shape of the pin channel relative to the pin*

   – Greater the coincidence between these two shapes the better will be the retention.

3. *Number of pins*

   – Pin location and its proximity relative to displacing forces (not the total no. of pins per tooth) affects the retention.

   – Pins placed closer than 2 mm to each other in a tooth results in the loss of retention.

4. *Surface texture of pins*

   – Pins with surface serrations or threading have good retention.

5. *Type of Dentin*

   – The decreasing order of pin retention of different types of dentin is primary dentin > tubular secondary dentin > scleorosed dentin > calcific barrier > dehydrated dentin (non-vital dentin).

6. *Bulk of the dentin around the pin*

   – Greater the amount of dentin separating pins from the pulp, tooth and root surface, the greater will be the retention.

7. *Types of cement (For cemented pins)*

   – The decreasing order of retention for different types of cement is copper-phosphate cement > Zn PO_4 > polycarboxylate > ZOE.

SLOT RETAINED AMALGAM RESTORATIONS

– *Slot is a retention groove in dentin whose length is in a horizontal plane.*

– Slots are particularly indicated in short clinical crowns and in cusps that have been reduced 2 to 3 mm for amalgam. Compared to pin placement more tooth structure is removed in preparing slots.

– Slots are less likely to create microfractures in the dentin and to perforate the tooth or penetrate into the pulp.

Tooth Preparation

– Slot length depends on the extent of the tooth preparation.

– Slots are usually placed on the facial, lingual, mesial and distal aspects of the preparation.

– The slot may be continuous or segmented, depending on the amount of missing tooth structure and whether pins were used.

– Slots are generally 0.5 to 1mm in depth and the width of the no. 33 1/2 bur. Their length is usually 2 to 4 mm, depending on the distance between the remaining vertical walls. No. 33 1/2 bur is used to place a slot in the gingival floor 0.5 mm axial of the DEJ.

– Slots can be used in combination with pins to generate additional retention and resistance forms.

AMALGAPIN

– Introduced by Shavell in 1980 for complex amalgam restorations.

– A round end bur is used for placing 2 to 3 mm deep holes.

– Amalgam is then condensed into the holes and the remainder of the restoration is condensed and carved.

– These amalgapin chambers are much larger by volume than the pinholes.

– The shear strength of the amalgapin is weaker than an amalgam with self threaded pins.

Indication

– Weak gingival areas.

Disadvantage

– Associated with greater tooth substance removal.

CHAPTER 08

ESTHETIC RESTORATIONS

ESTHETIC RESTORATIVE MATERIALS

1. **FUSED PORCELAIN**
   - Refer 'DENTAL CERAMICS'.

2. **SILICATE CEMENT**
   - First translucent material, introduced in 1878 by Fletcher in England.
   - Recommended for small restorations in anterior teeth of patients with high caries activity.
   - Linear or base required to protect pulp tissue from irritation due to initial low pH of material.

   Advantages
   - Tooth matching ability
   - Ease of manipulation
   - Anticariogenic
   - Good insulator

   Disadvantages
   - Discoloration
   - Loss of contour

3. **ACRYLIC RESINS**
   - Developed in Germany in 1930.

   Uses
   - As a restoration, most successful in protected areas of teeth where temperature change, abrasion and stress are minimal.
   - Esthetic veneer on facial surface of class 3 and class 4 metal restorations.
   - Temporary restorations in operative and fixed prosthodontic indirect restoration procedures.

   Disadvantages
   - Poor wear resistance.
   - Low strength and would flow under load.
   - Discoloration at the margins because of polymerization shrinkage and microleakage.

4. **GLASS IONOMERS**
   1. **Conventional glass ionomers**
      - Developed first by Wilson and Kent in 1972.

      Advantages
      - Anticariogenic effect
      - Favourable coefficient of thermal expansion
      - Tooth coloured
      - Chemical adhesion
      - Less soluble compared to silicate cement

Disadvantages

  – Low resistance to wear.

  – Low strength compared to composite or amalgam.

2. **Resin Modified Glass Ionomers**
  – Refer `DENTAL CEMENTS'.

3. **Compomers (Poly acid modified composites)**
  – Refer `DENTAL CEMENTS'.

5. COMPOSITES

COMPOSITES

– Composite resins are becoming the most widely accepted materials of choice by dentists and patients. They are placed mainly in the anterior teeth because of their esthetic (a term used for an artistically pleasing appearance) qualities, but with a new advances in their manufacturing, they are increasingly being placed in posterior teeth as well.

– Introduced by Bowen in 1962.

COMPOSITION

1. **Resin matrix :** A plastic resin material that forms a continuous phase and binds the filler particles Ex: BIS-GMA, TEGDMA.

2. **Fillers :** Reinforcing particles and/or fibers that are dispersed in the matrix, Ex: Silica.

  Purpose

  (i). Increases strength, hardness and wear resistance.

  (ii). Reduces polymerization shrinkage.

  (iii). Reduces thermal expansion and contraction.

  (iv). Improves workability.

  (v). Reduces water sorption, softening and staining.

  (iv). Increased radiopacity.

3. **Coupling agent :** Bonding agent that promotes adhesion between filler and resin matrix, Ex. Organosilanes, zirconates, titanates, etc.

4. **Activator :** Generates free radicals; chemical activator is tertiary amine; external energy activation is by heat, light or microwave.

5. **Initiator :** Initiates the polymerization, Ex: Benzylperoxide.

6. **Inhibitor :** Minimizes or prevent spontaneous or accidental polymerization of monomers, Ex: Butylated Hydroxy Toluene (BHT).

7. **Opacifiers:** Ex: Titanium dioxide, Aluminium oxide.

INDICATIONS

1. Class 1, 2, 3, 4, 5 and 6 restorations.
2. Pit and fissure sealants.
3. Esthetic enhancement procedures, i.e. veneers, tooth contour modifications, diastema closures, etc.
4. Core buildups
5. Splinting purpose
6. Cements (for indirect restorations)
7. Temporary restorations

CONTRA INDICATIONS

1. Grossly destructed tooth
2. Areas difficult to isolate

Advantages

1. Esthetics
2. Conservation of tooth structure
3. Bonded to tooth structure
4. Good retention
5. Minimal interfacial staining
6. Repairable
7. Insulative

Disadvantages

1. polymerization shrinkage
2. technique sensitive
3. difficult to finish and polish
4. difficult to establish proximal, axial contours and embrasures
5. greater occlusal wear
6. time consuming
7. not economic

CLASSIFICATION

I. **Based on filler particle size and size distribution (see Table 8.1)**

II. **Based on curing mechanism**

  1. Chemically activated
  2. Light activated
    i. U.V. Light
    ii. Visible light

1. CONVENTIONAL/TRADITIONAL/MACRO FILLED COMPOSITES

– *Contain 75 to 80% inorganic filler by weight.*

– *Average particle size is 8 μm.*

Disadvantages

– Rough surface texture.

Table 8.1

Sl. no.	Type	Size
1.	Traditional (large particle)	1–50 μm
2.	Hybrid (large particle)	0.04–20 μm
3.	Hybrid (mid filer)	0.04–10 μm
4.	Hybrid (minifiller/small particle filled)	0.04–2 μm
5.	Packable hybrid	Midfiller/minifiller hybrid with lower than fraction.
6.	Flowable hybrid	Midfiller hybrid with finer particle size distribution.
7.	Homogenous microfill	0.04 μm
8.	Heterogeneous microfill	0.04 μm

– Resin matrix wears at faster rate than filler particles.

– More susceptible to discoloration from extrinsic staining.

– Higher amount of initial wear at occlusal contacts.

2. MICRO FILLED COMPOSITES (Polishable Composites)

– Designed in 1970 to replace rough surface characteristic of conventional composites with a smooth lustrous surface similar to tooth enamel.

– *Particle size: 0.01 to 0.04 μm.*

– *Inorganic filler: 35 to 60% by weight.*

– Soft or friable glass such as strontium and/or barium-composite is made radioopaque.

Advantages

– Produces smoothest restorative surface.

– Low modulus of elasticity allow microfill composite restorations to flex during tooth flexure thus better protecting bonding interface.

– Clinically very wear resistant.

Disadvantages

– Inferior physical and mechanical properties.

3. HYBRID COMPOSITES

Definition

– *A particle-filled resin that contains a graded blend of small and colloidal silica filler particles to achieve an optimal balance among the properties of strength, polymerization shrinkage, wear resistance and polishability.*

– *Filler content : 75 to 85% by weight.*

– *Average particle size : 0.4 to 1.0 μm.*

Classification and uses

– *Based on filler size*

  1. *Hybrid (large filler)*

  – For high stress areas requiring improved polishability (class 1, 2, 3 and 4).

  2. *Hybrid (Mid filler)*

  – For high stress areas requiring improved polishability (class 3 and 4).

  3. *Hybrid [minifiller/small particle filled (SPF)]*

  – For moderate stress areas requiring optimal polishability (class 3 and 4).

Advantages

1. Smooth surface
2. Good strength
3. Can be used for stress-bearing and posterior restorations.

Disadvantages

– inferior mechanical properties than SPF composites.

4. FLOWABLE COMPOSITES

Definition

– *A hybrid composite with reduced filler level and a more narrow particle size distribution that increases flow and promotes intimate adaptation to prepared tooth surfaces.*

– *Filler content : 40 to 60% by weight.*

– *Average particle size : 0.6 to 1.0 μm.*

Uses

1. Preventive resin restorations
2. Cavity liners
3. Restoration repairs
4. Cervical restorations
5. Small class 1 restorations
6. Low stress bearing restorations

Advantages

1. Easy to use
2. Favourable wettability
3. Good handling properties

Disadvantages

1. Lower filler content
2. Inferior physical properties
3. Higher polymerization shrinkage
4. Lower wear resistance

5. PACKABLE COMPOSITES

Definition

- *A hybrid resin composite designed for use in posterior areas, where a stiffer consistency facilitates condensation in posterior teeth.*
- *Filler content : 65-81% by weight.*
- *Size: Fibrous form.*

Uses

- For use in class 1, 2 and 4 cavity preparations.

Advantages

1. High depth of cure
2. Low polymerization shrinkage
3. Radiopacity
4. Low wear rate

Disadvantages

1. Increased viscosity
2. Resistance to packing

COMPOSITES FOR POSTERIOR RESTORATIONS

- These are available in two forms,
  1. Direct posterior composites.
  2. Indirect posterior composites.

1. DIRECT POSTERIOR COMPOSITES

Indications

1. Esthetics
2. Need for conservation of tooth structure
3. To minimize thermal conduction

Contraindications

1. Not to be used for cuspal coverage.
2. Large restorations exceeding one-third the buccolingual width of the tooth.
3. Patients with parafunctional habits.

Types of composites used

1. Traditional composites
2. Hybrid composites
3. Microfilled composites
4. Packable composites

2. INDIRECT POSTERIOR COMPOSITES

- Indirect composites for fabrication of onlays are polymerized outside the oral environment and luted to the tooth with a compatible resin cement.

Methods of Resin Inlay fabrication

1. **Direct fabrication**
   - Application of the separating medium to the prepared tooth.
   - The restorative resin pattern is then formed, light cured and removed from the preparation.
   - The rough inlay is then exposed to additional light for approximately 4 to 6 min or heat activated at approximately 100°C for 7 min.
   - Then the preparation is etched.
   - Now the inlay is cemented into the place with a dual cure resin and it is then polished.

2. **Indirect fabrication**
   - Indirect inlay resin requires an impression and is fabricated in the laboratory.
   - In addition to conventional light and heat curing, laboratory processing may employ heat (150° C) and pressure (0.6 Mpa for 10 min) for the fabrication.

POLYMERIZATION OF COMPOSITES

Methods of Polymerization

A. *Self cured composites*

- Contains catalyst and base.
- Since components are mixed, there is greater chance for air inclusion in mixture and therefore greater internal porosity.
- Working time to insert self cured material is restricted by speed of chemical reaction.
- Requires increased finishing time.
- Less colour stable because of eventual breakdown of polymerization initiating chemical ingredients, tertiary amines.
- Direction of polymerization shrinkage of self cured materials is generally centralized (towards center of mass). This may help maintain marginal adaptation to prevent microleakage.

B. Light cured materials

- Provide increased working time.
- Require less finishing time.
- Exhibit greater colour stability and less internal porosity.
- Effects of polymerization shrinkage can be partially compensated by an incremental insertion technique and positioning light source close to material.
- Light curing mechanisms
    - Quartz / tungsten / halogen
    - Light curing units
    - Plasma arc curing
    - Argon laser curing
    - Blue light emitting diodes Less polymerization shrinkage more efficient, cooler, portable.

Polymerization Shrinkage

- Composites shrink while hardening, it is referred to as polymerization shrinkage.
- Polymerization shrinkage usually does not cause significant problems with restorations cured in preparations having all enamel margins.
- However, when a tooth preparation has extended onto a root surface, polymerization shrinkage can cause a gap formation at the junction of composite and root surface.
- The V-shaped gap occurs because of the force of polymerisation of composite is greater than the initial bond strength of composite to dentin of the root.
- The V-shaped gap is probably composed of composite on restoration side and hybridized dentin on root side.

ACID ETCHING

- It was conceived by Michael Buonocore in 1950's.

Purpose

1. Increases the mechanical retention of the restoration.
2. Better wetting of the resin.
3. Increases surface area which inturn increases the potential for bonding.

Indications

1. Support of class 1 and 2 posterior restorations.
2. Class 3 restorations.
3. Class 4 incisal angles of anterior teeth.
4. Class 5 in occlusal or incisal enamel as added retention.

Mechanism of Action

- The acid leaves a clean enamel surface which permits the increased wetting of the surface by resin.

- The acid attacks the enamel surface leaving microscopic surface irregularities with peaks and valleys in the enamel which allow for mechanical interlocking.

Procedure

1. Dentin and Pulp Protection

- Prior to the application of acid for etching, the dentin must be protected by placing a liner. If a liner is not placed, the acid causes irritation to the pulp.
- For this purpose light activated glass ionomer is the preferred liner.

2. Method

- Phosphoric acid may be brush applied or injected in viscous gel form.
- Brush is recommended because, 1. The fine tip confines the acid to the enamel periphery, 2. The soft bristles prevent a heavy rubbing or scrubbing mode of acid application which may result in decreased retention caused by the fracture of interstitial enamel surrounding the micropores.

3. Time

- The acid should be applied for a period of 15 to 20 seconds.
- Prolonged etching does not improve the bond.
- The application time should be increased to 1 minute for fluorosed or deciduous enamel because both are relatively resistant to the etching procedure.

4. Acid concentration

- 30-40% concentration is most reliable, effective.

5. Type of Acid

i. Aqueous solutions are easy to apply but difficult to control because of their free flow nature.

ii. High viscosity gels can be readily controlled clinically; particularly used in the treatment of cervical erosion lesions by means of dentin bonding materials and in posterior composite restorations.

6. Post etch cleaning

- After acid etching, the enamel surface should be thoroughly cleaned by means of a copious water lavage for atleast 15 or 30 seconds.
- Failure in thorough cleaning results in bond failure.

7. Drying the enamel surface

- Drying should never be accomplished with a dual air water syringe because this cause microcontamination of enamel surface with microdroplets of water.
- Warm air drying is preferred though chemical drying agents are also in use.
- After drying the enamel surface should present a chalky white opaque appearance and this is the

critical state because it is most sensitive to contamination.

– If contamination occurs, it should be cleaned by the application of phosphoric acid for a period of 15 to 20 seconds.

Special Considerations

1. Teeth of patients rinsed on a fluoride water supply possess enamel that is resistant to decalcification and often require reapplication of the acid etching procedure.

2. Immature enamel in a child is more rapidly etched than mature enamel in the adult patient.

CONDITIONING OF THE CAVITY (Fig. 8.1)

Purpose

– Removes the smear layer.

– Opens the dentinal tubules, increases dentin permeability and decalcification of the intertubular and peritubular dentin, exposing collagen fibres there by formation of smear plugs which increases bonding.

Conditioning agents

1. Orthophosphoric acid (37%) for composites.
2. Polyacrylic acid (10%) for GIC.
3. Citric acid (50%) for root conditioning.
4. Pumice wash.

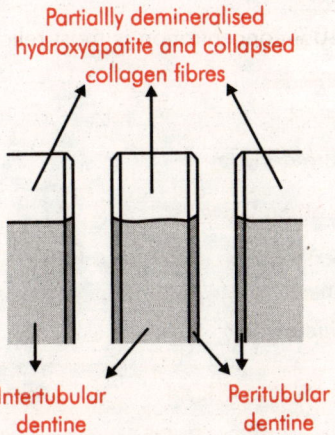

Partiallly demineralised hydroxyapatite and collapsed collagen fibres

Intertubular dentine

Peritubular dentine

Fig. 8.1

DENTAL ADHESION

CONCEPTS OF ADHESION

Adhesion

– "The state in which two surfaces are held together by interfacial forces which may consist of valence forces or interlocking forces or both". (Definition given by the American Society for Testing and Materials (ASTM) SP No. D 907).

Adherend

– Materials substrate that is bonded to another material by means of an adhesive.

Adhesive

– A substance that promotes adhesion of one substance or material to another.

Mechanism of Adhesion

– There are four different mechanism of adhesion, i.e.

1. *Mechanical Adhesion:* Interlocking of the adhesive with irregularities in the surface of the substrate or adherend. Ex: Amalgam restoration.

2. *Adsorption Adhesion:* Chemical bonding between the adhesive and the adhesion. Ex: GIC.

3. *Diffusion Adhesion:* Interlocking between mobile molecules. Ex: Adhesion of two polymers.

4. *Electrostatic Adhesion:* An electrical double layer at the interface of a metal with a polymer.

Classification

– Based on the type of atomic interactions.

1. *Physical bonding :* It involves vander wall or electrostatic interactions. Bonding occurs if surfaces are smooth and dissimilar.

2. *Chemical bonding :* Bonding occurs between adhesive and adherend. Ex : Glass Ionomer Cement.

3. *Mechanical bonding :* It is due to the interface that involves undercuts and other irregularities that form interlocking of materials. Ex : Amalgam restoration occlusal convergence.

4. *Micromechanical bonding :* Mechanical roughness produces a microscopically interlocked adhesive and adherend, this situation is called Micromechanical adhesion/Micromechanical retention. Ex : Composites.

Requirements for Good Adhesion

– Good wetting (close contact).

– The surface tension of the adhesive must be lower than the surface energy of the enamel and dentin.

ENAMEL BONDING AGENTS

– The bond agent is usually a low viscosity, unfilled BIS - GMA resin.

– The theory is that the use of such an intermediate resin will ensure maximum tag formation and therefore better bond strength of the composite restoration to the enamel.

– The exact additive effect of the bond agent is not yet defined.

SMEAR LAYER (Fig. 8.2)

– *It is an amorphous microcrystalline layer of cutting debris on freshly cut dentinal tooth surface.*

– It is a few micrometers thick.

– Composed of denatured collagen, hydroxyapatite and other cutting debris.

– Smear layer serves as natural bandage on freshly cut dentinal surface and it occludes with dentinal tubules, forming smear plug.

– It acts as good protective layer or barrier and has weak attachment to the dentin.

– During Glass Ionomer Cement (GIC) restoration, smear layer has to be removed as it tends to inhibit effective ionic exchange and bonding of the glass ionomer to the underlying tooth surface.

– Agents for removal of smear layer : Citric acid, EDTA, Tannic acid.

– Most effectively used is polyacrylic acid.

Smear plug

– *The micro structure which forms when the cutting debris is forced into the dentinal tubules.*

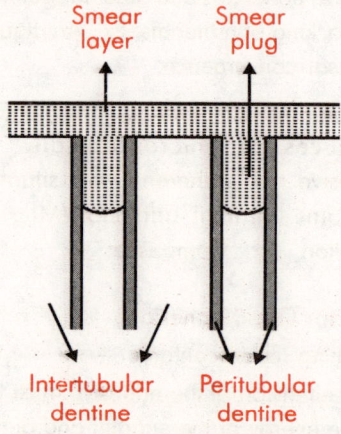

Fig. 8.2

HYBRID LAYER

– *An intermediate layer of resin, collagen, and dentin produced by acid etching of dentin and resin infiltration into the conditioned dentin (Fig 8.3).*

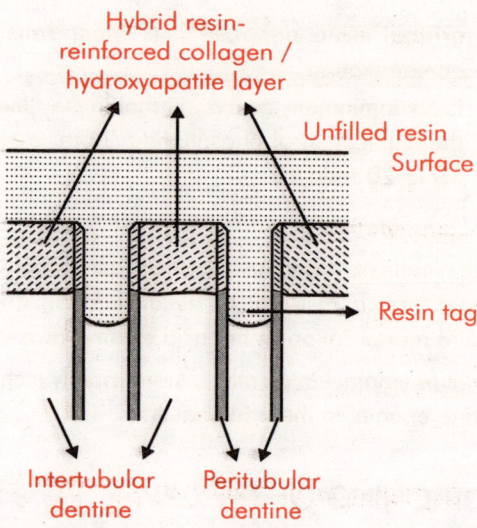

Fig. 8.3

CLASSIFICATION OF DENTIN BONDING AGENTS

I.   **Based on Generation:** *(DEEWEY'S classification)*

1.   I - Generation
2.   II - Generation
3.   III - Generation
4.   IV - Generation
5.   V - Generation
6.   VI - Generation

II.   **Based on Composition**

1.   Oxalates
2.   Phosphates
3.   Isocyanides
4.   4 - META
5.   Glutaraldehyde

III.   **Based on Smear Layer**

1.   Removed
2.   Retained
3.   Modified

DEEWEY'S CLASSIFICATION

I.   **Generation : NPG - GMA**

– *Mechanism of Adhesion :* Phosphate group of GMA chelates with the calcium ion in tooth which is bonded chemically to the tooth structure.

– But carbon B Analysis shows no chemical bond.

– *Bond strength :* 2-3 Mpa and which is poor.

II.   **Generation: Phosphate ester 4 HEMA**

– *Mechanism of Adhesion:* By polar attraction between negatively charged phosphate groups and positively charged calcium ion in the tooth.

– *Bond strength: 4–6 Mpa.*

– Ex: Scotch Bond, Clearfil, Universal Bond.

III. Generation

– In this modification of the smear layer, component used PENTA.

– Here some system of acid etching was used which had hydrophobic monomer resulting in no penetration into dentinal tubules and resulted in modified smear layer.

– Ex: Gluma, Scotch bond tooth.

– *Bond Strength:* 10 Mpa.

IV. Generation

– It is a 2 component system.

   #### 1. Primer

   – It acts as water chaser and enhances adhesive penetration.

   #### 2. Adhesive

   – It is acetone based.

   – Hydrophobic - BISGMA

   – Hydrophillic - HEMA

   – Acid etching was done, removed the smear layer thus increased dentinal permeability.

   – *Bond strength : 17–24 Mpa.*

V. Generation

– It is a single component with primer and adhesive together.

– Thus less clinical steps are required.

– *Bond strength:* 17 - 30 Mpa.

– Ex: Prime bond, Single bond, Sintacsprint.

VI. Generation

– These are self etching primers.

– The primer includes phosphorated resin which includes etching and bond simultaneously.

– No separate etching is required.

– It reduces rinsing, over wetting, overdrying which has negative influence on bond strength.

– Ex : PROMPT L - TOP.

PULPAL PROTECTION

– Pulpal protection is an attempt to create an environment within the pulp that lessen the immediate insult of preparation and restoration of the tooth.

– Application of liners and bases serve as a barriers to an irritating chemical; Aids in the attainment of healthy pulpal response.

Pulpal Protection Beneath Composite Resin

– A cavity prepared to minimum depth can be treated by application of thin paste like consistency of Glass Ionomer to the exposed dentin as a cavity liner.

– The lining cement is placed against the axial wall of the cavity.

– If a prepared cavity extends into a dentin to an extent that a pulp exposure is evident or less than 0.5mm thickness of dentin, then a thin layer of calcium hydroxide is placed as medicament.

– Upon this, liner of Glass Ionomer is placed.

– Other cements used are light activated calcium hydroxide, polycarboxylate cements.

– Note: *Zinc oxide eugenol cement and cavity varnish are contraindicated beneath filled and unfilled resin.*

– In zinc oxide eugenol cement, eugenol interferes with the polymerization of resin system and leaves the resin soft at the interface between resin and cement.

– A varnish is not acceptable as the monomer portion of resin dissolves the varnish, thus removes the protective barrier.

GLASS IONOMER CEMENT RESTORATIONS

Indications

1. Root surface caries in class V locations.

2. Slot like preparations in either class II or class III cervical locations (Not involving proximal contact).

3. Notched cervical defects of idiopathic erosion or abrasion origin.

4. As temporary treatment of anterior teeth where caries is not controlled.

Instrumentation and Cavity Preparation

– Rubber dam

– Mouth mirror

- Explorer
- Cotton pliers
- Matrix material
- No. 330, 1/4, 1/2, 1 and 2 burs
- Curved chisel
- Monangle hoe
- GMT
- Wooden wedge

Procedure

- Application of rubber dam for isolation. Cavity design is similar to that for resins.

- The cavity outlines are extended only to facilitate removal of grossly weakened tooth structure.

- The burs and instruments used to make the preparation are identical to those used for resin preparations.

- If the pulp is less than 2.0 mm from the preparation, a fast setting calcium hydroxide preparation is placed in the deep portion.

- Most conventional GI systems require etching dentinal surfaces to remove smear layer, there by effecting improved adhesion of glass ionomer to dentin.

- To etch dentin, mild acid such as 10% polyacrylic acid is placed in preparation for approximately 20 secs followed by rinsing and removal of excess water leaving dentin moist.

- Additionally, some RMGI's and all compomers use an intermediary bonding agent to facilitate bonding.

- Original GIC's require careful mixing of powder and liquid within 30 sec to optimize powder incorporation.

- If conventional type of GIC is used, place a thin coat of light cured resin bonding agent on surface immediately after placement to prevent dehydration and cracking.

- If RMGI is used, cure for minimum time of 40 secs.

- RMGI can be contoured and polished immediately after light curing.

- For conventional type, final contouring and finishing is done after 24 hours, as it requires 24 hours for polymerization.

- Contouring and finishing done with micron finishing diamonds used with petroleum lubricant or flexible abrasive discs are used.

- A fine grit Al_2O_3 polishing paste applied with prophylaxis cup is used to impart a smooth surface.

VENEERS

Definition

- It is a layer of tooth coloured material which is applied to a tooth to restore localized or generalized defects and intrinsic discolorations.

Materials for Veneers

- Chairside composite, processed composite, porcelain and pressed ceramic, etc.

Indications

1. Teeth with facial surfaces that are malformed, discoloured, abraded, eroded.
2. Teeth with faulty restorations.

Types of Veneers

I. **Based on the extent of coverage**

   1. Partial Veneers
   - Indicated for the restoration of localized defects or areas of intrinsic discoloration.

   2. Full Veneers
   - Indicated for the restoration of generalized defects or areas of intrinsic staining involving the major portion of the facial surface of the tooth.

II. **Based on the method of fabrication**

   1. Direct technique
   2. Indirect technique

1. DIRECT TECHNIQUE

Indications

1. When a small number of teeth are involved.
2. When the entire facial surface is not defective.

Advantages

1. Single appointment.
2. Useful for single discoloured tooth.
3. Useful in young patients.
4. Useful when the limited time period is available.
5. Economic.

Disadvantages

1. Time consuming
2. Labour intensive

2. INDIRECT TECHNIQUE

Indication

– Used when the multiple teeth are to be veneered.

Advantages

1. Less sensitive to operator technique.
2. When multiple teeth are to be veneered.
3. Lasts longer.

Disadvantages

1. Tooth preparation is necessary.
2. Expensive
– To achieve esthetic and physiologically sound tooth, an intraenamel preparation and location of the gingival margin of the preparation are important.

1. Intraenamel Preparation

– It is the roughening of the surface in under contoured areas of the tooth.

Significance

1. To provide space for veneering material.
2. To remove the fluoride rich layer of enamel which is more resistant to acid etching.
3. To create a rough surface for improved bonding.
4. To create a definite finish line (important for placing indirectly fabricated veneers).

2. Location of the Gingival Margin

– If the defect or discoloration does not extend subgingivally, then the margin of the veneer should not extend subgingivally.

MISCELLANEOUS

ABFRACTION / IDIOPATHIC EROSION

Definition

– "The loss of tooth surface at the cervical areas of teeth caused by tensile and compressive forces during tooth flexure, which begins as microfracture of thin enamel tooth structure occlusal to CEJ and produces a notched defect when combined with abrasive tooth brushing".

Etiology

– Has been found in association with parafunctional habits such as clenching or bruxism.

Clinical Features

– Seen in adults.
– Seen as a wedge-shaped notching at the cervical areas of involved teeth.

Treatment

– Restoration of the defective area.
– Adjustment of the bite for the evenly distribution of chewing forces.

GOLDEN PROPORTION

– It results from the division of a straight line in such a way that the shorter part (S) is to the longer part as the longer part (L) is to the whole.
– Each ratio equals to 0.618.

$$\frac{S}{L} = \frac{L}{(S+L)} = 0.618$$

– Linear progressions and surface division by the same number are common in nature both geometrically and arithmetically.
– *The geometrical progressions can be obtained by multiplying each term by 1.618 or dividing by 0.618:*

$1.000 \times 1.618 = 1.618$ OR $1.000 : 0.618 = 1.618$

$1.618 \times 1.618 = 2.618$ OR $1.618 : 0.618 = 2.618$

$2.618 \times 1.618 = 4.236$ OR $2.618 : 0.618 = 4.236$

– *In the arithmetic progression, each term is the sum of the preceding two terms:*

$0.618 + 1.000 = 1.618$

$1.000 + 1.618 = 2.618$

$1.618 + 2.618 = 4.236$

– As can be seen here, the progression using the golden number is unique because three different methods produce the same results.
– Obviously, the golden proportion is not the only parameter that defines harmony and therefore beauty.
– However, numerous studies and experiments have demonstrated that this surface division creates an esthetic appeal, independently from ethnic or civilization factors.

Golden Proportions in Facial and Dental Elements (Fig. 8.4)

–   The nasal height (A) is related to the maxillary height (B) as 1.000 : 0.618. The sum of nasal height and maxillary height (A + B) are related to the mandibular height (C) as 1.618 : 1.000.

–   The mandibular height (C) is related to the maxillary height (B) as 1.000 : 0.618.

–   The orofacial height (A + B) is related to the nasal height (A) as 1.618 : 1.000.

–   Note that each ratio is 1.618.

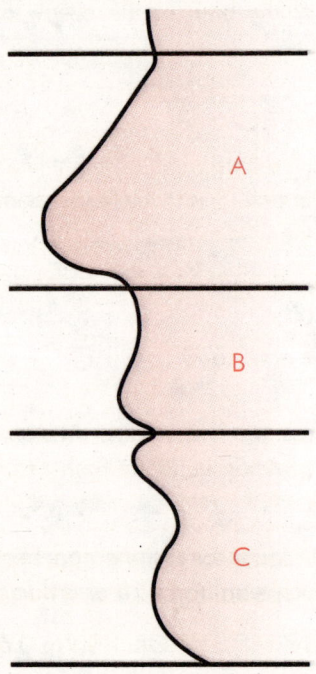

Fig. 8.4

Dental Proportions (Fig. 8.5)

–   The width of the central incisor is in golden proportion to the width of the lateral incisor (from the labial view), which inturn is in golden proportion to the part of the canine that is visible from the front.

–   The dark space between the corners of the mouth and the outer surface of the canines during a smile (line 1.0) is called negative space. The negative space is in golden proportion with one half of the width of the upper anterior segment (line 1.618).

–   Even though the negative space escapes the attention of the public, it cannot be ignored.

–   It creates a balance between cohesive and segregative forces in a smile and provides a harmonious relationship between the smile and other facial features.

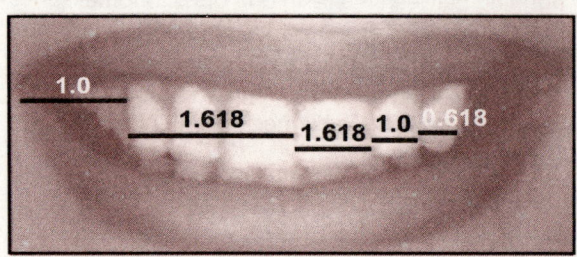

Fig. 8.5

SANDWICH TECHNIQUE (Fig. 8.6)

–   Also called as *Bilayered Restoration.*

–   *It consists of placing the glass ionomer cement as an intermediate layer between the tooth structure and a resin based composite.*

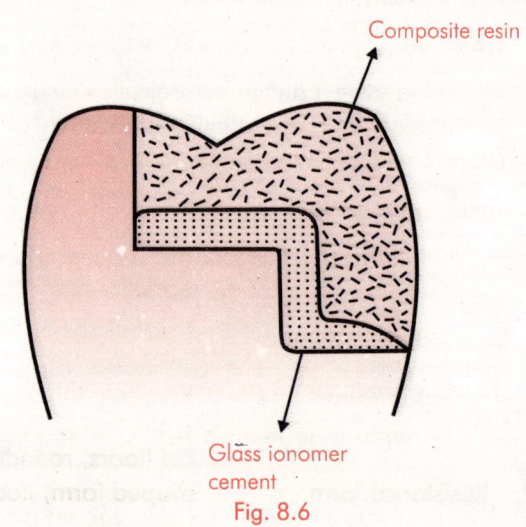

Composite resin

Glass ionomer cement

Fig. 8.6

Advantages

1.   Chemical bonding of GIC to tooth structure.
2.   Fluoride releasing ability of GIC to minimize caries.
3.   Esthetic quality of composite.
4.   Durability of composite.
5.   Better seal with increased retention.

Technique

–   It involves the placement of glass ionomer in the cavity at a thickness of about 1 mm.

–   The materials is placed like a conventional lining for a class V or class II cavity except that it is extended out to the aproximal margin in case of the class II cavity, and to the gingival margin for the class V cavity.

–   Then the surface of the glass ionomer is etched and dried.

–   Apply the composite resin.

– Bonding between the resin and glass ionomer surface is through penetration of resin into the surface irregularities of the etched cement surface.

– Setting of the resin is by mechanical interlocking.

DIFFERENCES BETWEEN CLASS 2 CAVITY PREPARATION FOR AMALGAM AND COMPOSITE RESTORATIONS

Features	Amalgam	Composite
1. Outline form:	– include defects. – may extend to break proximal contact – includes adjacent suspicious area	– same – same – does not include
2. Pulpal depth:	– uniform 1.5 mm	– usually not uniform
3. Axial depth:	– uniform 0.2 – 0.5 mm into DEJ	– usually not uniform
4. Cavosurface margin:	– 90 degree	– 90 or more than 90 degrees
5. Bevels:	– only gingival	– given
6. Texture of the prepared walls:	– smoother	– rough
7. Primary retention form:	– occlusal convergence	– none (bonding/roughness)
8. Secondary retention form:	– grooves, slots, locks, pins, bonding	– bonding; grooves for very large or root – surface preparation.
9. Resistance form:	– flat floors, rounded angles, box-shaped form, floors are perpendicular to occlusal forces	– same for large preparations; no special form for small to moderate size preparations.

CHAPTER 09

DIRECT FILLING GOLD (DFG)

INDICATIONS

1. Occlusal, buccal and lingual pit and fissure cavities on teeth (Class I).
2. Gingival third cavities on bicuspids, cuspids and incisors where access and esthetics permit (Class V).
3. Incipient interproximal lesions of the anterior teeth (Class V).
4. Cuspal and incisal areas of all teeth.
5. Limited numbers of interproximal cavities on bicuspids and mesial of first molars (Class II).
6. Small eroded areas on the facial surface of premolars, canines and on incisors.
7. Small, less conspicuous circular and irregular areas such as hypoplasias, white spots or defective pits.
8. DFG is used to repair defective inlay or crown margins and vent holes in crowns.

CONTRAINDICATIONS

1. Inaccessibility
2. Isolation of difficult areas
3. Grossly destructed tooth
4. Uncooperative patients
5. Extensive periodontal involvement
6. Esthetically important areas
7. Undesirable occlusal stress

Advantages

1. It can last as long as the tooth if restored properly.
2. No tarnish and corrosion.
3. Insoluble in the oral fluids.
4. Perfect adaptability to cavity walls if restored properly.
5. Great density, crushing resistance and edge strength.
6. No cementing medium is necessary for retention.
7. Capability of receiving and maintaining a high polish.
8. Perfect weldability in a cold state.
9. Low tendency to molecular change.

Disadvantages

1. Inharmoneous colour
2. High thermal conductivity
3. Difficulty of manipulation

FORMS / TYPES OF DFG

1. Foil (or fibrous gold)

   i. Sheet
      a. Cohesive
      b. Non-cohesive

ii.   Ropes

iii. Cylinders

iv.   Laminated foil

v.   Platinized foil

2. **Electrolytic precipitate (or crystalline gold)**

   i.   Matgold

   ii. Mat foil (Mat gold + gold foil)

   iii. Gold calcium alloy

3. **Granulated gold (encapsulated powdered gold)**

I.   GOLD FOIL

– Oldest form of gold and is the most durable.

– Standard no. 4 gold foil is supplied in 4 × 4 inch (100 × 100 mm) sheets that weigh 4 grains (0.259 g) and are about 0.51 µm thick. The numbering system refers to the weight of a standard sheet and reflects the thickness. Thus, no. 3 foil weighs 3 grains (0.194 g) and is about 0.38 µm thick.

– Gold foil is supplied in the following forms,

   i.   *Plain gold foil:* Which is the product of the cold working procedure without any modifications.

   ii. *Corrugated gold foil:* Which is manufactured by placing a thin leaf of paper between two sheets of gold foil and after which the whole unit is ignited. As the paper leaves are burnt out, they shrivel and impart a corrugated shape to the gold foil. It is more cohesive than plain ones; it is the outcome of great Chicago Fire in 1871.

   iii. *Platinum gold foil:* Which is produced by sandwiching platinum foil between two leaves of gold foil; platinum increases the hardness of the finished restoration. Therefore, it is used in areas of excessive stress such as the incisal edge of anterior teeth.

   iv. *Laminated gold foil:* Which has directional properties, i.e. resistant to stresses in one direction better than the other. It is to combine two or three leaves of gold, each from different ingots which have been cold worked in different directions. So they can be resistant in different directions when combined together.

   v.   *Gold foil cylinder:* Which is produced by rolling cut segments of no. 4 foils into a desired width, usually 3.2 mm, 4.8 mm and 6.4 mm using a modified no. 22 tapestry needle.

Cohesive and Non-cohesive Gold

– Although the forms of DFG can be supplied in both the cohesive and the non-cohesive forms only the sheet foil is typically furnished in either of these two forms.

Cohesive Gold

– *The gold foil which is free of surface contaminants is called* **Cohesive Gold**.

– Gases like oxygen are absorbed at the surface of the gold, thus prevents bonding of gold during compaction.

– Only if gold surface is free from impurities it can be welded at room temperature.

Non-cohesive Gold

– Ammonia treated foil is called Non-cohesive gold.

– *Intentional coating:* Is treating of gold with 18 percent of ammonia.

– This acts as a protective film to prevent adsorption of non-volatile gases and premature cohesion of pellets in their container.

– Non-cohesive gold can also have adsorbed agents like iron salt or an acidic gas on its surface.

– This volatile film is readily removed by heating at 350°C there by restoring the cohesive character of the foil.

– Non-cohesive gold is rarely used nowadays.

– But may be used to build up the bulk of a direct gold restoration.

II. ELECTROLYTIC PRECIPITATE

A. *Mat gold :* It is a crystalline, electrolytically precipitated gold form that is formed into strips. It is used to form the core of the restoration because of its ease in compaction. It is used in combination technique along with regular cohesive gold.

B. *Mat Foil :* It is manufactured by sandwiching a ribbon of mat gold between two regular cohesive gold sheets.

C. *Gold-calcium alloy (Alloyed Electrolytic Precipitate):* Newest form, Electralloy R V is alloyed with calcium. The calcium content is 0.1%. Its purpose is to produce stronger restorations by dispersion strengthening. The alloy is sandwiched between two layers of gold foil.

III. POWDERED GOLD : (SPONGY GOLD)

– It is a blend of atomized and precipitated powder embedded in a wax like organic matrix. From this material various sized pellets are cut and encased in gold foil wrappers and packed prior to use. The matrix is burnt away to leave only pure gold.

CHARACTERISTICS OF GOLD

1. *Fibrous gold foil :* It is best suitable for restricted cavity preparations such as small pits and narrow fissures and also used to veneer other forms of cohesive gold.

2. *Mat foil :* Is used as a bulk filler for single surface restorations such as class I and class V. It is not used on the surface of a restoration since it has a tendency to become pitted afterwards when some minor abrasion takes place.

3. *Encapsulated powdered gold :* Used as a bulk filler and for the restoration surface. It is used for the restoration of all classes of cavities where cohesive gold may be indicated.

4. *Alloyed filling gold :* Is used for restoring all classes of cavities where cohesive gold is used most frequently. It is used for class I, II, III and V cavity restorations.

MANIPULATION OF DFG

– It consists of two stages, i.e.
    1. Annealing / Heat treatment / Degassing.
    2. Condensation / Compaction.

1. ANNEALING

– *Cleansing of the gold surface by heating is referred to as 'annealing'.*

– *Purpose:* Annealing removes all of the volatile contaminants, thereby restoring or assuring the cohesive characteristics of the gold.

– There are of two methods for the purpose of annealing, i.e.

A. Bulk method

– Accomplished by using an electric or gas source of heat.

– The required number of pellets of gold is placed on the surface of the annealer. A mica slab is held over an open glass flame until the gold shows a dull red colour. Then the slab is removed from the heat and foil is ready for use.

– *Precaution :* DFG should never be annealed directly in an open gas flame.

Advantage : Convenient method.

Disadvantages
1. Danger of over annealing.
2. Waste formation due to the contamination of unused gold.
3. Inability to select a suitable desired piece from annealed gold.

B. Piece method

– It is the most practical method.

– Annealing is accomplished using a simple alcohol lamp and a gold foil carrier.

– Acetone: Free alcohol must be used to avoid contamination.

– The wick of the lamp should be about 1/4 inch long and be pointed.

– Gold is picked-up with the point of the carrier and brought to the `hot' cone of the flame and heated until to a dull red colour.

– *Precaution:* Pliers should not be used for the piece method to avoid uneven heating.

Advantages
1. Elimination of the chance of contamination between annealing and compaction.
2. Lack of waste
3. Ability to select a piece of desired size.

2. CONDENSATION / COMPACTION

– *Condensation is the procedure used to harden the gold inside the preparation.*

A. Objectives
1. To wedge initial pieces between dentinal walls- especially at starting points.
2. To weld together the pieces of gold.
3. To adapt the gold intimately to the walls and margins of the prepared cavity.
4. To gain a uniform compactness by eliminating voids between the gold pieces.
5. To develop strength within the restoration.

B. Modes of Condensation

i. *Hand Instrument Condensation:* Can be used only as a first step in a two-step condensation process as the condensation energy produced by this method is not sufficient to fill the cavity.

ii. *Pneumatic Condensation:* Involves the use of vibrating condensers which work by using compressed air. Though this is the efficient method, but cannot be controllable.

iii. *Electronic condensation :* It is the most efficient and controlled way of condensation.

iv. *Hand condenser and mallet :* Oldest method of condensation.

C. Gold Condensers

– They are of the following types:

i. *Round condensers (Bayonet condenser):* Used in initial restoration phase and to establish `ties' in the inner parts of the restoration.

ii. *Foot Condensers :* Used mainly for cavosurface condensation, surface hardening of the restoration and for bulk build-up.

iii. Parallelogram and Hatchet Condensers: Used for preliminary condensation and to create the bulk of restoration.

D. Procedure / Principles of condensation

- After the pellet or piece is placed in the tooth, it is compacted to develop hardness and to produce adaptation of the material to the cavity wall.

- When the gold is condensed slip planes develop between the anatomic structure and restoration and the resultant stress produces the hardness.

- Thorough condensation results in a dense, non-porous gold restoration.

- Regardless of the type of condensation employed the force should be at least 15 lb /sq. inch.

1. Line of force / Angle of force (Fig. 9.1)

- *It is the direction of force exerted by the condenser.*

- It follows and is parallel to an extension of the long axis of the shaft of the instrument regardless of the deflection or angle of the working point.

- *According to black, the line of force must be directed at an angle of 45° to cavity walls and floors, i.e should bisect line angles and trisect point angles formed by the cavity walls.*

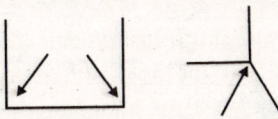

Fig. 9.1

- *Forces of condensation must be directed at 90° to previously condensed gold to avoid shear components which can displace or loosen the already condensed pieces of gold.*

- A building shelf is produced with the first layer of powdered gold for proximal restorations and a gold bank is developed from then on.

2. Bridging

- *When an improper building shelf is produced a bridging occurs, i.e. the gold bulges and produces a convexity in the material, preventing the condenser from reaching the cavity wall, causing porosity.*

- Bridging prevents the proper lines of force from being applied and thus resulting in poor adaptation.

- Bridging is prevented by uniform placement of the material and adequate condensation using the proper lines of force.

- The most important rule is to keep the gold banked against the walls until the cavosurface margin is reached thus creating a concavity.

3. Stepping of the condenser (Fig. 9.2)

- *Refers to the overlapping (by one fourth of its diameter) of the previous area of the condenser's stroke both in individual steps and in lines of steps.*

- Stepping can be done in two ways either;

  a. In rows parallel to the wall being approached moving toward this wall, row by row and wedging the last row between the already condensed gold and the wall.

  b. In rows perpendicular to the wall being approached.

- Stepping always start at a point on one side and proceed in a straight line to another point on the opposite side then back to the original side on a different straight line. This ensures that the condenser has covered the entire surface of that piece of gold.

Significance

1. Ensures that each portion of the gold increment has been welded and cold worked.
2. No voids.
3. Maximal adaptation.
4. Denser restoration.

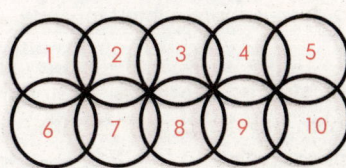

Fig. 9.2

4. Pellet placement.

- *It refers to the exact location at which each pellet of gold foil is placed in order to ensure correct building of the gold.*

- Each pellet should be placed where needed to be condensed, not moved around after original placement. If it is moved it becomes harsh and difficult to handle.

- Accurate placing is essential to correct gold building.

- *Convenient points or starting points are refined retention forms placed in the corners of the tooth preparation to accept the first pellets and can be placed in the preparation to facilitate starting the gold.* They are usually pyramidal or triangular and prevent slippage of the pellet or mass of mat or powdered gold. They are often used in proximal class III restoration because these preparations do not have four confining walls.

Condensation of Mat Gold or Mat foil

- Condensation of Mat gold is different from that of regular cohesive gold.

- The metal is condensed by hand and spread thoroughly into the retention forms.

- Mat golds are spongy and thick and require a rocking motion for adaptation.

- If the gold is too thick, the surface strain hardens, preventing the condensation forces from properly forcing the material against the tooth.

- Therefore, if the layer is too thick, the mat gold must be `broken up' to prevent bridging and for obtaining proper adaptation and condensation.

- Even though adaptation is difficult (because of thickness), mat golds are easy to start in the cavity because they are spongy.

- *Mat golds can be used on axial walls of Class - V and III restorations and pulpal walls of Class - I and II restorations.*

Condensation of Powdered gold

- Powdered gold is manipulated in same way as the mat gold.

- More pressure is required for the hardening of encapsulated powdered gold because of varying sizes and density of pellets.

- There are special condensers with special working points are available.

- The powdered pellets are placed in the cavity and the envelops are ruptured with the face of the condenser.

- The gold is placed in the deepest part of the prepared cavity, and it is spread into the retention forms and line angles. Then pressure is exerted with a rocking motion for gradual hardening.

- The advantage of powdered golds over the mat golds is that they will produce a less porous surface, which does not require a veneer of gold foil.

STEPS FOR INSERTION OF DFG

1. Three step build - up

i. *Tie formation :* It is the connecting of two opposing point angles or starting points filled with gold with a transverse bar of gold. It forms the foundation for the restoration.

ii. *Banking of walls :* It is the covering of each wall from its floor or axial wall to the cavosurface margin with the direct gold. A wall should be banked in such a way that, it will not obstruct tie formation or banking of other walls in the cavity.

iii. *Shoulder formation :* It is the connecting of two opposing walls with the direct gold to complete the build up.

2. Paving of the Restoration

- It is the individual covering of every area of cavosurface margin portion with excess cohesive gold foil. A foot condenser is used for this purpose.

3. Surface hardening

- Done to fulfill the rest of the condensation objectives and to strain harden the surface gold.

4. Burnishing

- Should be done from gold to tooth surface. It enhances surface hardening, adapts restoration to the margins and eliminates voids.

5. Margination

- Done with sharp instruments like knives and files moving from the gold surface to the tooth surface to eliminate excess material.

6. Burnishing

- It follows margination to close marginal discrepancies and to strain harden the surface.

7. Contouring

- Done to create the proper anatomy of the restoration to coincide with that of the tooth. Done with knives, files or finishing burs.

8. Additional Burnishing

- Done to fulfill previously mentioned objectives.

9. Finishing and Polishing

- Done by using precipitated chalk or tin oxide powder on soft bristle brushes or rubber cups.

10. Final Burnishing

- Done to ensure closure of marginal voids and other surface discrepancies.

PRINCIPLES OF TOOTH PREPARATION FOR DIRECT GOLD RESTORATIONS

1. Outline form

   – Margins must not be ragged.

   – Margins should be established on sound areas of the tooth, which can be finished and polished.

   – Outline form must include all structural defects.

   – It should be pleasing esthetically.

   – *Failure to give proper outline form results in an unsightly restoration.*

2. Resistance form

   – Pulpal floor should be flat and perpendicular to occlusal forces.

   – All the enamel must be supported by sound dentin.

   – *Poor resistance form can result in the fracture of the tooth.*

3. Retention form

   – Can be established by parallelism of some walls and by strategically placing converging walls.

   – Walls must be smooth and flat (to provide resistance to loosening).

   – Internal line angles must be sharp (to resist movement).

   – *Poor retention form results in loosened restoration.*

4. Convenience form

   – It requires suitable access and a rubberdam isolation.

   – Sharp internal line and point angles are created to allow convenient "starting" gold foil as compaction begins.

   – Rounded form is allowed when E - Z gold is used to begin the restorative phase.

   – *Improper convenience form can make the tooth preparation unrestorable.*

5. Final cavity preparation

   – Removal of remaining carious dentin, final planing of cavosurface margins and debridement complete the tooth preparation for direct gold.

CHAPTER 10

CAST RESTORATIONS

INLAY

– *An indirect restoration involving proximal, occlusal surface (not more than two surfaces), may cover one or more cusps but not all.*

CLASS II INLAY

– *An indirect restoration involving proximal and occlusal surfaces and may cover one or more cusps but not all (Fig. 10.1).*

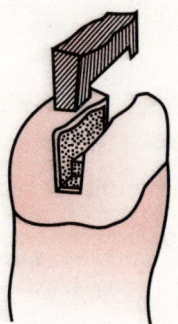

Fig. 10.1

INDICATIONS FOR INLAYS

1. A cavity whose width does not exceed one-third the intercuspal distance.
2. Strong, self resistant cusps should be remained.
3. Indicated teeth have minimal or no occlusal facets.
4. The tooth is not to be an abutment for a fixed or removable prosthesis.

ONLAY

– *An indirect restoration, involving entire occlusal surface which covers all the cusps.*

CLASS II ONLAY

– *An indirect restoration which involves proximal surfaces of posterior tooth and caps all of the cusps* (Fig. 10.2).

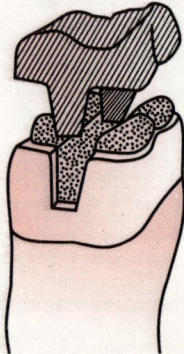

Fig. 10.2

INDICATIONS FOR ONLAYS

1. A cavity whose width is one-third to one-half of the intercuspal distance.

2. In the tooth preparation, if the length: width ratio of the cusp is more than 1:1, but not exceeding 2:1, onlay can be considered.

3. In the tooth preparation, if length: width ratio of a cusp is more than 2:1 onlay is mandated.

4. Replacement of defective amalgam restorations.

5. When the restoration needs to splint the buccal and lingual cusps.

6. Restoration of posterior interproximal caries.

7. Restoration of posterior teeth with heavy occlusal wear.

CAST RESTORATIONS

INDICATIONS

1. Extensive tooth involvement.

2. Restoration of endodontically treated tooth.

3. Cracked teeth (vertically or diagonally).

4. Esthetics.

5. Repeated failures of amalgam restoration.

6. Worn teeth.

7. Fixed and removable denture retainers.

8. Low incidences of plaque accumulation and decay.

9. Patient preference.

CONTRAINDICATIONS

1. Developing and deciduous teeth.

2. High plaque / caries indices.

3. Occlusal disharmony.

4. Dissimilar metals.

ADVANTAGES

1. High strength.

2. Capable of reproduction of minute details also.

3. No significant tarnish and corrosion.

4. Very much biocompatible.

5. Long lasting.

DISADVANTAGES

1. Microleakage at the tooth cement casting junction.

2. Extensive tooth preparation.

3. Galvanism.

4. Needs multiple visits.

5. Some cast alloys have high abrasive resistance than that of enamel.

6. Not economical.

MATERIALS FOR CAST RESTORATIONS

Classification

1. Class I

– These are gold and platinum group based alloys.

– These are sub-divided into type I, II, III and IV gold alloys.

2. Class II

– These are low gold alloys with gold content less than 50%.

3. Class III

– These are non-gold palladium based alloys.

4. Class - IV

– These are nickel-chromium based alloys.

5. Class-V

– These are castable, moldable ceramics.

PRINCIPLES OF TOOTH PREPARATION FOR CAST RESTORATIONS

– Tooth preparation is divided into,

  i. *Intracoronal tooth preparation.*

  ii. *Extracoronal tooth preparation.*

– *Intracoronal preparations* are mortise shaped having definite walls and floors joined at line and point angles.

Extracoronal preparations are created by occlusal and axial surface reduction. In most of the cases, ends gingivally with no definite flat floor.

– There are 3 principles of tooth preparation,

  1. *Preparation path*

  2. *Apicoocclusal taper of the preparation*

  3. *Circumferential tie*

1. PREPARATION PATH (Fig. 10.3)

– The preparation should have a single insertion path, opposite to the direction of the occlusal load.

– *This path is usually parallel to the long axis of the tooth crown.*

– *This feature helps in the retention of restoration and decreases its micromovements during function.*

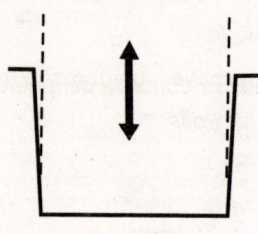

Fig. 10.3

2. APICOOCCLUSAL TAPER / INLAY TAPER (Fig. 10.4)

– *The concept is, intracoronally the cavity walls must diverge from the floor of the preparation to external surface and extracoronally walls must converge from the cervical to the occlusal surface.*

– *Taper permits an unobstructed removal of the wax pattern and seating of the subsequent casting.*

– Generally, the axis of taper for a class I or II preparation is parallel to the long axis of the tooth and for a class V, it is perpendicular to the long axis of the tooth.

– The taper should be on an average of 2–5° from the path of preparation.

– The amount of taper is influenced by certain factors, i.e. greater the wall length is the more taper will be but not to exceed 10° and greater the need for retention, the less taper will be.

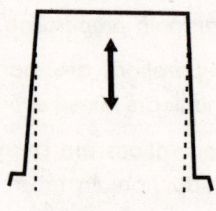

Fig. 10.4

3. CIRCUMFERENTIAL TIE

– *The peripheral marginal anatomy of the preparation is called circumferential tie.*

– If the margin ends on enamel, enamel walls should fulfill all requirements.

1. Enamel must be supported by sound dentin.

2. Enamel rods forming the cavosurface margin should be continuous with sound dentin.

3. Enamel rods forming the cavosurface margin should be covered with restorative material.

4. Angular cavosurface angles should be trimmed.

– *For the occlusal and gingival walls in intracoronal cavity preparations the tooth circumferential tie will be in the form of a bevel (which is a plane of a cavity wall or floor directed away from the cavity preparation).*

BEVELS

Definition

– Bevels are the flexible extensions of a cavity preparation allowing the inclusion of surface defects, supplementary grooves or other areas on the tooth surface (Fig. 10.5).

Types

– According to their shape and type of tissue involvement they are divided into,

1. *Partial Bevel*

   – Involves the part of the enamel wall, not exceeding two-thirds of its dimension.

   – *Usually not used in cast restorations.*

   – *Used to trim weak enamel rods from margin peripheries.*

2. *Short Bevel*

   – Includes the entire enamel wall, but not dentin.

   – *Used mostly with class I alloys especially for type I and II.*

3. *Long Bevel*

   – Includes all of the enamel wall and up to one half of the dentinal wall.

   – It is the most frequently used bevel for the first three classes (Class I, II and III) of cast materials.

   – *Advantage :* Preserves the internal 'boxed-up' resistance and retention features of the preparation.

4. *Full Bevel*

   – Includes all of the dentinal and enamel walls of the cavity wall or floor.

   – It's use should be avoided except in cases where it is impossible to use any other form of bevel.

   – *Disadvantage :* Deprives the preparations internal resistance and retention form.

5. *Counter Bevel*

- Given opposite to an axial cavity wall, on the facial or lingual surface of the tooth with the gingival inclination facially or lingually.

- It is used for the capping of cusps to protect and support them.

6. *Hollow ground (concave) bevel*

- It is prepared in a concave form. This allows more space for cast material bulk; a design feature needed in special preparations to improve materials castability retention and better resistance to stresses.

- It is ideal for class IV and V cast materials.

Functions

1. Produce obtuse angled marginal tooth structures which is the bulkiest and strongest configuration of any marginal tooth anatomy.

2. Producing an acute angled margin will be most amenable to burnishing for that alloy.

3. Reduce the error factors (space between cast and tooth substances).

4. Major retention forms for cast restoration.

5. Gingival bevels bring the gingival margins as cleansable or protected areas.

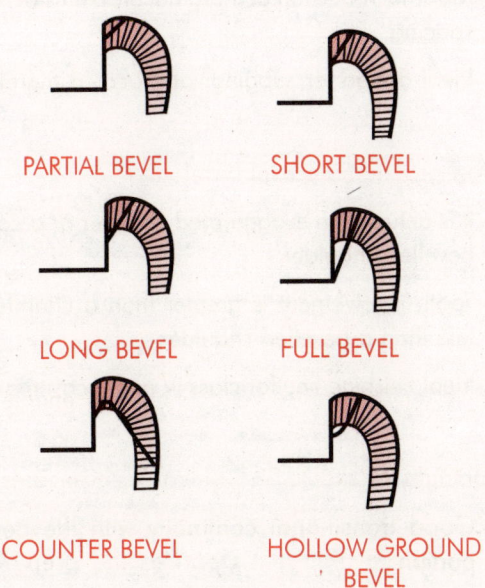

PARTIAL BEVEL   SHORT BEVEL

LONG BEVEL   FULL BEVEL

COUNTER BEVEL   HOLLOW GROUND BEVEL

Fig. 10.5

FLARES

Flares are the flat or concave peripheral portions of the facial and lingual walls (Fig. 10.6).

Types of flares

1. **Primary Flare**

- It is the conventional and basic part of the circumferential tie facially and lingually for an intra-coronal preparation.

- It always has a specific angulation, i.e. 45° to the inner dentinal wall proper.

- It may be a hollow ground in the preparation for a nonnoble alloy or cast ceramics.

Functions and Indications

- Perform the same functions as bevels.

- They bring the facial and lingual margins of the cavity preparations to cleansable, finishable areas.

- Indicated for any facial or lingual proximal wall of an intracoronal cavity preparation.

2. **Secondary Flare**

- It is a flat plane superimposed peripherally to a primary flare.

- It can be prepared in a hollow ground form also.

- Unlike primary flares, secondary flares may have different angulations, involvement and extent depending on their function.

Functions and Indications

- Perform the same functions as bevels.

- In addition,

  - Provide obtuse angulation of the marginal tooth structure in a teeth with very widely extended lesions buccolingually.

  - Bring the facial and lingual margins to finishable, cleansable areas in the teeth with very broad contact areas or malposed contact areas.

  - Avoid marginal failures due to peripheral marginal undercuts in ovoid teeth.

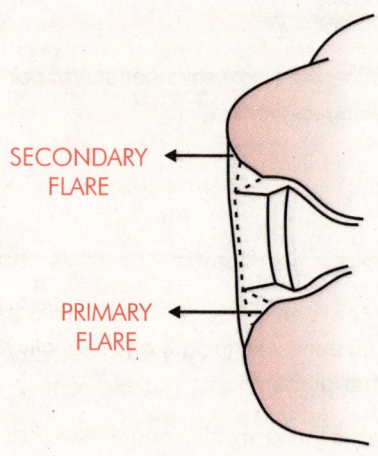

SECONDARY FLARE

PRIMARY FLARE

Fig. 10.6

CIRCUMFERENTIAL TIE CONSTITUENTS FOR EXTRACORONAL PREPARATIONS : (FINISHING LINES)

– *For extracoronal preparations, circumferential tie will be in one of the following forms.*

1. Chamfer finishing line

– A concave extracoronal finish line that possesses greater angulation than a knife edge with less width than a shoulder.

– Is an obtuse angled gingival termination.

– Most universally used design for class I, II and III cast materials.

– Most practical type of finishing line for subgingival extracoronal preparations.

– *Contraindicated for Class IV and V cast materials due to their poor castability.*

Advantages

1. Assures bulk.
2. Definite marginal termination with little tooth involvement (0.5 mm maximal depth).

Disadvantage

– Limited burnishability of the marginal cast alloy.

2. Knife edge (feather edge) finishing line

– Circumferential tie consistent with the involvement of least tooth structure.

– If the margin is on enamel, it involves part of the enamel only.

– Used only for very castable burnishable type of alloy (preferably type II gold alloys).

– It should be located on accessible areas of the tooth surface for proper finishing.

– Indicated when minimal axial depth is required for biologic or anatomic purposes.

– *Contraindicated for Class III, IV and V cast materials.*

Advantages

1. Involvement of least tooth structure.
2. Blends easily and efficiently with bevelled constituents.

Disadvantages

– Possibility for indefinite termination for the casting.

3. Bevelled shoulder finishing line

– Most tooth structure is involved.

– It can be used for any class of cast materials.

– It is indicated when (i) a definite gingival floor, with all its components (wall proper and bevel) is needed for resistance, retention purposes, (ii) maximum bulk of the cast is needed marginally for materials that are limited in their castability and difficult to burnish.

Advantages

1. Blends easily with bevelled constituents.
2. Maximal reduction of marginal problems of internal spacing.
3. Ideal design for subgingivally located margins.

4. Hollow ground (concave) bevel

– It is actually an exaggerated chamfer or a concave bevelled shoulder.

– Tooth involvement is greater than a chamfer and less than a bevelled shoulder.

– Ideal finishing line for class IV and V cast materials.

Advantages

1. Good transitional continuity with the bevelled portion.
2. Helps in stabilization of the casting.

DIFFERENCES BETWEEN THE CLASS II CAVITY PREPARATION FOR *SILVER AMALGAM AND CAST RESTORATIONS*

Preparation Feature	Silver Amalgam	Cast Restoration
1. Outline form:	– Narrow	– Wide
2. Cavity width:	– 1/4th of intercuspal distance.	– 1/3rd of intercuspal distance.
3. Cavity depth:	– More	– Less
4. Cavity walls:	– Converge occlusally.	– Parallel or diverge occlusally.
5. Cavosurface bevel:	– Not given (Butt joint)	– Given (Lap joint)
6. Line and point angles:	– Rounded and axiopulpal line angle is bevelled.	– well-defined and axiopulpal line angle is slightly rounded.
7. Reverse bevel:	– Not given	– Given
8. Secondary retention:	– Only locks are given	– Only grooves are given.

CHAPTER 11

NON-CARIOUS LESIONS

– Non-carious lesions may be classified into,
1. Attrition
2. Abrasion
3. Erosion
4. Localized non-hereditary enamel hypoplasia
5. Localized non-hereditary enamel hypocalcification
6. Localized non-hereditary dentin hypoplasia
7. Localized non-hereditary dentin hypocalcification
8. Discolorations
9. Malformation
10. Amelogenesis imperfecta
11. Dentinogenesis imperfecta
12. Trauma

– In this chapter, we have described about the three most common lesions of teeth among the above said.

ATTRITION

– *Attrition is defined as the loss of surface tooth structure resulting from direct frictional forces between contacting teeth.*

– Attrition affecting occlusal surfaces results in flattening of their inclined planes, in facet formation and reverse cusp formation.

– Attrition affecting proximal surfaces results in flat, faceted proximal contours and sometimes concave proximal surfaces.

– Attrition increases in patients with parafunctional mandibular movements, i.e. bruxism.

– *Attrition is a physiologic process.*

EFFECTS OF ATTRITION

1. **Occluding surface attrition (Occlusal wear)**

   The effects are,

   – Loss of vertical dimension of the tooth
   – Cheek biting
   – Gingival irritation
   – Decay
   – Tooth sensitivity

2. **Proximal surface attrition (proximal surface faceting)**

   The effects are,

   – Increased susceptibility to caries
   – Hindering of cleansability
   – Drifting of teeth

– Overall reduction of the length of dental arch

– Decreased interproximal space

CAUSES OF ATTRITION

– They are of two types, i.e.

1. Physiological attrition
2. Pathological attrition

1. Physiological attrition

– Attrition is constant and is proportionate to the age of individual.

– Attrition also occurs in proximal surface in the contact point areas.

2. Pathological attrition

i *Abnormal occlusion*. Ex: crowding of teeth and malposed teeth.

ii *Abnormal chewing habits*. Ex: Bruxism and chronic persistent chewing of coarse and abrasive foods or other substance.

iii *Structural defects* in teeth. Ex: Amelogenesis imperfecta, dentinogenesis imperfecta.

TREATMENT

1. For pulpally involved teeth, endodontic therapy or extraction depending on its restorability and role in the stomatognathic system.

2. Treating of parafunctional activities.

3. Resolving of myofunctional, TMJ or any other symptoms in the stomatognathic system.

4. Occlusal equilibration is performed after the reliving of all notable symptoms.

   – Occlusal equilibration is defined as the selective grinding of tooth surfaces which include rounding and smoothening of the peripheries of the occlusal tables and also the creation of adequate overlap between the working inclines.

5. Protection of exposed sensitive dentinal areas and obliteration of actual carious lesions. Protection is by fluoride solution and obliteration is by proper temporary restoration.

6. *Restorative modalities* : Metallic restorations are used to replace lost tooth structure due to attrition which is at high stress concentration areas.

ABRASION

– *Abrasion is defined as the mechanical wearing away of the teeth.*

– Occurs most frequently on incisal and occlusal surfaces.

– *Abrasion is a pathologic process which is usually inseparable from attrition and/or erosion.*

TYPES OF ABRASION (CAUSES)

– Based on the etiologic factor,

1. Toothbrush abrasion (most predominant).
2. Pipe smoking 'depression abrasion'.
3. Abrasion due to tobacco chewing.
4. Proximal abrasion due to the forcing of a tooth pick, inter dental stimulator, etc.
5. Abrasion due to professional habits such as cutting of sewing thread with incisors, holding and pulling of nails with anterior teeth.
6. Iatrogenic tooth abrasion, i.e. between porcelain teeth and opposing natural teeth; between cast alloy restoration of high abrasion resistance and opposing natural teeth.

1. Toothbrush Abrasion

– Occurs cervically, mostly on the facial surface of canines and bicuspids. It is usually on the left side for right handed persons and vice versa for left-handed people.

The extent of abrasion is depend on the following,

– Horizontal direction of brushing is most **detrimental.**

– The larger and more irregular the abrasive particles the more the abrasion will be.

– The higher the percentage of abrasives in the dentifrice, the more the abrasion will be.

– Silica abrasives are much more abrading than phosphate and carbonate ones.

– The greater the diameter of brush bristles, the more the abrasion will be. Natural bristles are more abrasive than synthetic bristles.

– Type of tooth tissues being abraded: The most resistant tissues to abrasion are enamel especially occlusally and the least resistant is cementum. Dentin abrades very easily at cervical region.

SIGNS AND SYMPTOMS

1. Lesion is linear shape in outline.
2. Peripheries of the lesion are angularly demarcated from the surrounding tooth surface.
3. Surface of the lesion is extremely smooth and polished.
4. The surrounding walls of the lesion make a V-shape by meeting at an acute angle axially.
5. Stimulating (with hot, cold or sweets) or probing of the lesion can elicit the pain.

2. Pipe smoking `depression abrasion'

   – An abrading depression on the occlusal surfaces of teeth at anterolateral portion of the arch coinciding with the intraoral location of the pipe stem.

   Pica-syndrome

   – It is due to the habit of chewing clay (mud), has a specific occlusal abrasion pattern and other systemic disorders.

TREATMENT

1. Preventive

   – Correct or avoid ill-fitting metal clasps and dentures.

   – Discontinuation of the habits of chewing tobacco, gum, toothpick, etc.

2. Restorative

   a. *Milder cases:* Limiting of the lateral extrusions of the mandible, excessive movements of the mandible by placing gold- foil restorations or inlays, building up of a cusp.

   b. *Moderate cases:* 'Shoeing' method is employed, i.e. cutting cavities in the abraded surfaces and placing gold-foil restorations, inlays or onlays, making no attempt to restore original tooth forms.

   c. *Extensive cases:* Operation of restoring vertical dimensions or `opening the bite' may be attempted, placing crowns or inlays on the posterior teeth, bridges or removable dentures in any existing spaces and building up and restoring to original form the anterior teeth with restorations or porcelain crowns.

EROSION

– Erosion is the chemical or chemico-mechanical wearing away in such a manner that broad, shallow, smooth, highly polished excavations or depressions are made in the enamel and dentin on surfaces not subject to mastication.

– Erosion is the pathologic process.

CAUSES

A. Mechanical Factors

   – The action of the muscles of the lips and cheeks and of the tooth brush against the affected surfaces.

B. Chemical factors

   1. Diseases of suboxidation or faulty metabolism resulting in excessive formation of acid sodium phosphate, acid calcium phosphate or both.

   2. Excess of lactic acid in the saliva.

   3. Excess of acid salts excreted from the blood by the salivary or mucous glands.

   4. Excess of alkaline salts or bases present in the saliva.

   5. Solution of the organic matrix by bacterial enzymes and later dissolution of the inorganic material.

   6. Excessive use of extraneous acids such as lemonjuice, vinegar, grapefruit and grapes.

   7. Acid vapours from nitric acid and sulfuric acids, acting in the mouths of workers in factories.

   8. Acidity from a local acidosis in the periodontal tissues as a result of traumatic occlusion.

SIGNS AND SYMPTOMS

1. No demarcation between the lesion and adjacent tooth surface.

2. Lesion's surface is glazed.

3. Erosion rate is same for enamel, dentin and cementum.

4. Adjacent gingiva and periodontium are almost always sound and healthy.

5. Presence of tooth sensitivity.

6. Carious lesions usually do not found on tooth surfaces attacked by erosion.

7. Erosion affects upper teeth more than lower teeth especially on the facial surface of cuspids and premolars; Facial surface of lower anterior teeth is a common location for erosion.

TREATMENT

A. Preventive

   i. *General*

   – Rx is directed against faulty metabolism including such features as regulation of the diet, exercise, fresh air, massage.

   – Plenty of pure water should be drunk or as a substitute some of the carbonated or `spring' waters.

   ii. *Local*

   – Prevention and cure of periodontal disturbances.

   – Stiff toothbrushes and gritty dentifrices should be abandoned.

B. Restorative

   – In the advanced cases, extend the cavity margins well beyond the eroded area and insert porcelain inlays, gold inlays, or gold foil restorations.

CHAPTER 12

DENTIN HYPERSENSITIVITY

DEFINITION

- `Sensitive or Hypersensitive dentin' implies an abnormal sensitiveness of an exposed area of dentin, exhibiting itself in the form of reflex or localized pains, sometimes in the absence of apparent external sources of irritation, or otherwise as a result of the contact of heat and cold, salt, sweet and acid substances or of foods and instruments.
- Pain is sharp, transient and well localized.

CAUSES

1. The action of caries, erosion, abrasion, cracks and fractures of the enamel.
2. The careless use of scalers.
3. Recessions of the gingivae.
4. Changes of temperature.
5. Action of salt, sweet and acid substances.

THEORIES OF DENTIN HYPERSENSITIVITY

1. Dentin innervation theory

- This theory states that dentin hypersensitivity occurs due to direct stimulation of nerve fibers present in dentin.

2. Odontoblast transmission theory

- It states that dentin hypersensitivity occurs due to direct stimulation of odontoblastic processes that are present in dentinal tubules.

3. Hydrodynamic theory of dentin sensitivity

- Proposed by BRANTHROM.
- Well accepted theory.
- Dential tubules contain dentinal fluid, odontoblastic processes, nerve fibers.
- Dentinal fluid composition is similar to tissue fluid and it fills the entire length of tubule.
- The odontoblastic cell processes and nerve fibers extend only very little distance into the dentinal tubules from their origin in the pulp.
- This theory states that the fluid in the dentinal tubules can be affected by mechanical, thermal and osmotic stimuli. Movement of the dentinal fluid within the tubules in either direction stimulates nerves in the dentin or pulp which result in a painful response.
- Various stimuli that can alter the dentinal fluid flow in an exposed dentin are,
    1. Temperature changes, i.e. hot/cold food
    2. Sweets

3. Dental drill
4. Compressed air
5. Chiselling

MANAGEMENT

– It depends on cause,
   1. Restorative method.
   2. Nonrestorative method.

1. Restorative method

– When hypersensitivity is associated with significant loss of tooth structure, restorative methods are used.

– Cervical defects like abrasion erosion and abfraction can be treated by using glass ionomer or composites with proper pulp protection if required.

– Dental caries can be treated with suitable metallic or non-metallic restoration.

– Cracked tooth syndrome is treated with full crowns.

– Faulty restorations should be removed and then restored temporarily. Once the symptoms of sensitivity subsides tooth is permanently restored.

2. Nonrestorative Method

– If the loss of tooth structure is insignificant and generalized, then nonrestorative methods are indicated.

Various treatment Modalities

1. Resin impregnation technique
2. Iontophoresis
3. Topical fluoride application
4. Application of calcium hydroxide
5. Chemical agents, i.e. potassium oxalate, silver nitrate
6. Medicated toothpaste
7. Dentin bonding agent
8. Lasers
9. Desiccation

1. Resin Impregnation Technique

– Exposed dentin surface is cleaned.

– Surface is etched with phosphoric acid for 5 sec.

– Rinsing and drying for 20 sec.

– Immediately an enamel bonding agent is applied on the surface which results in quick penetration of resin into the tubules and bonding resin is then cured.

2. Iontophoresis

– Iontophoresis is the transfer of ions under electrical pressure through electrodes having opposite charge.

– In this process, 1–2% sodium chloride or solution containing potassium, zincions, etc. are applied.

– These ions are forced into the tubules by applying electrical force through electrodes.

– Fluoride ions react with calcium, get precipitated in tubules and there by blocks the tubules.

– They also reduce the excitability of a delta nerve fibres and reduce dentin sensitivity.

3. Topical fluoride Application: (Fluoride Varnish)

– 30% sodium fluoride paste is used.

– Fluoride varnishes at regular intervals can reduce sensitivity by promoting remineralization and they also have antibacterial effects.

4. Application of Calcium hydroxide

– Used especially in root cementum exposures.

– A paste of calcium hydroxide is placed over exposure area and covered and protected by periodontal paste dressing.

5. Chemical Agents

– Potassium oxalate when applied on the dentinal tubules, calcium oxalate is formed within the tubules and blocks dentinal tubules.

– Single application will be effective for 6 months.

– Potassium ions also have the ability to reduce the alpha–delta nerve fibre excitation.

– Silver nitrate is rarely used.

6. Use of Medicated Toothpaste

A. *Toothpaste with strontium chloride*

– Strontium reacts with phosphate in the dentinal fluid to form strontium phosphate crystals and block the tubules.

– It also stimulates: (1) the formation of secondary dentin, (2) can bind to the collagen matrix of the tubules and there by reduces the diameter of tubules.

B. *Toothpaste with 5% potassium nitrate*

– Potassium reduces the excitability of peripheral A- delta nerve fibers.

– Promotes mineralization.

C. Toothpaste containing 0.7% sodium mono fluoro phosphate

- Promotes crystallization and mineralization inside the dentinal tubules.

Formalin

- Formalin combines with dentinal fluid which contains fluorine.
- Precipitates inside the tubules to occlude the dentinal tubules.

7. Use of Dentin Bonding Agents

- Various recently available dentin bonding agents have been found to be useful in treating hypersensitivity.
- These bonding agents contain resins like HEMA, META, etc.

8. LASERS

- LASERS are used to melt and recrystallize the surface tooth structure and there by occlude the dentinal tubules.
- This method provide the result which lasts quite long.
- Commonly used LASER is Nd-YAG.

9. Desiccation

- Dry heat is applied by the use of electrically heated blasts of compressed air.
- The cavity may be moistened first with absolute alcohol or acetone, then the heat is applied, until the cavity is thoroughly desiccated.

CHAPTER 13

MISCELLANEOUS

LASERS

– *LASER* stands for *Light Amplification by Stimulated Emission of Radiation*.
– Lasers are devices that produce beams of coherent and very high intensity light.
– Various types of lasers are used in dentistry.
– Most commonly used are, Nd:YAG and Er:YAG.

Uses

1. *Soft tissue applications*
   - i. Pulpotomy
   - ii. Pulp extirpation
   - iii. Apicoectomy
   - iv. Gingivectomy
   - v. Frenectomy
   - vi. Curettage
   - vii. Lesion excision
   - viii. Hemostasis
   - ix. Incision and drainage of abscesses

2. *Hard tissue applications*
   - i. Caries removal
   - ii. Cavity preparation
   - iii. Enamel etching
   - iv. Enameloplasty

3. *Non-surgical procedures*
   - i. Curing of materials
   - ii. Instrument sterilization

4. *Root canal procedures*
   - i. Access cavity preparation
   - ii. Biomechanical preparation
   - iii. Root canal debridement and cleaning

5. *Endodontic surgical procedures*
   - i. Flap preparation
   - ii. Cutting the bone to prepare a window access to the apex of the root.
   - iii. Root end preparation for retrograde filling.
   - iv. Removal of pathological tissues.

Advantages

1. Blood less
2. Painless

MICRO- and MACROABRASION

– It is an alternative for the reduction or elimination of superficial discolorations.

– They result in the physical removal of tooth structure and therefore, are indicated only for stains or enamel defects that do not extend beyond a few tenths of a millimeter in depth.

MICROABRASION

– *A technique involving the surface dissolution of the enamel by the acid along with the abrasiveness of the pumice to remove superficial stains or defects.*

Uses

– The following defects can be removed by microabrasion technique, i.e. incipient carious lesions, fluorosis discolorations extending with in the 0.2 to 0.3 mm deep, small localized idiopathic white or light-brown areas and developmental discolored spots to some extent.

Advantages

1. Better control of the removal of tooth structure.
2. Superior patient acceptance.

MACROABRASION

– *A technique of removal of the defect using a 12-fluted composite finishing bur or a fine grit finishing diamond in a high-speed handpiece.*

Precautions

1. Use light
2. Apply intermittent pressure
3. Careful monitoring of removal of tooth structure.
4. Use Air-water spray to maintain the hydrated stage of tooth.

Uses

– Technique is used for the removal of localized, superficial white spots (not subject to conservative, remineralization therapy) and other surface stains or defects.

Advantages

1. Faster
2. No need of rubberdam application
3. Easy removal of defect

Disadvantages

1. Technique sensitive.
2. Should be extreme cautious.

AIR ABRASION

Definition

– *A method of removal of tooth structure with the use of finely graded 27.5 μ alluminium oxide powder administered under compressed air through a fine tip.*

– Air abrasion uses the kinetic energy principle, in which particles bounce off the tooth and blasts the decay away.

Uses

1. To remove any stains or decay from teeth.
2. To expose hidden cavities, which can then be removed and a filling added.

Advantages

1. Virtually painless procedure.
2. Produce no vibration and no heat from friction.
3. No harm to soft tissues.
4. Preservation of tooth structure.
5. Little or no discomfort.
6. Shorter chair side time.
7. Operate very quitely (hence preferred in treating young patients who would normally be afraid of the dentist's drill).

Limitations

1. Cannot be used to remove interproximal caries.
2. Cannot be used to prepare a tooth for larger restoration such as amalgam.

MICROLEAKAGE

Definition

– *Flow of oral fluid and bacteria into the microscopic gap between a prepared tooth surface and a restorative material.*

Consequences

– The biocompatibility of a restoration is altered by the leakage process, which may cause a number of undesirable events, i.e.

　1. It may allow bacteria or bacterial products to reach the pulp and cause infection.
　2. It may encourage the breakdown of the material.
　3. It may discolour the margins of the restoration.
　4. Post operative sensitivity.

Detecting methods of Microleakage

- Dyes
- Chemical tracers
- Radioactive isotopes
- Neutron activation analysis
- Scanning electron microscopy
- Bacterial studies
- Electrochemical studies
- Air pressure
- Artificial caries
- Pain perception
- Reverse diffusion method

Microleakage around the Restorations

Amalgam

- If the restoration is properly inserted, leakage decreases as the restoration ages in the mouth. This may be caused by corrosion products that form along the interface between the tooth and the restoration sealing the interface and thereby preventing leakage. Accumulation of corrosion products is slower for high-copper alloys.

NANO LEAKAGE

- If the resin penetrates the collagen network of the dentin but does not penetrate it completely, a much smaller gap (< 0.1mm) will exist between the mineralized matrix of the dentin and collagen-resin hybrid layer. This much smaller gap allows *Nano leakage*.
- It reduces the longevity of the dentin-resin bond.
- This degradation process may gradually increase the gap size until microleakage begins to occur.
- Nano leakage is not known to occur between restorations and enamel because enamel does not contain organic mass and therefore no collagenous matrix into which a resin may be embedded.

FINISHING AND POLISHING OF THE RESTORATIONS

- *Finishing is the process of removal of excess and contouring the restoration, and which is done immediately after the placement of restoration.*
- Smooth surface does not tarnish, corrode, gives shiny appearance, no surface deposition. Hence, the polishing of restoration is done to achieve the smooth surface.

Goals

- The goals of finishing and polishing procedures are to obtain the,
  1. Desired anatomy
  2. Proper occlusion
- Reduction of roughness, gouges and scratches which were produced by contouring and finishing instruments.

Polishing Materials

- They are supplied in paste and powder.

Polishing Agents

- Rubber cup, Brittle brush, Diamond points, Abrasive points, wheels and cylinders, etc.
- Polishing pastes are applied with soft felt points, muslin (Woven cotton fabric) wheels, prophylaxis rubber cups or buffing wheels.
- A nonabrasive material should be used as an applicator while using polishing pastes.
- For polishing, initially coarse abrasives and finally fine abrasives are used.
- Polishing should be done at slow speeds only.
- High speed results in heat generation which causes damage to the pulp.
- Dry polishing is not advocated because it releases vapours from the restoration and generates frictional heat.

BENEFITS

- Finishing and polishing provide three benefits of dental care.

1. *Oral health*
   - A well contoured and polished restoration promotes oral health by resisting the accumulation of food debris and pathologic bacteria.

2. *Function*
   - Oral function is enhanced with a well-polished restoration because food glides more freely over occlusal and embrasure surfaces during mastications.
   - Smooth surfaces minimize wear rates on opposing and adjacent teeth.
   - Rough material surfaces lead to the development of high-contact stresses that can cause the loss of functional and stabilizing contacts between teeth.

3. *Esthetics*
   - Well finished and polished restoration gives pleasing appearance.

REACTION OF THE PULP TO IRRITATING STIMULI

– The reaction will be in one of the following ways,

1. **Healthy Reparative Reaction**

   – It is the most favourable response.

   – It consists of, formation of sclerotic dentin and/or calcific barrier. These are followed by normal secondary dentin.

   – It occurs without any disturbances in the pulp tissues.

2. **Unhealthy Reparative Reaction**

   – It is fairly favourable.

   – It consists of, degeneration of the odontoblasts, followed by the formation of the dead tracts.

   – It is accompanied by mild pathological clinical changes of reversible nature in the pulp, which results in the formation of tertiary dentin.

3. **Destructive Reaction**

   – Most unfavourable response.

   – It begins with the loss of odontoblasts and the outer protective layer of the pulp.

   – The resulting reaction will be inflammation, abscess formation, finally necrosis of the pulp.

   – In any event, pulp tissues cannot recuperate from these pathologic changes.

Pulpal Response During Cavity Preparation

– It depends on many factors,

1. Thermal injury
2. Frictional heat
3. Vibration
4. Desiccation of dentin
5. Pulp exposure
6. Smear layer
7. Remaining dentin thickness
8. Agents for cleaning, drying and sterilization
9. Acid etching

– Sharp hand cutting instruments are the most biologically acceptable cutting instruments.

– Rotary cutting instruments (burs) are also biologically acceptable if used over effective depth of 2 mm and more with proper coolants.

– Rotary abrasive instruments (stones) are not recommended for cutting in vital dentin as their abrasive action elevates the temperature of surrounding dentin.

– The less the effective depth, the more destructive reaction will be.

– Heat generation not only creates destruction of pulp, but it can also coagulate protoplasm and even char dentin and enamel.

– Desiccation creates a disturbance in the osmotic pressure of dentinal tubules, increases the permeability of the dentin.

– Excessive vibration can cause,

   – Disruption of the odontoblasts in the opposite side of the pulp chamber.

   – Edema.

   – Fibrosis of pulp tissues.

   – Change in ground substance of the pulp.

   – Reduction in the predentin formation.

   – Microcracks in enamel and in non-elastic dentin.

– Excessive frictional heat: Coronal dentin develops a pinkish hue very soon after the dentin is cut. This pinkish hue represents vascular stasis in the subodontoblastic capillary plexus blood flow. A dark colour indicates thrombosis.

Section II

Endodontics

CHAPTER 01

INTRODUCTION

DEFINITION

– *Endodontics is that branch of dental science which deals with the diagnosis, prevention and treatment of diseases and injuries of the pulp and associated periradicular conditions.*

– It includes the study of basic sciences like biology of normal pulp, etiology for the various diseases and pathology of human dental pulp along with morphology and physiology.

AIMS AND OBJECTIVES

1. Diagnosis of the diseases of the pulp.
2. To identify and determine etiological factors responsible for pulpal and periapical disease.
3. Measures to prevent diseases of the pulp and periapical tissues.
4. Selection of cases for treatment.
5. To provide care which is proper and consistent with the knowledge and experience.
6. To determine reasonable prognosis for the cases selected for the treatment.
7. To evaluate or assess the completed endodontic procedures.

SCOPE OF ENDODONTICS

– Formerly, endodontic treatment confined itself to root canal filling techniques by conventional methods, even endodontic surgery was considered to be in the field of oral surgery.

– Modern endodontics has a much wider field and includes the following,

1. Diagnosis of oral pain.
2. Protection of healthy pulp from disease or injury.
3. Pulp capping.
4. Pulpotomy.
5. Root canal treatment of infected root canals.
6. Surgical endodontics, which includes apicoectomy, hemi-section, root amputation and replantation.

"Father of Modern Endodontics"

– Dr. Louis Grossman

CHAPTER 02

DENTAL PULP AND PERIRADICULAR TISSUES

- The dental pulp consists of vascular connective tissue contained within the rigid dentinal walls.
- *Primary function* of the pulp is the elaboration of dentin to form the tooth and to protect against and to repair the effects of noxious stimuli.

ZONES OF PULP

- Pulp is divided into,
    1. odontoblastic zone
    2. cell-free zone
    3. cell-rich zone
    4. central zone

I. ODONTOBLASTIC ZONE

- The odontoblastic cell bodies form the odontoblastic zone.
- In this odontoblastic zone capillaries and unmyelinated sensory nerves are around the odontoblastic cell bodies.

1. Predentin layer

- It is the first formed dentin, located adjacent to the pulp tissue.
- It is 2 to 6 μm wide.
- It is uncalcified dentin.
- Dentinogenesis includes the production, deposition and calcification of a matrix. This matrix is the predentin layer deposited around the odontoblastic process and is found between the calcified dentin and the odontoblastic zone.
- This is a protein carbohydrate complex consisting of proteoglycans, phosphoproteins, plasma proteins, glycoproteins and collagen fibrils.

Primary Dentin

- Primary dentin is formed before the teeth erupts and is divided into mantle and circum pulpal dentin.
- a. *Mantle dentin*, the first calcified layer of the dentin deposited against the enamel; forms the dentinal side of the dentino enamel junction.
- b. *Circum pulpal dentin* is the dentin formed after the layer of mantle dentin.
- It forms initial shape.

2. Secondary Dentin

- It is a narrow band of dentin bordering the pulp and representing that dentin formed after root completion.

– Secondary dentin is elaborated after eruption of the teeth.

– It can be differentiated from primary dentin by the sharp bending of the tubules producing a line of demarcation.

– It is deposited unevenly on primary dentin and has incremental patterns and tubular structures less regular than those of primary dentin.

– For Ex : secondary dentin is deposited in greater quantities in the floor and roof of the pulp chamber than on the walls.

– This deposition of secondary dentin protects the pulp.

– It is also formed in response to calcium hydroxide cement due to its high pH.

3. Peritubular Dentin / Intratubular Dentin

– The dentin that immediately surrounds the dentinal tubules is termed peritubular dentin.

– It forms the walls of the tubules in all but the dentin near the pulp.

– It is hyper mineralised (about 40%) than intertubular dentin.

– It is twice as thick in outer dentin than in inner dentin.

– It differs from intertubular dentin,

    – in lacking collagenous fibrous matrix.

    – a zone of increased radiographic and electron density.

– When dentin is routinely demineralised, the peritubular dentin will be lost as it lacks the stabilizing feature of collagen.

– By its growth, it constricts the dentinal tubules to a diameter of 1 µm near the DEJ.

– It is the *most highly mineralised part of dentin*.

– It is not found in interglobular areas.

4. Intertubular Dentin

– The main body of dentin is composed of intertubular dentin.

– It is located between the zones of peritubular dentin.

– Organic matrix is the main content.

5. Interglobular Dentin

– Sometimes mineralization of dentin begins in small globular areas that fail to coalesce into a homogenous mass, which results in zones of hypomineralization between the globules. These zones are known as Interglobular dentin or Interglobular spaces.

6. Reparative Dentin

– *Also known as irregular or reactionary or tertiary dentin*.

– It is laid down by the pulp as a protective response to noxious stimuli.

– These stimuli can result from caries, operative procedures, restorative materials, abrasion, erosion or trauma.

– The reparative dentin is deposited in the affected area at an average rate of 1.5 µm per day.

– Deposition depends on the severity and duration of the injury to the odontoblasts.

– When there is mild stimulus for a prolonged period of time, produces slightly irregular tubules.

– Aggressive carious lesion or abrupt stimulus stimulates the production of reparative dentin with fewer and more irregular tubules.

7. Dead Tracts

– Dentin areas characterized by degenerated odontoblast process give rise to dead tracts.

– They appear black in transmitted and white in reflected light.

– Those areas show decreased sensitivity and more seen in older teeth.

– They are probably the initial step in the formation of sclerotic dentin.

8. Sclerotic / Transparent / Translucent Dentin

– Dentin that has more mineral content than normal dentin is called sclerotic dentin.

– It occurs ahead of *demineralization*.

– It is seen in slowly advancing carious lesion or under old restoration and in the roots of elderly people.

– It is shiny and more dark in colour.

– It reduces the permeability of the dentin and thus prolong the pulp vitality (decreases the tubular lumen diameter).

– Therefore, it is difficult to bond a restorative material to sclerotic dentin.

II. `CELL FREE ZONE (Zone of Weil)

- It is a acellular zone of the pulp located centrally to the odontoblastic zone.

- This zone contains some fibroblasts, mesenchymal cells and macrophages although called `cell free'.

- Main constituents of this zone are plexus of capillaries, the nerve plexus of Raschkow and the ground substance.

- This zone is more prominent in the coronal pulp.

III. CELL RICH ZONE

- This zone is located central to the cell free zone.

- Its main components are ground substance, fibroblasts with their product the collagen fibers, undifferentiated mesenchymal cells and macrophages.

IV. CENTRAL ZONE

- The central zone or pulp proper contains blood vessels and nerves that are embedded in the pulp matrix together with fibroblasts.

- From their central location blood vessels and nerves send branches to the periphery of the pulp.

ANATOMY OF THE PULP CAVITY

PULP CAVITY (Fig. 2.1 A and B)

- *It is the central cavity within a tooth and is entirely enclosed by dentin expect at the apical foramen.*

- Pulp cavity may be divided into *coronal portion, pulp chamber, radicular portion* and *root canal.*

- In anterior teeth the pulp chamber gradually merges into the root canal and this division becomes indistinct.

- In multirooted teeth the pulp cavity consists of a single pulp chamber and usually three root canals although the number of canals can very from one to five.

- *Roof of the pulp chamber* consists of dentin covering the pulp chamber occlusally or incisally.

- A *pulp horn* is an accentuation of the root of the pulp chamber directly under a cusp or developmental lobe.

- The *floor of the pulp chamber* runs parallel to the roof and consists of dentin bounding the pulp chamber near the cervix of the tooth particularly dentin forming the furcation area.

- The *canal orifices* are openings in the floor of the pulp chamber leading into the root canals. These are continuous with both the pulp chamber and root canals.

- The *walls of a pulp chamber* derive their names from the corresponding walls of the tooth surface, such as the buccal wall of a pulp chamber.

- The *angles of a pulp chamber* derive their names from the walls forming the angle such as the mesio buccal angle of a pulp chamber.

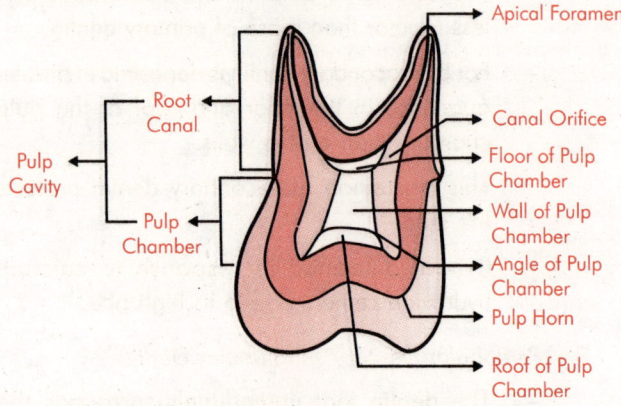

Fig. 2.1 A

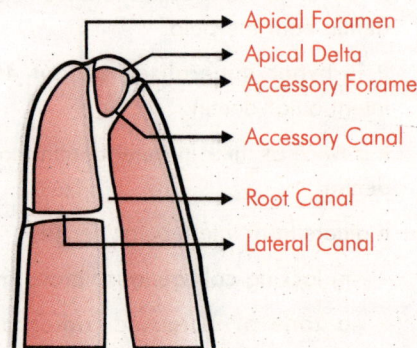

Fig. 2.1 B

ROOT CANAL

- *It is that portion of the pulp cavity from the canal orifice to the apical foramen.*

- It is divided into three sections, i.e. coronal, middle and apical thirds.

Accessory Canals or Lateral Canals

- These are lateral branchings of the main root canal generally occuring in the apical third or furcation area of a root.

- Sometimes a distinction can be made between an accessory canal and a lateral canal.

- Lateral canal is an accessory canal that branches to the lateral surface of the root and may be visible on a radiograph.

Apical Foramen

– *An aperture at or near apex of a root through which the blood vessels and the nerves of the pulp enter or leave the pulp cavity.*

Accessory Foramina

– *An orifice on the surface of the root communicating with a lateral or accessory canal.*

– *The periodontal vessels curve around the root apex of a developing tooth and become entrapped in Hertwig's epithelial root sheath which resulting in formation of the lateral and accessory foramina during calcification.*

Apical Stop

– *A barrier at the preparation end is an apical stop.*

Apical Seat

– *Lack of a complete barrier but the presence of a constriction represents an apical seat.*

Open Apex

– *The apical preparation resembles an open cylinder, i.e. neither barrier nor constriction.*

– *No apical seat will be created.*

Apical Constriction
(Minor apical diameter or apical stop)

– *It is the apical portion of the root canal having the narrowest diameter.*

– *This position may vary but is usually 0.5 to 1.0 mm short of the center of the apical foramen.*

– *The minor diameter widens apically to the foramen (major diameter) and assumes a funnel shape.*

TYPES OF ROOT CANAL CONFIGURATIONS

1. Weine's Classification

1. Type I : Single canal from the pulp chamber to the apex.

2. Type II : Two separate canals leaving the chamber but merging short of the apex to form only one canal.

3. Type III : Two separate canals leaving the chamber and exiting the root in separate apical foramina.

4. Type IV : One canal leaving the pulp chamber but dividing short of the apex into two separate and distinct canals with separate apical foramina.

2. Vertussi's Classification (Fig. 2.2)

– They are of 8 types,

1. Type I : Single root canal which exits as one single canal.

2. Type II : There will be two canals which exit as single canal.

3. Type III : Single canal which divides into two at the coronal 1/3 and rejoin at apical 1/3 and exit as one.

4. Type IV : Two canals which are exiting as two canals.

5. Type V : Single canal splitting into two.

6. Type VI : Two canals joining together at cervical 1/3 as one and again dividing into two in the apical 1/3.

7. Type VII : Single canal splitting and joining and again splitting into two.

8. Type VIII : Single canal splitting into three.

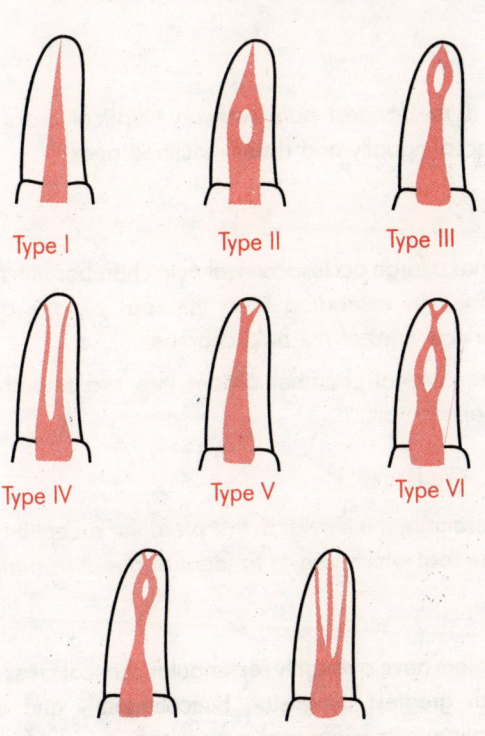

Type I Type II Type III

Type IV Type V Type VI

Type VII Type VIII

Fig. 2.2

– *The pulp horns that are most likely to be exposed during cavity preparation are,*

1. *mesiobuccal horn of upper molars.*

2. *mesiolingual horn of lower molars.*

NORMAL PERIRADICULAR TISSUES

- The periradicular tissues consists of, the cementum which covers the teeth. Alveolar process which forms the bony troughs containing the roots of the teeth.
- Periodontal ligament whose collagen fibers embedded in the cementum of the roots to the surrounding tissues.

MORPHOLOGY OF THE PULP

PULPS OF MAXILLARY TEETH

Central Incisor

- *It is shovel shaped coronally with three short horns on the coronal roof.*
- Tapering down to a triangle root in cross-section with the point of the triangle pointing lingually.

Lateral Incisor

- It is small and spoon shaped coronally changing to a round evenly tapering root to the apex.

Cuspid

- It is *the longest pulp* with an elliptical cross-section buccolingually and distally inclined apex.

First Premolar

- It has a large occlusocervical pulp chamber with a mesial concavity extending from the root surface onto the cervical third of the pulp chamber.
- The coronal chamber divides into two smooth funnel shaped roots.

Second Premolar

- Coronally, it is similar to first premolar except it has only one root which begins to taper at about its midpoint.

Molars

- Molars have a roughly rectangular cervical cross section with greatest dimension buccolingually and demonstrating a mesiobuccal prominence.
- There are 3 roots:
  - The lingual is longest.
  - The distobuccal is shortest and straight.
  - The mesiobuccal is curved and flattened buccolingually with its convex meisal surface.
  - From the first to third molar the coronal pulp chambers get smaller and roots get closer together.

PULPS OF MANDIBULAR TEETH

Central Incisor

- *It is the smallest pulp in the dentition.*
- It is long and narrow with a flattened elliptical shape in cross-section buccolingually.

Lateral Incisor

- It is similar to central incisor but smaller in all dimensions.

Cuspid

- It is similar to, but shorter than the maxillary canine.
- Its root begins tapering at about its midpoint ending in a distally inclined apex.

First Premolar

- It looks like a small mandibular canine with an insignificant or missing lingual pulp horn.

Second Premolar

- The lingual horn is smaller than the buccal horn and is about the dimension of the mandibular canine.
- In cross-section it is often roundly triangular or sometimes rectangular.

Molars

- The coronal cross-section is rectangular with the mesiodistal dimension greatest.
- Displays a mesiobuccal prominence.
- The horn heights from highest to lowest are mesiobuccal, mesiolingual, distobuccal, distolingual.
- There are two roots,
  - Distal is shorter and straighter and singular.
  - Mesial is longer, curved and often double.
  - From first to third the roots get smaller and closer together.

APICAL CLOSURE

- While calcification and cementum deposition at the apex continue throughout life, apices can be considered as fully formed several years after eruption, and approximate ages are given below:

TOOTH		APICAL CLOSURE (Years)
I – PRIMARY TEETH:		
Upper	CI	1 ½
	LI	2
	C	3 ¼
	M_1	2 ½
	M_2	3
Lower	CI	1 ½
	LI	1 ½
	C	3 ¼
	M_1	2 ¼
	M_2	3

TOOTH		APICAL CLOSURE (Years)
II – PERMANENT TEETH:		
Upper	CI	10
	LI	11
	C	13 – 15
	I_{PM}	12 – 13
	II_{PM}	12 – 14
	I_M	9 – 10
	II_M	14 – 16
	III_M	18 – 25
Lower	CI	9
	LI	10
	C	12 – 14
	I_{PM}	12 – 13
	I_{PM}	13 – 14
	I_M	9 – 10
	II_M	14 – 15
	III_M	18 – 25

CHAPTER 03

DISEASES OF THE DENTAL PULP AND PERIRADICULAR TISSUES

CAUSES OF PULP DISEASE
- According to Grossman,

I. PHYSICAL
   A. Mechanical
      1. Trauma
         a. Accidental
         b. Iatrogenic dental procedures
      2. Pathologic wear
      3. Crack through the body of tooth
      4. Barometric changes
   B. Thermal
      1. Heat during cavity preparation.
      2. Exothermic heat during setting of cement.
      3. Conduction of heat and cold through deep restorations without a protective base.
      4. Frictional heat during the polishing of restorations.
   C. Electrical
      - Galvanic shock.

II. CHEMICAL
   A. Phosphoric aid, acrylic monomer, etc.
   B. Erosion (acids).

III. BACTERIAL
   A. Toxins associated with caries.
   B. Direct invasion of pulp from caries or trauma.
   C. Anachoresis

- According to Ingle,
   I. BACTERIAL
      A. Coronal Ingress
         1. Caries
         2. Fracture
            i. Complete
            ii. Incomplete
         3. Non-fracture trauma
         4. Anamolous tract,
            i. dens invaginatus
            ii. dens evaginatus
            iii. radicular lingual groove
      B. Radicular ingress
         1. Caries

2. Retrogenic infection
   i. periodontal pocket
   ii. periodontal abscess
3. Hematogenic

II. TRAUMATIC

A. Acute
1. Coronal fracture
2. Radicular fracture
3. Vascular stasis
4. Luxation
5. Avulsion

B. Chronic
1. Adolescent female bruxism
2. Traumatism
3. Attrition or abrasion
4. Erosion

III. IATRAL

A. Cavity preparation
1. Heat of preparation
2. Depth of preparation
3. Dehydration
4. Pulp horn extensions
5. Pulp haemorrhage
6. Pulp exposure
7. Pulp incertion
8. Impression taking

B. Restoration
1. Insertion
2. Fracture
   i. complete
   ii. incomplete
3. Force of cementing
4. Heat of polishing

C. Intentional extirpation and root canal filling
D. Orthodontic movement
E. Periodontal curettage
F. Electrosurgery
G. Laser burn
H. Periradicular curettage
I. Rhinoplasty
J. Osteotomy
K. Intubation for general anesthesia

IV. CHEMICAL

A. Restorative materials
1. Cements
2. Plastics
3. Etching agents
4. Cavity liners
5. Dentin bonding agents
6. Tubule blockage agents

B. Disinfectants
1. Silver nitrate
2. Phenol
3. Sodium fluoride

C. Desiccants
1. Alcohol
2. Ether
3. Others

V. IDIOPATHIC

A. Aging
B. Internal resorption
C. External resorption
D. Hereditary hypophosphatemia
E. Sickle cell anemia
F. Herpes zoster infection
G. HIV and AIDS

CLASSIFICATION OF PULP DISEASES
- According to Grossman,
- Based on clinical features,

I. Pulpitides (Inflammation)

A. *Reversible*
1. Symptomatic (acute)
2. Asymptomatic (chronic)

B. *Irreversible*
1. Acute
   a. Abnormally responsive to cold
   b. Abnormally responsive to heat
2. Chronic
   a. Asymptomatic with pulp exposure
   b. Hyperplastic pulpitis
   c. Internal resorption

II. Pulp degeneration
A. Calcific (Radiographic diagnosis)
B. Others (Histopathologic diagnosis)

III. Necrosis

BARODONTALGIA (AERODONTALGIA)

– Toothache occurring at low atmospheric pressure experienced either during flight or during a test run in a decompression chamber.

– Barodontalgia has generally been observed in altitudes over 5,000 feet but it is more likely to occur at 10,000 feet or above.

– A tooth with chronic pulpitis can be symptomless at ground level, but it may cause pain at high altitude because of reduced pressure.

Treatment

– Lining the cavity with a varnish or a base of zinc phosphate cement, with a subbase of ZOE cement in deep cavities helps to prevent barodontalgia.

PATHWAYS OF BACTERIAL INVASION OF THE PULP

BACTERIA

– The most common cause of pulp injury is bacterial.

– Once bacteria have invaded the pulp, the damage is almost always irreparable.

– The bacteria most often recovered from infected vital pulps are streptococci, but many other microorganisms from diphtheroids to an aerobes have also been isolated.

– Microorganisms reach the dental pulp in various ways

1. *Through the open cavity*, i.e. by dental caries, traumatic injuries or operative procedures.

2. *Through the dental tubules* following carious invasions, restorative procedures.

3. *Through the lymphatic or haematogenous route (Anachoresis)*.

4. *Through the gingival sulcus or periodontal ligament,* i.e. microorganisms and other irritants from the periodental tissue through exposed dental tubules reach the lateral and accessory canals or apical and lateral foramina.

5. *Through a broken occlusal seal* or faulty restoration of a tooth previously treated by endodontic therapy.

6. *Through extension of a periapical infection* from adjacent infected teeth.

ANACHORESIS

– It is the transportation of microbes through the blood or lymph to an area of inflammation such as a tooth with pulpitis.

CLASSIFICATION OF PERIRADICULAR DISEASES

1. Acute periradicular diseases

    – Acute alveolar abscess.

    – Acute apical periodontitis,

        i. Vital

        ii. Non-vital

    – Acute exacerbation of a chronic lesion (Phoenix abscess).

2. Chronic periradicular diseases with areas of rarefaction

    – Chronic alveolar abscess

    – Granuloma

    – Cyst

3. Chronic periradicular disease with area of condensation

    – Condensing osteitis

4. Other periradicular lesions

    – External root resorption

    – Diseases of the periradicular tissues of non-odontogenic origin.

CHAPTER 04

CLINICAL DIAGNOSTIC METHODS

HISTORY AND RECORD

- To avoid irrelevant information and to prevent errors of omission in clinical tests, the clinician must establish a routine for examination.
- Questions concerning the patients chief complaint, past medical history and past dental history are reviewed.

I. SUBJECTIVE SYMPTOMS

- The symptoms which are felt by patient like pain, swelling, lack of function or esthetics.
- Whatever may be the reason but patients chief complaint is best starting point for a correct diagnosis.

Pain

- One should ask the patient about:
  - The kind of pain
  - Its location
  - Its duration
  - What causes it
  - What alleviates it
  - Whether it is referred to any site or not.
  - It is important to know whether the pain is localized to particular teeth (or) diffuse type of pain surrounding areas.
  - Generally, pulpal pain is described by a patient in one of 2 ways.

1. *Sharp, Piercing and Lancinating Pain*

- Consistent with those usually associated with excitation of the 'A Delta' nerve fibers in the pulp.
- Usually localized.
- Response promptly to cold.

2. *Dull, boring, gnawing and excruciating pain*

- Consistent with those resulting from exitation and slower rate of transmission of the 'C' nerve fibers in the pulp.
- Usually diffused.
- Responds abnormally to heat more than to cold and with symptoms that can be referred to other sites.

Duration of Pain

- The duration of pain is also diagnostic.
- At times pulpal pain lasts only as long as irritant is present.
- At other times, it lasts for minutes to hours.
- The pain may be either intermittent or constant.

- A tooth with fleeting pulpal pain that disappears on removal of the irritant has an excellent chance of recovery without the need for endodontic treatment.

- *Acute Reversible Pulpitis (Hyperemia)* is characterized by pain of short duration, caused by a specific irritant that disappears as soon as the irritant is removed. The pain is usually localized and is more responsive to cold than to heat.

- If the pain persists or if it occurs without any apparent cause the pulpitis usually be irreversible and the patient will require endodontic therapy.

- Abnormal dental pain caused by heat usually requires endodontic treatment.

- Pain that occurs on changing the position of the head, awakens the patient from sleep or occurs during mastication of food in a cariously exposed tooth usually indicates a need for endodontic treatment.

- Spontaneous pain and pain of long duration are symptoms of irreversible pulpitis.

II. OBJECTIVE SYMPTOMS

- Are determined by tests and observations performed by the clinicians.

- These tests are as follows,

    1. Visual and tactile inspection
    2. Percussion
    3. Palpation
    4. Mobility and depressibility
    5. Radiographs
    6. Electric pulp test
    7. Thermal tests (hot and cold)
    8. Anesthetic test
    9. Test cavity preparation
    10. Occlusal pressure test

1. VISUAL AND TACTILE INSPECTION

- Simplest clinical test.

- A thorough visual, tactile examination of the hard and soft tissue relies on checking the three 'C's, i.e.

    - Colour
    - Consistency
    - Contour

- In soft tissue such as gingiva, deviation from the healthy pink colour is readily recognized when inflammation is present.

- A change in contour occurs with swelling and the consistency of soft, fluctuant or spongy tissue differs from that of normal, healthy, firm tissue and is indicative of a pathologic condition.

- Similarly teeth should be visually examined using the three 'C's.

- A normal appearing crown has a life like translucency and sparkle that is missing in pulpless teeth.

- Staining may be caused by old amalgam restorations, root canal filling materials and medicaments or systemic medications such as Tetracycline Staining.

- Many discolorations are the result of diseases commonly associated with necrotic, gangrenous pulps, internal or external resorption and carious exposure.

- Crown fractures should be examined because fractures, wear facets and restoration change the crowns contour.

Technique

- One uses ones eyes, fingers, an explorer and the periodontal probe.

- The patient's teeth and periodontium should be examined in good light under dry conditions.

2. PERCUSSION

- This test enables one to evaluate the status of the periodontium surrounding a tooth.

- The tooth is struck a quick, moderate blow initially with low intensity by using the handle of an instrument to determine whether the tooth is tender.

- A sensitive response differing from that of the adjacent teeth, usually indicates the presence of periodontitis.

- Although percussion is a simple method, it may be misleading if used alone.

- To eliminate bias on the part of the patient one must change the sequence of the teeth percussed on successive tests.

- And also one should change the direction of the blow from the vertical occlusal to the buccal or lingual surface of the crown and strike separate cusps in a differing order.

- One must not percuss a sensitive tooth beyond the patient tolerance.

3. PALPATION

- Act of determining by tactile sense which will dictate the consistency of tissues.

- Done with the fingertip, using light pressure to examine tissue consistency and pain response.

- Its value lies in locating the swelling over an involved tooth and determining the following,

    - Whether the tissue is fluctuant and enlarged sufficiently for incision and drainage.

    - The presence, intensity and location of pain.

    - The presence and location of adenopathy.

    - The presence of bone crepitus.

- Diagnostically, when the posterior teeth are infected the submaxillary lymphnodes become involved.

- Infection of the lower anterior teeth may cause swelling of the submental lymphnodes.

- Percussion, palpation, mobility depressibility are tests of the periodontium rather than of the pulp.

4. MOBILITY TEST

- Used to evaluate the integrity of the attachment apparatus surrounding the tooth.

- *Objective:* To determine whether the tooth is firmly or loosely attached to its alveolus.

- The test consists of moving a tooth laterally in its socket by using the fingers or preferably the handles of two instruments.

- The amount of movement is indicative of the condition of the periodontium, the greater the movement the poorer the periodontal condition.

5. DEPRESSABILITY TEST

- It consists of moving a tooth vertically in its socket.

- The test is done with the fingers or with an instrument.

- When depressability exists, the chance for retaining the tooth ranges from poor to hopeless.

- *First Degree Mobility:* A noticeable movement of the tooth.

- *Second Degree Mobility:* Movement of a tooth with in a range of 1mm.

- *Third Degree Mobility:* Movement greater than 1 mm or when the tooth can be depressed.

- Endodontic treatment should not be carried out on teeth with third degree mobility unless mobility is reduced when pressure in the peridontium has been relieved. For Ex: this situation could occur in the case of an acute apical abscess if sufficient drainage was established and pus escaped after the root canal was opened sufficiently enlarged and left patent.

6. RADIOGRAPHY

Uses

- Shows the presence of caries that may involve or may threaten to involve the pulp.

- Number, course, shape, length and width of root conals.

- The presence of calcified material in the pulp chamber or root canal.

- The presence of internal and external root resorption.

- The calcification or obliteration of the pulp cavity.

- The thickening of the periodontal ligament.

- The resorption of cementum.

- The nature and extent of periapical and alveolar bone destruction.

- Thus radiographs provide pertinent information concerning diagnosis, prognosis, case selection, instrumentation, obturation and repair of bone and cementum.

Limitations

1. Pulpal status (Ex: Necrosis) cannot be determined in the radiograph.

2. Radiographic differentiation of different periapical lesions is difficult like periapical granuloma, chronic periapical abscess or cyst; to be accurate, histologic examination is necessary.

3. Lesion in the cancellous structure of bone cannot be detected radiographically until it is penetrated or reached the cortical bone.

4. Periapical radiolucency does not indicate diseased tooth all the time.

5. It cannot give a true picture of bacteriologic or pathologic conditions.

Periapical osteofibrosis cementoma, ossifying fibroma cementoblastoma	→	Lead to misinterpretation, though the pulp is healthy without any disease

7. OCCLUSAL PRESSURE TEST

- Most frequent complaint from the patients is pain on biting or chewing.

- The test which stimulates the pain on biting or chewing is the occlusal pressure test.

– The pain may be due to apical periodontitis, apical abscess and incomplete tooth fractures.

Method

– It can be tested by biting on an orange wood stick, a Burlew rubber disc or a wet cotton roll.

8. PULP VITALITY TESTS

1. Electric pulp testing
2. Thermal testing
   i. Heat testing
   ii. Cold testing
3. Anesthetic testing
4. Test cavity preparation
5. Thermography
6. Transillumination

1. ELECTRIC PULP TESTING

– It is one of the most useful tool in endodontics.

– Pulp testers are designed to elicit response by electrical excitation of neural elements in the pulp.

– They only suggest whether a tooth is *vital-non vital*.

Technique

– Describe the test to the patient in such a way, that will reduce anxiety and will eliminate a biased response.

– Isolate the area of teeth to be tested with cotton rolls and saliva ejector and air dry all the teeth.

– Check the electric pulp tester for function and determine that current is passing through the electrode.

– Apply an electrolyte (tooth paste) on the tooth electrode and place it against the dried enamel of the crowns on the occlusobuccal or incisolabial surface.

– It is important to avoid contacting any restoration in the tooth or the adjacent gingival tissue with the electrolyte or the electrode or else this would cause a false and misleading response.

– Retract the patients cheek away from the tooth electrode with the free hand. When this hand contacts with the patients cheek, it completes the electrical circuit.

– Turn the rheostat slowly to introduce minimal current into the tooth and increase the current slowly. Ask the patient to indicate when sensation occurs

by using such words as tingling or warmth. Record the result according to the numeric scale on the pulp tester.

– Repeat the foregoing for each tooth to be tested.

– *Accuracy depends on,*

1. Accuracy of apparatus.
2. State of mind of the patient whether the patient is apprehensive or relaxed.
3. Individual threshold response.
4. Patient under sedative medication.
5. Recently erupted teeth with incomplete root formation.
6. Recently traumatized teeth.
7. Teeth with extensive restoration and a pulp protecting base.

False Positive Response

1. Conductor / Electrode contact with a large metal restoration (Bridge, class II restoration) or the gingiva.
2. Patient anxiety.
3. Liquefaction necrosis.
4. Inadequate isolation.
5. Multirooted tooth.

False Negative Response

1. Patient premedicated with analgesics, narcotics, alcohol tranquilizers.
2. Inadequate contact of electrode with the enamel.
3. Recently traumatized tooth.
4. Excessive calcification in the canal.
5. Dead batteries or forgetting to turn the pulp tester.
6. Recently erupted tooth with an immature apex.
7. Partial necrosis.
8. Clinician wearing surgical gloves.
9. Presence of pulp protecting materials under restoration.
10. Patient's high pain threshold.

Disadvantages

1. No indication is given of the state of the vascular supply, which would give a more reliable measure of the vitality of the pulp.
2. Readings taken from posterior teeth may be misleading since the chances of presence of some combination of vital and non-vital root canal pulps.
3. Cannot be used on crowned tooth. In such a case we have to prepare a cavity and use the pulp tester.

4. False positive readings may be due to stimulation of nerve fibres in the periodontium.

5. Anxiety can cause false positive response.

6. It may elicit response from the periodontium.

7. False positive response may be seen in liquefaction necrosis of the pulp due to transmission of current from the liquid.

Examples of Electric Pulp Testers

1. Digilog pulp tester (battery operated).

2. Pelton-Crane Compact (Transistorized battery operated electric pulp tester).

3. Battery operated parkell pulp tester.

4. Analytic technology pulp tester.

5. Neotest ADP (Automatic digital pulp tester).

Precaution

– *Electric pulp testers should not be used on patients who have a pacemaker because of the possible electrical interference.*

2. THERMAL TESTING

– *It involves the application of cold and heat to a tooth to determine sensitivity to thermal changes.*

– A response to cold indicates a vital pulp regardless of whether that pulp is normal or abnormal.

– An abnormal response to heat usually indicates the presence of a pulpal or periapical disorder requiring endodontic treatment.

i. Heat Testing

– Usually done by using a hot gutta-percha / hot burnisher / hot air / hot water.

Procedure

– 3.0 mm of the end of a stick of pink gutta-percha is heated in a flame for 2 seconds and is applied to the suspected tooth.

Precautions

– Tooth surface is lightly coated with vaseline to prevent the sticking of gutta-percha.

– First a normal contralateral tooth should be tested and then the affected tooth is tested.

Observation

1. *No response—necrosis, gangrene, chronic abscess.*

2. *Mild to moderate response—normal pulp.*

3. *Painful response which subsides after the removal of stimulus—reversible pulpitis.*

4. *Painful response which continues even after the removal of stimulus—irreversible pulpitis, acute alveolar abscess, acute pulpitis.*

ii. Cold Testing

– It is done by using an air blast, cold drink, ethylene chloride, fluori-methane, sticks of ice, carbon dioxide snow (dry ice).

– Excess cold may cause pulpal damage or crazing lines in the enamel.

– The CO_2 dry ice stick is preferred for testing as it does not affect adjacent teeth.

– When testing with a cold stimulus, one must begin with the most posterior tooth and proceeds towards the anterior teeth because such sequence will prevent melting of ice water from dripping in a posterior direction and possible excitation of non-tested tooth by giving false response.

Observations

1. *No response—Nonvital or false negative.*
   Examples of negative response
   – Calcification of immature opening.
   – Recent trauma to the tooth.
   – Patient is premedicated.

2. *Moderate response—normal pulp.*

3. *Painful response which subsides immediately after the stimulus is removed—reversible pulpitis / hyperemia.*

4. *Painful response which may remain even after removal of stimulus—irreversible pulpitis.*
   – In case of hyperemia, there may be a quick response and in chronic pulpitis, may be a delayed response.

– However, thermal tests are not as accurate as an electric pulp test.

3. ANESTHETIC TESTING

– This test is restricted to patients who are in pain at the time of the test, when the usual tests have failed to enable one to identify the tooth.

Objective

– To anesthetize a single tooth at a time until the pain disappears and is localized to a specific tooth.

Technique

– Using either infiltration or intraligamentary injection, inject the most posterior tooth in the area suspected of being the cause of pain.

– If pain persists when the tooth has been fully anesthetized, anesthetize the next tooth mesial to it and continue to do so until the pain disappears.

– If the source of pain cannot be determined, whether in maxillary or mandibular teeth, an inferior alveolar injection should be given.

– Cessation of pain naturally indicates involvement of a mandibular tooth and localization of the specific tooth is done by the intraligamentary injection when the anesthetic has spent itself.

– This test is a last resort and has an advantage over the *test cavity preparation* during which iatrogenic damage is possible.

4. TEST CAVITY PREPARATION

– It is performed when the other methods of diagnosis are failed.

– The test cavity is made by drilling through the enamel dentin junction of an unanesthetized tooth.

– The drilling should be done at slow speed and without a water coolant.

– Sensitivity or pain felt by the patient is an indication of pulp vitality. If so, no endodontic treatment is indicated. A sedative cement is then placed in the cavity and the search for the source of pain continues.

– If no pain is felt, cavity preparation may be continued until the pulp chamber is reached.

– If the pulp is completely necrotic endodontic treatment can be continued painlessly in many cases without anesthesia.

5. THERMOGRAPHY

– Not widely used.

– It uses crystal to determine the vitality.

– It determines vitality by measuring the temperature of the tooth.

– A non-vital tooth has no blood supply so there is lower surface temperature than a vital tooth.

– But this test is impractical and so not used.

6. TRANSILLUMINATION

– Strong fibre optic light helps to distinguish both vital and necrotic pulp in young patients.

– It will also help in diagnosing vertically fracture crowns when a beam of strong fibre optic light is passed.

– The light does not pass across the fracture line so that the part of the tooth nearest to the light is bright and beyond fracture remains dark.

– Necrosed tooth appear opaque and dark because of breakdown by blood in the pulp chamber.

CHAPTER 05

ENDODONTIC ARMAMENTARIUM

CLASSIFICATION OF ENDODONTIC INSTRUMENTS

I. GROSSMAN'S CLASSIFICATION

– Root canal instruments are divided into 4 types according to their function.

1. Endodontic Explorers (Exploring Instruments)

– To locate the canal orifice.
– To determine or assist in obtaining patency of the root canal.

Ex: 1. Smooth broaches
2. Endodontic explorers

2. Debridement Instruments (Extirpating Instruments)

– To extripate the pulp.
– To remove debris and other foreign material.

Ex: Barbed broach.

3. Root canal shaping Instruments

– To shape the root canal laterally and apically.

Ex: 1. Reamers
2. Gates-Glidden drill
3. Files

4. Obturating Instruments

– To cement and pack gutta-percha into the root canal.

Examples

1. Pluggers (flat end-for vertical condensation)
2. Spreaders (pointed end-lateral condensation).
3. Lentulospirals (to deliver sealer or paste to the root canal).

II. I.S.O. AND FDI CLASSIFICATION

1. Group I : Hand Use Only

– Hand operated instruments such as barbed and smooth broaches, reamers, K,H, and R files, plugger, spreaders, etc.

2. Group II : Engine Driven Instruments

– Same instruments as described above. But the handles of these instruments have been replaced by latch type adapter for insertion into low speed handpieces.
– These instruments consist of two parts.

1. An operative cutting head
2. Latch type of attachment

3. Group III : Engine driven latch type-drills

– Similar to Group II these instruments have latch attachment but are fabricated from a single piece of metal. So latch, shaft and cutting head are made of a single piece. Ex: Gates glidden drill, Peeso reamer.

4. Group IV : Root canal points

   – They are usually the materials used. Ex: Gutta-percha points, Absorbable points.

STANDARDIZATION OF ENDODONTIC INSTRUMENTS

– Earlier, root canal instruments were manufactured according to the manufacturer's wish with no definite specifications regarding length, diameter, shape and length of the cutting instrument.

– *Ingle and Levine* using a electrode microcomparator found variations in diameter and taper for the same sizes of instruments and later suggested some recommendations to maintain uniformity.

Ingle and Levine Recommendations   (Fig. 5.1)

1. *Instruments shall be numbered from 10 to 100–150. The numbers advance by 5 units, to size 60 and then by 10 units to size 100.*

2. *Each number shall be representative of the diameter of the instrument in hundredths of a millimeter at the tip.*

   Ex: No: 10 is 10/100 or 0.1 mm at the tip

   No: 25 is 25/100 or 0.25 mm at the tip

   No: 90 is 90/100 or 0.9 mm at the tip

3. *The working blade (flutes) shall begin at the tip, designated site D_1 and shall extend exactly 16 mm up the shaft, terminating at designated site D_2. The diameter of D_2 shall be 32/100 or 0.32 mm greater than of D_1.*

   Ex: A no: 20 reamer shall have a diameter of 0.20 mm at D_1 and a diameter of 0.20 plus 0.32 or 0.52 at D_2.

   This sizing ensures a constant increase in taper of 0.02 mm per mm for every instrument regardless of size.

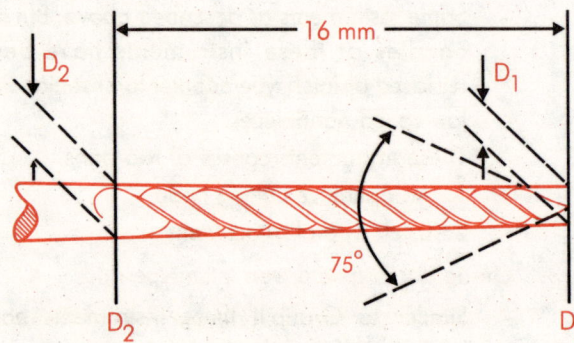

Fig. 5.1

D_1 *diameter at the tip,*

D_2 *diameter at the tip end of the cutting blade,*

The tip angle of the instrument should be 75 ± 5°.

Other Specifications (were added later)

1. *The tip angle of an instrument should be 75 ± 15°.*

2. *Instrument sizes should increase by 0.05 mm at D_1 between numbers: 10 and 60. Ex: Numbers: 10,15 and 20. They should increase by 0.1 mm from Numbers: 60 to 150. Ex: Numbers 60, 70 and 80.*

3. *06 and 08 have been added for increased instrument selection.*

4. *In addition, instrument handles have been colour coded for easier recognition.*

– Stainless steel root canal instruments are used more often today than carbon steel instruments because of heir more flexibility, less likely to fracture, less susceptible to corrosion.

– The finer sizes of reamers and files have low resistance to torque (pressure used to rotate instrument for cutting and shaping) and break using less force than larger instruments when they bind in a root canal.

– As a result small instruments are manufactured from square blanks, which are more resistant to torque, fractures, and large instruments are manufactured from triangular blanks, to improve their cutting efficiency.

– Instruments are available in lengths of 21, 25, 28 and 30 mm.

– Ordinarily, instruments of 25 mm long are used, but occasionally 21mm instruments are needed for molars especially when the patient cannot open the mouth wide and 28 and 30 mm instruments are necessary for cuspids and other teeth in which a 25 mm instrument cannot reach the apical foramen.

– Reamers are also available in 40 mm lengths for use in preparing root canals for endodontic treatment.

Colour Coding of Handles of Instruments

6	– Pink	30	– Blue
8	– Grey	35	– Green
10	– Purple	40	– Black
15	– White	45	– White
20	– Yellow	50	– Yellow
25	– Red		
		150	

EXPLORING INSTRUMENTS

1. ENDODONTIC EXPLORER

- A double ended instrument with long tapered tines at either a right or an obtuse angle. This design facilitates the location of canal orifice (Fig. 5.2).
- These instruments are very stiff and should not be inserted into canals or used for condensing guttapercha.
- Explorers should never be heated.

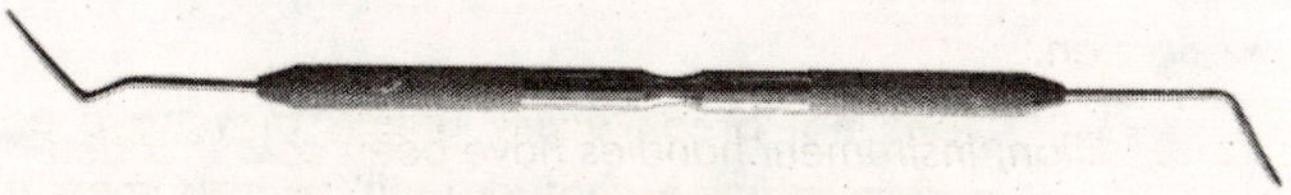

Fig. 5.2

EXTRIPATING INSTRUMENTS

1. BARBED BROAC   H (Fig. 5.3 A and B)

Uses

- To extripate the pulp.
- To remove debris and other foreign material, absorbent points, cotton pellets, etc.

Manufacture

- It is manufactured from a tapered, round, soft iron wire in which angle cuts are made into the surface to produce barbs.

Available as

- A variety of sizes from *triple extra fine to extra coarse*.
- Barbs are used to engage the pulp as the broach is carefully rotated within the canal until it begins to meet resistance against the walls of the canal.
- Barbed broaches break easily especially if they bind in the root canal hence root canal should be enlarged before insertion of the broach.

Selection

- By comparing the size of the broach with the size of the last instrument used in the root canal or an estimated size of the image in a radiograph. One should select a barbed broaches that fits loosely into the apical third of the root canal.
- A barbed broach that is too wide does not permit removal of all the pulp tissue or it may force the pulp apically as the broach is inserted in the canal.

Technique

- The root canal is irrigated with a 5.2% solution of sodium hypochlorite and the barbed broach is introduced until one notes unforced contact with root canal walls.
- The broach is withdrawn about 1 mm and is rotated 360° to engage the pulp tissue and it is withdrawn again to remove this tissue.
- When the root canal is unusually wide as in young teeth even a coarse barbed broach may not be able to engage and remove the massive pulp tissue.
- In such cases, two fine barbed broaches are inserted into the canal and are rotated at the same time until the pulp tissue is engaged and removed.

Sterilization

- A barbed broach can be cleaned by scrubbing with a bur brush.
- To clean a broach which has tissue tags or necrotic debris, place it in a 5.2% sodium hypochlorite solution for half an hour and then broach is rinsed in running water, air dried and is sterilized in dry heat.

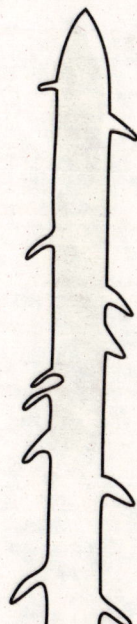

Fig. 5.3 A

Fig. 5.3 B

2. RASPS or R-Type Files

- This is similar in design to barbed broach, but have shallower and more rounded barbs.

– Used to enlarge the root canal but usually produce rough wall of the root canal. So it is not preferred often.

INSTRUMENTS FOR CLEANING AND SHAPING OF ROOT CANALS

I. REAMERS (Fig. 5.4)

1. **Physical Characteristics**

   – Manufactured from stainless steel triangular blank.

   – Has less number of flutes.

   – Do not break easily unless they have an undetected steel shaft or until the instrument is strained or deformed.

   – Flutes are loosely twisted.

2. **Functional Characteristics**

   – Used with a rotating-pushing motion limited to a quarter-to a half turn to engage their blades into the dentin and withdrawn—penetration, rotation and retraction.

   – The cut is made during retraction.

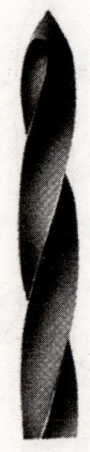

Fig. 5.4

II. **FILES**

1. **K-file (Kerr manufacturing company)**

   – Has got the name from its manufacturing company (Fig. 5.5).

   – Manufactured from stainless steel square blank.

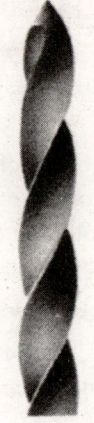

Fig. 5.5

   – Does not break easily unless they have an undetected steel shaft or until the instrument is strained or deformed.

   – Flutes are tightly twisted.

   – K-files can be used as `PATHFINDER' (to locate the root canal orifices)

2. **K-Flex Files**

   – Manufactured from rhomboidal or diamond shaped blanks.

   – Designed for more flexibility and cutting efficiency.

   – Has alternating high and low flutes for more efficiency.

3. **Hedstroem Files (H-Files)** (Fig. 5.6)

   – Manufactured from a round stainless steel wire machined to produce spiral flutes resembling cones or as crew or christmas tree appearance.

   – When placed in contact with the root canal wall the cutting edges contact the wall at angles approaching 90 degrees and when the instrument is withdrawn exert an effective honoring action. Cut in one direction only retraction.

   – Used in wide opened canals (Blunder bluss canals).

   – Used to flare the canal from the apical region to the occusal or incisal orifice.

   – Fragile and fractures easily.

   – Higher cutting efficiency than K-Instruments.

   – Also used to engage and remove retained instruments, gutta-percha and silver points.

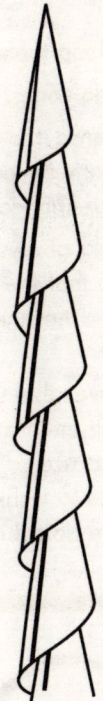

Fig. 5.6

4. Uni Files (Modification of H-File)

- Manufactured from round stainless steel wire by cutting two superficial grooves to produce flutes in a double helix design.
- Resemble H-file in appearance.
- Less subject to fracture.
- Less efficient.

5. S-File (Modification of H-File)

- Manufactured from a solid piece of stainless steel wire that produces a sharp cutting edge.
- Has a double cutting edge.
- Similar to unifile except that the angles of the flutes remain uniform where as pitch and depth of the flutes increases from the tip to the handle.
- Stiffer than H-files.
- Has 90° cutting tip.
- Can be used for straight or curved canals.
- Used either as a reamer or file.

6. Flexofile

- Manufactured by Dentsply maillefer.
- Manufactured in the same way as the K-file but using a more flexible stainless steel alloy.
- It has more flutes than K-file.
- It has a non-cutting (Batt) tip and a triangular cross-section so the cutting flutes are sharper and there is more scope for debris removal.

Advantages

1. More cutting efficiency
2. Resistance to fracture

7. Niti Files (Nitinol Files)

- The name Nitinol was derived from the elements that make up the alloy, i.e. Nickel and Titanium and 'nol' for the Naval ordinance Laboratory (who manufactured it for the first time).
- Nitinol instruments should be used with a rotational or reaming motion and are effective in the shaping of root canals.

Advantages

1. More flexible
2. Better conformation to canal curvature
3. Resistance to fracture
4. Less wear
5. Super elasticity
6. Enhanced canal negotiation
7. Faster instrumentation
8. No need to pre curve

8. GT (Greater Taper) hand files

- Were designed by Buchanan.
- Are made from Ni-Ti.
- The set of four hand files of varying tapers, 0.12–0.16, all have a tip size of ISO 20.
- They have pear-shaped handles and each file is designed for different areas and types of canals. For example, 0.12 GT file is suited to canal orifices of relatively straight canals of large apical diameter, 0.06 GT file is suited to the apical third in a thin or curved canal.
- Used in a sequence of counter clockwise and clockwise rotations.
- They are intended to allow the creation of a predetermined funnel-shaped canal with fewer instruments than using the ISO series.

9. Series 29 Files

- In accordance with ISO specifications for traditional hand instruments sizes, the percentage difference between tip diameters of sizes 10–15 is 50%, whilst between sizes 55 and 60 is 9%. This variable percentage changes are leading for procedural errors such as ledging, difficulty in negotiating narrow and curved canals.

– These instruments are based on a constant percentage change of diameter at *D*, instead of the variable linear dimensional changes.

– These are made with a constant 29% increase in tip diameter between successive sizes.

Functional Characteristics of Files

– Inserted into the root canal to the apex laterally pressed against one side of the canal wall and withdrawn with a pulling motion or respiring motion.

– The cutting action of the file can be effected in either a filing (rasping) or reaming (drilling).

COMPARISION BETWEEN REAMERS AND FILES

	Reamers		Files
1.	Made of stainless steel.	1.	Made of stainless steel.
2.	Used with push motion and rotation quarter to half turn.	2.	Used with pull or rasping motion.
3.	Has less number of flutes.	3.	Has more number of flutes.
4.	Flutes are loosely twisted.	4.	Flutes are tightly twisted.
5.	Manufactured from triangular blanks.	5.	Manufactured from square blanks.

OBTURATING INSTRUMENTS

1. PLUGGERS (Condenser) (Fig. 5.7)

– Have smooth and flat apical tips.

– These are used for condensation of gutta-percha during obturation.

– Used primarily for vertical condensation.

Selection of pluggers

– 3 or 4 pluggers to be used in the coronal, middle and apical thirds of the canal must be persecuted to ensure their lose fit.

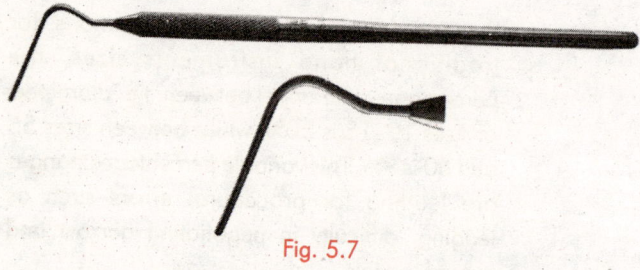

Fig. 5.7

2. SPREADERS (Fig. 5.8)

– Spreaders are long tapered pointed instruments.

– Available in wide variety of lengths and taper.

– Used to condense the filling material laterally against the canal walls creating space for insertion of additional auxiliary cones.

– Spreaders should always be fit into the an empty canal to ensure that the force is absorbed by the gutta-percha and not the canal walls selection of spreaders.

– Spreaders are available that have been numbered to match the instrument size. Spreader of the same apical instrument size or one size larger is chosen so that it reaches to within 1.0 to 2.0 mm but will not penetrate the apical orifice.

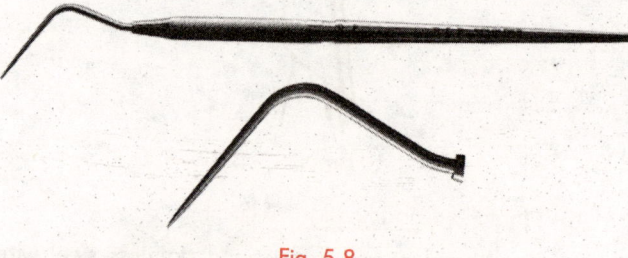

Fig. 5.8

3. LENTULO SPIRALS (Fig. 5.9)

– Used for coating sealer on root canal walls.

– Used in clockwise rotary motion.

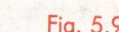

Fig. 5.9

MOTIONS OF INSTRUMENTATION

– These are also referred to as *envelops of motion*.

– They are useful for generating or controlling the cutting activity of an endodontic file.

– The motions are,

1. Filing
2. Reaming
3. Turn and Pull
4. Watch - Winding
5. Watch - Winding and Pull
6. Balanced force instrumentation

1. Filing (Fig. 5.10)

– *It indicates a push-pull action with the instrument.*

– Filing is an effective technique with hedstroem type instruments since they do not engage during the insertion and cut efficiently during the withdrawal motion. The *disadvantage* is that it can cause stripping of the canals.

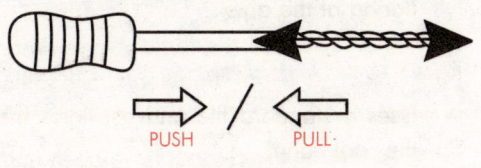

PUSH / PULL

Fig. 5.10

2. Reaming (Fig. 5.11)

– *It indicates clockwise or right-hand rotation of an instrument.*

– The instrument must be restrained from insertion to generate a cutting effect.

– *Disadvantage* of this motion is increased instrument fracture.

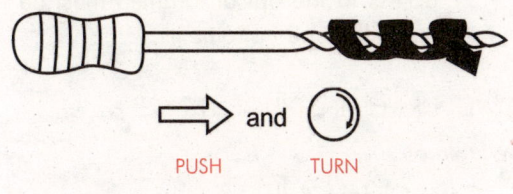

PUSH and TURN

Fig. 5.11

3. Turn and Pull (Fig. 5.12)

– *It is a combination of reaming and filing.*

– The file is inserted with a quarter turn clockwise and inwardly directed hand presure (i.e. reaming) positioned into the canal. By this action the file is subsequently withdrawn (i.e. filing).

– It is an effective motion where the instrument is not forcefully pushed towards the apex and the preparation depths are allowed to diminish with each subsequent instrument.

– *Disadvantages* are, the process is tedious and time consuming.

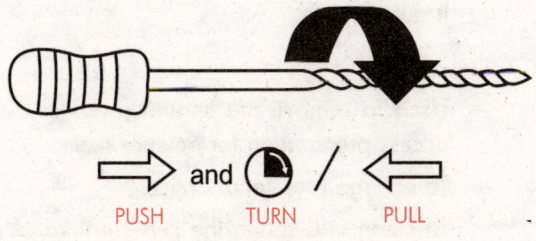

PUSH and TURN / PULL

Fig. 5.12

4. Watch-Winding (Fig. 5.13)

– It is the back and forth oscillation of a file (30 to 60) right and (30 to 60) left as the instrument is pushed forward into the canal.

– The back and forth movement of k-type files and reamers causes them to plane dentinal walls efficiently.

– This motion is very useful during shaping.

Advantages

1. Less aggressive than turn and pull motion.

2. Reduced apical ledge formation.

3. It is effective with all k-type files.

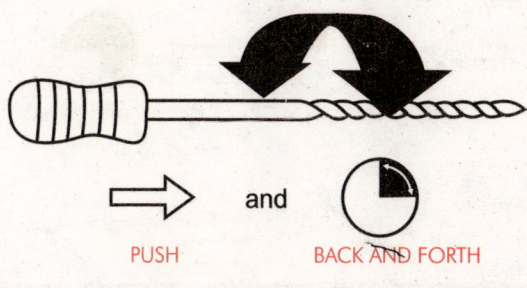

PUSH and BACK AND FORTH

Fig. 5.13

5. Watch-Winding and Pull (Fig. 5.14)

– It is used primarily with Hedstroem files.

– An inward pressure is mentioned while the file is gently rocked right and left, when that insertion stops, all rotation is ceased and the instrument is withdrawn from the canal.

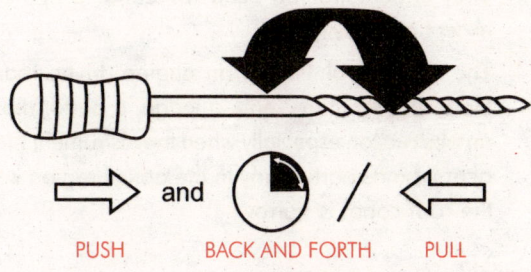

PUSH and BACK AND FORTH / PULL

Fig. 5.14

6. Balanced force instrumentation (Fig. 5.15)

– It is the most efficient way to cut dentin.

– It is specifically designed to operate k-type endodontic instruments and should not be used with Broach type or Hedstroem type instruments, since either possesses left hand cutting capacity.

– It is introduced by *Roane et al* in 1985.

– *He described the technique as "positioning and pre-loading an instrument through a clockwise rotation and then shaping the canal with a counter clockwise rotation".*

– The technique is, the file is pushed inwardly and rotated one quarter-turn clockwise. It is then rotated more that one half-turn counter clockwise. These alternate motions are repeated until the file reaches working length.

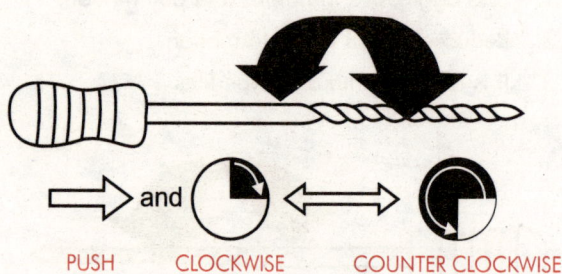

PUSH **and** CLOCKWISE ⟷ COUNTER CLOCKWISE

Fig. 5.15

MECHANICAL INSTRUMENTATION

1. Engine Driven Instruments.
2. Power Driven Instruments.
3. Ultrasonic and sonic Instruments.

1. ENGINE DRIVEN INSTRUMENTS

– Can be used for opening root canals.
– They should not be used for canal preparation except as a last resort.
– The rapid revolution of an engine driven reamer, file or broach can create a ledge, a perforation or an obstruction especially when the instrument breaks after it binds particularly in the apical region where the root canal is narrow.

Available as

– Two engine driven cont a angle handpieces namely,
   1. Giromatic
   2. Racer

1. Giromatic

– Activates a stainless steel barbed broach or reamer in the root canal through a 900 reciprocating arc at a speed up to 1000 cycles/min.

Disadvantages

– It may pack the dentinal shavings in the canal.
– Less effective for preparing root canals.
– Longer time is needed for preparation.
– Had a tendency to create ledges and to produce flaring at the apex.

2. Racer

– Uses a standard file and oscillates the file in the root canal.
– The instruments length can be adjusted to the working length using this contra angle.

Disadvantages

– Debris may be forced ahead of the instrument with resulting clogging of the canal or pushing of debris into periapical tissue.

Precaution

– When engine driven instruments are used, access to the apical foramen must be made first with hand instruments.

2. POWER DRIVEN INSTRUMENTS

Available as

1. Gates Glidden drills
2. Peeso reamers

1. Gates Glidden Drill

– *Has a long thin shaft ending in a flame shaped head with a safe tip to guard against perforations.*
– The flame head cuts laterally and is used with gentle, apically directed pressure.
– The long shaft is designed to break at the neck, i.e. narrowest diameter that lies adjacent to the handpiece.
– If the drill binds during use, it will fracture at the neck of the shaft and extrude from the tooth.
– The fractured segment is easily removed by grasping the broken shaft with pliers and pulling it out of tooth.

Uses

– Used to remove the lingual shoulder during access preparation for anterior teeth.
– To enlarge root canal orifices.
– To clean and shape the cervical third of root canals in the step back preparation.

2. **Peeso Reamer**

   – Has long, sharp flutes connected to a thick shaft.

   – It cuts laterally and is primarily used for the preparation of post space when gutta-percha has been removed from the obturated root canal.

   Precaution

   – Both gates glidden and peeso reamers are made of hardened carbon steel that corrodes easily.

   – These aggressive cutting instruments are inflexible and should be used with slow speed and with extreme caution to prevent overinstrumentation and perforations.

3. **ULTRASONIC AND SONIC INSTRUMENTS**

   – Have been developed for cleaning and shaping root canals.

   – Ultrasonic instrument consists of a piezoelectric ceramic unit that generates ultrasonic waves which activate a magneto strictive stack hand piece.

   – The handpiece holds a k-file or a specially designed diamond file that when activated produces movements of the shaft of the file between 0.01 and 0.004 at a frequency of 20000 to 25000/sec.

   – The oscillating movements produces cutting action of the file and creates a ultrasonic wave of sodium hypochlorite irrigant solution, which is delivered along the side of the file into the root canal.

   – Before ultrasonic instrumentation the apical third of the root canal should be hand instrumented to at least the size of a no: 15 file.

   – In curved root canals, a precurved no: 15, endosonic file is introduced into the canal to working length (1mm short of the apical foramen) and is activated.

   – After activation, the file is moved in a circumferential manner with a smooth push-pull stroke along the walls of the canal for a period of 1 min.

   – The procedure is repeated with no: 20 and 25 files.

   – The ultrasonic file should be inserted into the root canal to the working length before activation to prevent ledge formation.

   – The apical third of the canal should be filed cautiously to prevent transportation of the apical root canal and foramen.

Sonic Hand Pieces

   – Sonic hand pieces operate at 1500 to 6500 cycles/min when filing inside root canals.

   – They are similar in shape and weight to dental handpieces and are attached to existing air and water lines.

   – These instruments are used in a manner similar to the ultrasonic system in instrumentation of the root canals.

   – The only difference is that the sonic system uses water as an irrigant and does not usually require diamond files for the flare of the preparation.

MISCELLANEOUS

1. **ENDODONTIC IRRIGATING SYRINGE** (Fig. 5.16)

   – Used to carry and dispense irrigating solution into canal for cleansing during debridement of canal.

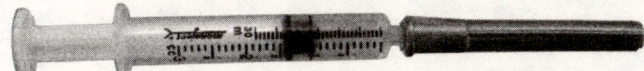

Fig. 5.16

2. **STERILE ABSORBENT PAPER POINTS** (Fig. 5.17)

   – Used to dry pulp chambers of canal.

   – Size of the point corresponds to width of the canal.

   – Sizes are available from extra fine to extra coarse.

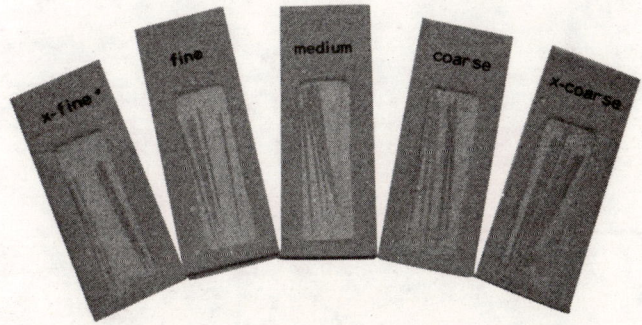

Fig. 5.17

3. **ENDODONTIC STOPPERS** (Fig. 5.18)

   – Used to place on file or reamer to help in determining the length of the canal.

   – Files or reamers are measured from stopper to apex of root to determine the length of the canal.

   – Stoppers are colour coded to correspond to a particular file or reamer or a single a colour of stopper is used for all files or reamers.

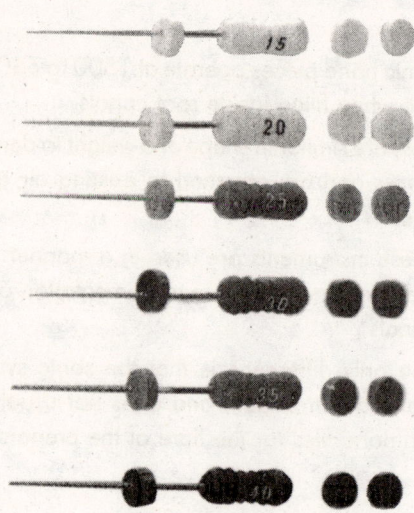

Fig. 5.18

SOTOKAWA'S CLASSIFICATION OF INSTRUMENT DAMAGE

– Sotokawa classified the types of damage to instruments as,

1.	Type I	:	Bent instrument.
2.	Type II	:	Stretching or straightening of twist contour.
3.	Type III	:	Peeling-off metal at blade edges.
4.	Type IV	:	Partial clockwise twist.
5.	Type V	:	Cracking along axis.
6.	Type VI	:	Full fracture.

– He found that no. 10 file is the most frequently damaged instrument.

– He described the progression of breakage as "first a starting point crack develops on the file's edge and then metal fatigue fans out from that point, spreading towards the file's axial center".

CHAPTER 06

RATIONALE OF ENDODONTIC TREATMENT

According to Grossman

- Any injury to the pulp (due to caries trauma chemicals) can produce many changes.
- Microorganisms in the root canal multiply sufficiently to grow out of root canal or the toxins produced by root canal flora may diffuse into periradicular area.
- As the microorganisms are virulent, the host defence decreases and they destroy PMN leukocytes and leads to chronic abscess.
- The proteolytic enzymes released by the dead PMN leukocytes produce pus.
- Following changes occur due to noxious stimuli from the diseased dental pulp,
  - Periapical infection causing lesion peripical radiolucency at the apex.
  - Cellular changes like infiltration of lymphocytes, macrophages, PMN lymphocytes, phagocytes, osteoclasts, fibroblasts which causes so many changes.
  - These changes in periradicular area due to the diffusion of toxins from root canal flora are experimentally demonstrated by FISH.
- Hence, it is necessary to go for endodontic treatment to remove the toxins in the root canal and which leads to healing, repair and establishment of tooth function and saving the tooth.

FISH ZONES

- Fish established experimental foci of infection in the jaws of guinea pigs by drilling openings in the bone and packing in wool fibres saturated with a broth culture of microorganisms.
- He found 4 well defined zones of reaction.
- They are,
  1. Zone of infection
  2. Zone of contamination
  3. Zone of irritation
  4. Zone of stimulation

1. Zone of Infection

- *Characterized by PMN Leukocytes.*
- Infection is present in the centre of the lesion.

2. Zone of Contamination

- *Characterized by Round Cell Infiltration.*
- Around the central zone, fish observed cellular destruction not from bacteria themselves but also from toxins discharged from the central zone.

– Empty lacunae are appeared as the bone cells had died and had undergone autolysis.

– Lymphocytes were prevalent.

3. Zone of Irritation

– *Characterized by macrophages and osteoclasts.*

– Fish found evidence of irritation further from the central lesion as the toxins became more diluted.

– The collagen framework is digested by phagocytic cells and the macrophages while the osteoclasts destroy the bone tissue.

– Some amount of repair has seen histopathologically.

4. Zone of stimulation

– *Characterized by Fibroblasts and Osteoblasts.*

– At the periphery the toxin was mild enough to be a stimulant.

– In response to this stimulation collagen fibres were laid down by the fibroblasts, which acted both as a wall of defense around the zone of irritation and as a scaffolding on which the osteoblasts built new bone.

– The new bone is built in a irregular fashion.

According to Cohen,

– The rationale of endodontic treatment is based on simple biologic principles (Fig. 6.1).

– Because the pulp is surrounded by dentin it can not benefit fully from the body's natural inflammatory response.

– First, the microcirculatory system of the pulp lacks a significant collateral circulation, second the pulp consists of a relatively large volume of tissue for a relatively small blood supply. And finally, the pulp of the root canal system is locked into the unyielding walls of surrounding dentin.

– Because of caries, restorative producers or trauma, a vascular pulp may degenerate into a vascular necrosis.

– The necrotic material then seeps out of the portals of exit (POE) of the root canal and into the supporting vascular attachment apparatus, generating lesions of endodontic origin (LEO).

– If the root canal system is sealed permanently in three dimensions, then the resolution can be expected.

– Longevity of a tooth is not based on the pulp, but on the healthy attachment apparatus.

– Therefore, treatment must be based on the effectiveness of cleaning shaping and packing the root canal with a permanent, biologically inert root canal filling.

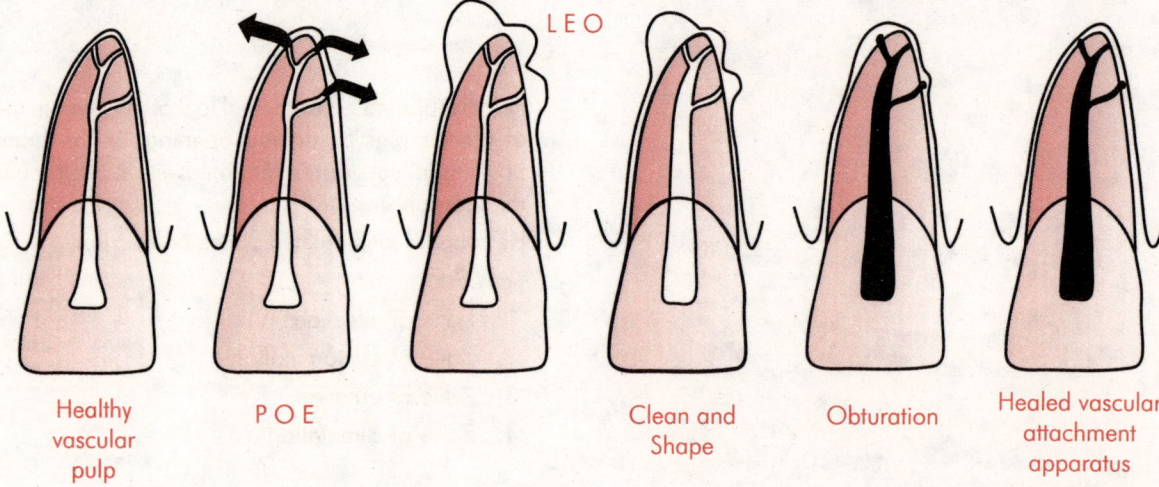

LEO

Healthy vascular pulp   P O E   Clean and Shape   Obturation   Healed vascular attachment apparatus

Fig. 6.1

CHAPTER 07

RCT AN OVERVIEW

– Once upon a time, if you had a tooth with a diseased nerve, you'd probably lose that tooth. Today with a special dental procedure called Root Canal Therapy you may save that tooth. Inside each tooth is the pulp which provides nutrients and nerves to the tooth, it runs like a thread down through the root. When the pulp is diseased or injured, the pulp tissue dies. If you don not remove it, your tooth gets infected and you could lose it. After the dentist removes the pulp the root canal is cleaned and sealed off to protect it. Then your dentist places a crown over the tooth to help make it stronger.

– Most of the time a root canal treatment is a relatively simple procedure with little or no discomfort, involving one to three visits.

– Best of all, it can save your tooth and your smile !

– The procedure for RCT is described below in brief.

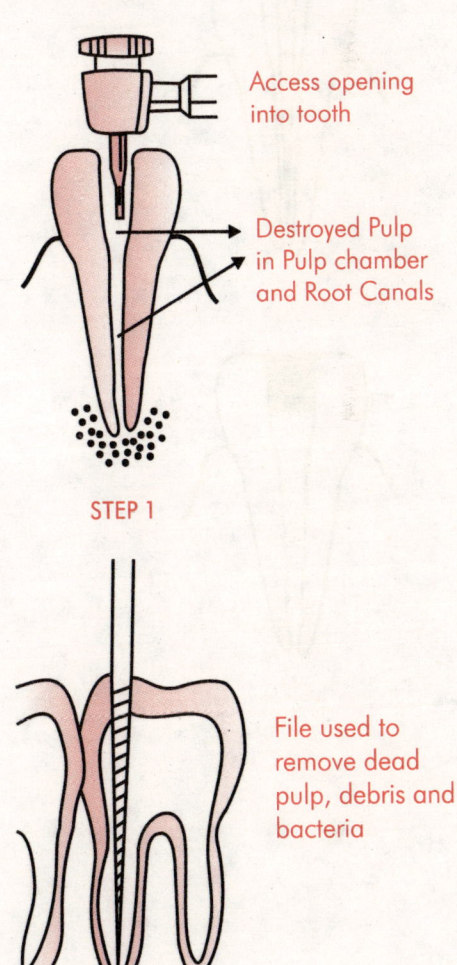

Access opening into tooth

Destroyed Pulp in Pulp chamber and Root Canals

STEP 1

File used to remove dead pulp, debris and bacteria

STEP 2

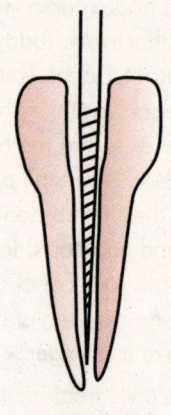

Examine by radiographs to ensure the instruments go exactly to the end of the root and not beyond root

STEP 3

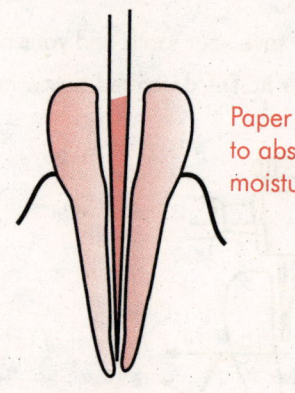

Paper point to absorb moisture

STEP 4

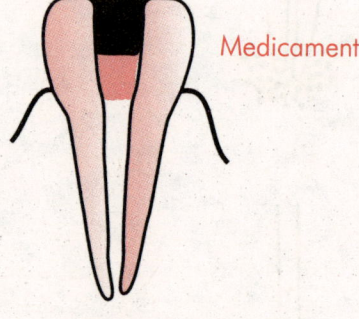

Medicament

STEP 5

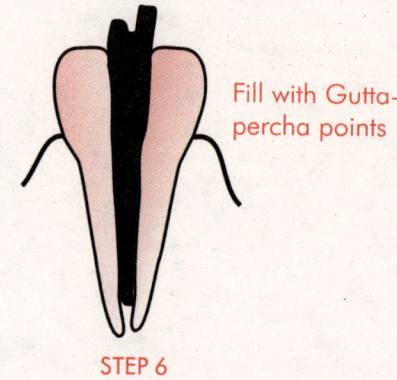

Fill with Gutta-percha points

STEP 6

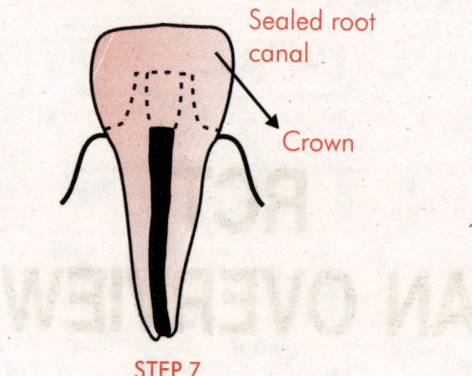

Sealed root canal

Crown

STEP 7

CHAPTER 08

PRINCIPLES OF ENDODONTIC CAVITY PREPARATION

– Here also Black's basic principles of cavity preparation are applied.

I. Endodontic coronal cavity preparation

1. Outline form
2. Convenience form
3. Removal of the remaining carious dentin
4. Toilet of the cavity

II. Endodontic radicular cavity preparation

1. Outline form
2. Convenience form
3. Toilet of the cavity
4. Retention form
5. Resistance form

A. CORONAL CAVITY PREPARATION

1. Outline form

– The outline form of the endodontic cavity must be correctly shaped and positioned to establish complete access for instrumentation from cavity margin to apical foramen.
– Access is obtained by drilling into the space and working the bur from within inside to the outside maintaining the circumferential contact all over.
– Dentinal wall overlying the pulp chamber should be removed.

Factors affecting outline form

i. *Size of pulp chamber*

– In young patients more extensive preparation is required than older patients where the pulp chamber has receded and it is small in all the three dimensions.
– A small orifice in the crown will not allow proper sized instruments and filling materials to pass through them.
– The access cavity preparation should be wider than the root canal.

ii. *Shape of the pulp chamber*

– It varies from tooth to tooth.

Anterior teeth

– The access preparation should diverge from the orifice towards the external surface of the tooth (Fig. 8.1).

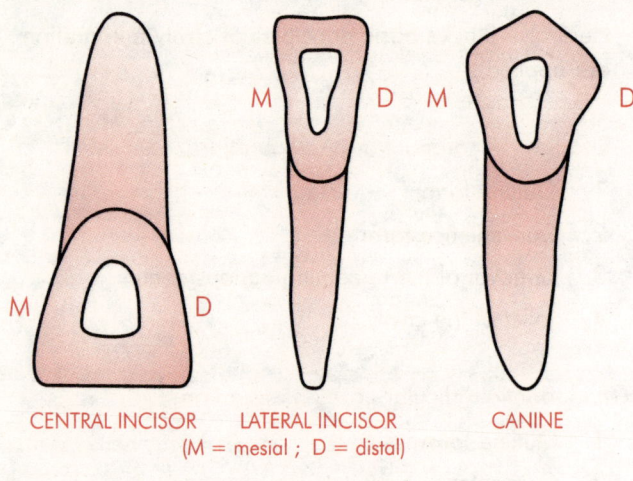

CENTRAL INCISOR   LATERAL INCISOR   CANINE
(M = mesial ; D = distal)

Fig. 8.1

Upper and lower premolars (Fig. 8.2)

– The access preparation should be oval shaped.

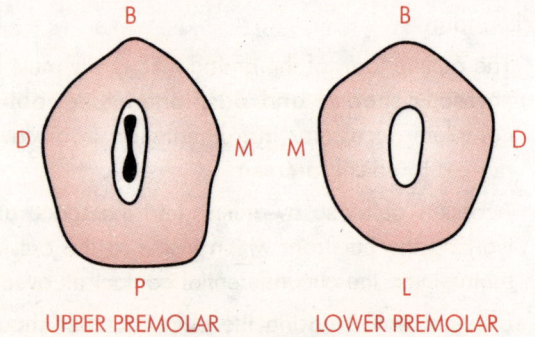

UPPER PREMOLAR   LOWER PREMOLAR

(M = mesial ; D = distal ; P = palatal ; B = buccal; L = Lingual)

Fig. 8.2

Maxillary molars (Fig. 8.3)

– Normally triangular in shape.

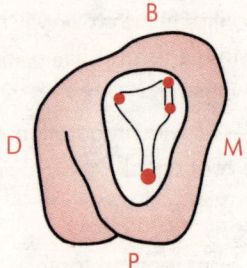

Fig. 8.3

Mandibular molars (Fig. 8.4)

– Normally square shaped.

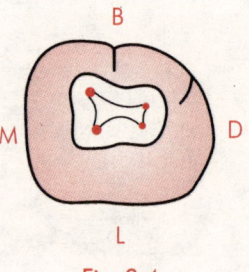

Fig. 8.4

iii. Number and curvature of root canals

– In order to instrument each canal efficiently without interference cavity walls have to be extended to allow the instruments to approach the apical foramen.

– When cavity walls are extended to improve instrumentation, the outline form is materially affected.

2. Convenience form

– Refers to convenient preparation and obturation of root canal.

– *Benefits of proper convenience form are:*

1. Unobstructed access to canal orifices.

2. Direct access to the apical foramen.

3. Cavity expansion to accommodate the filling material.

4. Complete authority over enlarging instruments.

– Luebke has made the important point that an entire wall need not be extended in the event that instrument impingement occurs owing to a severely curved root or an extracanal.

– In extending only that portion of the wall needed to free this instrument, a cloverleaf appearance may evolve as the outline form. Hence, Luebke has termed this a *Shamrock Preparation*.

3. Removal of remaining carious dentin and defective restorations

– Caries and defective restorations remaining in an endodontic cavity preparation must be removed for three reasons:

– To eliminate mechanically as many bacteria as possible from the interior of the tooth.

– To eliminate the discolored tooth structure, that may ultimately lead to staining of the crown.

– To eliminate the possibility of any bacteria laden saliva leaking into the prepared cavity.

4. Toilet of the Cavity

- After the removal of most of the debris any remaining necrotic debris should be flushed out during the toilet of the cavity.

- If the debris is carried out the root canal it may increase the bacterial population of the canal.

- Irrigation is done with sodium hypochlorite solution or hydrogen peroxide.

- The pulp chamber is dried with cotton rolls and use of air to dry the canal should be avoided.

- Even if air is used it should not be directed against the apex.

- If blasts of air escape from the apex, it may cause `emphysema'.

Objectives / Advantages of Ideal Access Cavity Preparation

1. Permits complete debridement of the pulp chamber.

2. Permits visualisation of its floor.

3. Permits unimpeded placement of instruments into the root canals (straight line access).

4. Permits conservation of tooth structure.

- An axiom of canal preparation is the instruments should physically contact and plane the walls in order to loosen the tissue and debris for removal.

B. RADICULAR PREPARATION

1. Retention form

- Obtained in the apical third where 3—5 mm of walls are parallel to ensure firm seating of the primary cone or one should get a 'tugback' or resistance when the primary cone is inserted and with drawn. This is known as preparation of APICAL COLLAR.

2. Resistance form

- Obtained by maintaining natural apical constriction which is that key to successful therapy. It prevents the over extension of the filling material following condensation.

Objectives

- Debridement of the root canal.

- Shaping of the root canal to receive a filling.

CHAPTER 09

ROOT CANAL IRRIGANTS

– Irrigant is a liquid used to lubricate the canal walls and flushout the debris and microorganisms from the root canals.

ADVANTAGES

1. Rinses out the debris.
2. Lubricant facilitates instrumentation.
3. Dissolution of organic matter.
4. Smear layer removal.
5. Penetrates into inaccessible areas to instruments-extending the cleaning process.
6. Antibacterial properties.

IDEAL PROPERTIES

– It should,
   1. Be a tissue or debris solvent.
   2. Be able to dissolve or disrupt soft tissue, hard tissue remnants.
   3. Be nonreactive to periapical tissues.
   4. Be a good lubricant.
   5. Act as disinfectant.
   6. Remove smear layer.
   7. Have low surface tension, i.e. promotes its flow into inaccessible areas.

IRRIGATING SOLUTIONS

1. Stream of hot water (140–170° F).
2. Physiologic saline
3. 30% solution of urea
4. Urea peroxide solution in glycerin
5. Sodium hypochlorite 5.2%
6. Hydrogen peroxide
7. Anesthetic solution
8. Solution of chloramines
9. Chlorhexidine gluconate (0.2%)
– Among these most commonly used are,
   – Sodium hypochlorite 5.2%
   – Hydrogen peroxide

In case of Acute Abscess

– Hydrogen peroxide is contraindicated.
– Distilled water or physiologic saline is used.
– *The most popular and most advocated irrigant is sodium hypochlorite in various concentrations.*

– Alternate irrigation of sodium hypochlorite and H_2O_2 (3%) helps in producing Effervescence.

– Interaction produces transient but energetic effervescence that mechanically forces the debris and microorganisms out of the canal.

SODIUM HYPOCHLORITE (5.2%)

– Most widely used root canal irrigant.

– It is a reducing agent.

– *It contains 5% available chlorine.*

– It is less effective in narrow root canals than in wide root canals.

Mechanism of action

– The effervescent reaction of sodium hypochlorite pushes debris out of the root canal through the least resistant orifice.

– It has both antimicrobial and tissue solvent properties.

– It destroys the bacteria by two phases,
  1. Penetration into the bacterial cell.
  2. Chemical combination with the protoplasm of the bacterial cell that destroys it.

Disadvantages

– Potential toxicity causes tissue damage so all round isolation of tissues with a rubber dam is necessary.

Prevention of procedural errors with NaOCl

1. Avoid the forceful injection.
2. Using of specially designed side - venting needles.
3. Careful use in the presence of resorbed or open apices and perforation areas.

COMBINATION SOLUTIONS

1. EDTA (Ethylene Diamine Tetraacetic Acid)

– EDTA is used in conjunction with sodium hypochlorite.

– It is a chelating agent.

– EDTA removes the smear layer of dentin.

– In some instances reactions of the pulp to inflammation causes calcification and blockage of the root canal orifice. The blockage orifice can be opened by sharp endodontic explorer or by using slow speed small burs.

– If these procedures are not effective a chelating agent, i.e. EDTA is sealed in the pulp chamber for 24 hours.

– EDTA softens the dentin, calcified tissue and it can be removed and orifice opened by packing with an endodontic explorer.

– EDTA has distant antimicrobial properties.

– It is capable of causing mild irritation.

– EDTA is inserted by depositing a few drops in the pulp chamber with a syringe or pipette and then carefully pumping the solution into the canal.

2. RC-PREP

– It is a gel like commercial preparation developed by Stewart and collegues.

Composition

– EDTA - 15%

– Urea Peroxide - 10%

– Propylene glycol

– It is an effective lubricating and cleaning agent.

– It allows deeper penetration of medicament into the dentin.

CHAPTER 10

WORKING LENGTH DETERMINATION

Definition

– The distance from a coronal reference point to the point at which canal preparation and obturation should terminate (Glossary of Endodontics).

I. Objectives

1. To establish the length at which canal preparation and obturation has to be done.
2. Optimum length has been established at 1–2 mm short of the apex.

– *Over instrumentation* causes apical perforation, overfilling and pain.

– *Failure* to determine correct working length leads to,

(i) Incomplete instrumentation

(ii) Ledge formation

(iii) Underfilling with apical percolation

(iv) Persistent pain and discomfort from retained pulp tissue.

II. Methods

1. *Radiographic Methods*

(i) Grossman's method

(ii) Ingle's method

(iii) Xeroradiography

(iv) Radiovisiography (RVG)

2. *Non Radiographic Methods*

(i) Electrical resistance method

(ii) Audiometric method

(iii) Paper point method

Anatomic apex

– It is the tip or the end of the root determined morphologically.

Radiographic (major apical diameter) apex

– It is the tip or the end of the root determined radiographically.

RADIOGRAPHIC METHODS

1. GROSSMAN'S METHOD

Technique

– An instrument extending to the apical constriction is placed in the root canal which can be determined by digital tactile sense and a radiograph is taken.

– Stopper is placed at the level of incisal or occlusal reference point.

– Measure the length of the X-ray images of both the tooth and measuring instrument as well as actual length of the instrument in the canal.

Formula

$$\frac{A}{D} = \frac{C}{D} \Rightarrow \frac{\text{Actual length of the tooth (A)}}{\text{Actual length of instrument (B)}} = \frac{\text{Radiographic length of tooth (C)}}{\text{Radiographic length of instrument in the tooth (D)}}$$

$$\text{Actual length the tooth }(A) = \frac{\text{Radiographic length of tooth (C)}}{\text{Radiographic length of instrument in the tooth (D)}} \times \text{Actual length the instrument }(B)$$

$$A = \frac{C}{D} \times B$$

2. INGLE'S METHOD (Fig. 10.1 A to D)

– Preoperative radiographs are taken.

– From these the approximate length of the root canal is found by adjusting a occlusal rubber stop on the shaft of a file.

– From this, a length of atleast 1mm is reduced by moving the rubber stopper on the shaft.

– This is a safety measure.

– According to ingle, it is to be observed for possible image distortion on the X-ray.

– After adjusting this, a radiograph is taken with the instrument in position.

– On the X-ray the difference between the tip of the instrument and the tip of the root is added to safety measure if it is short of the apex.

– If the instrument has gone beyond the apex, the measurement that is obtained is subtracted from the original measurement.

– Finally, 1 mm is reduced from final measurement so that the tip of the instrument will correspond to the apical foramen.

– In this method it is assumed that apical foramen is 0.5 mm away from the radiographic root tip.

Example

Initial measurement	-	23 mm
Safety measure	-	(–) 01 mm
Tentative working length	-	22 mm
After taking radiograph, if it is short of 1.5 mm	-	(+) 1.5 mm
		23.5 mm
Adjustment for apical termination	-	(–) 1.0 mm
Final working length	-	22.5 mm

– **Wein's** modifications for Ingle's method,

1. If radiographically, there is no resorption of the root end or bone, shorten the length by the standard 1mm.

2. If periapical bone resorption is apparent, shorten by 1.5 mm.

3. If both root and bone resorption are apparent shorten by 2 mm.

– This is because if there is root resorption, the apical constriction is probably destroyed hence the shorter move back up the canal. Also when bone resorption is apparent, probably there is also root resorption, even though it may not be apparent radiographically.

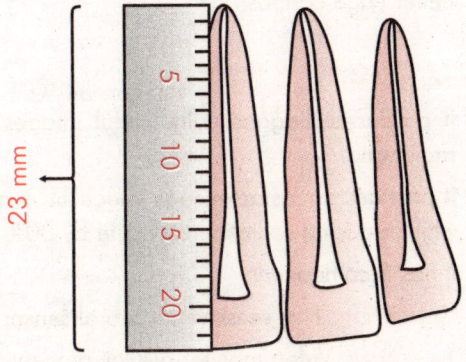

Fig. 10.1A Initial measurement

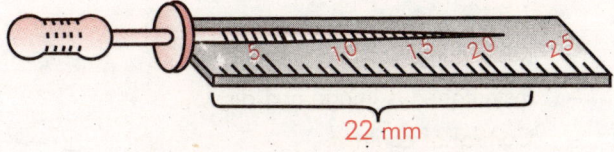

Fig. 10.1B Tentative working length

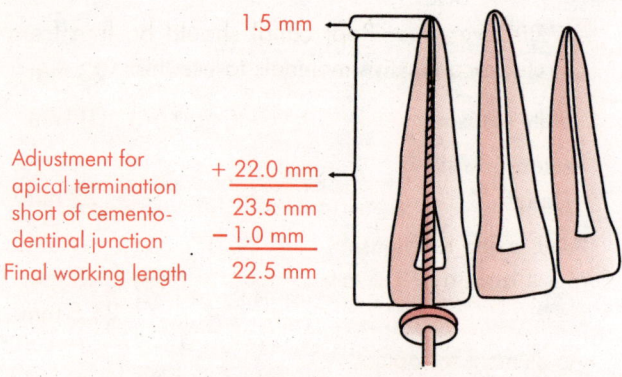

1.5 mm

Adjustment for
apical termination
short of cemento-
dentinal junction
Final working length

+ 22.0 mm
23.5 mm
− 1.0 mm
22.5 mm

Fig. 10.1C Final working length

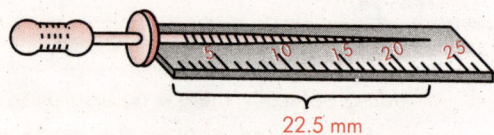

22.5 mm

Fig. 10.1D Setting the instruments at final working length

3. XERORADIOGRAPHY

– Not widely used in endodontics.

– They record images produced by an X-ray but differ from conventional radiography is that it does not require a wet chemical processing or dark rooms.

– Xeroradiographs are superior to conventional radiographs in that,

– Soft tissue and bone abnormalities are visible.

– Periapex is seen with greater sharpness.

– Better edge contrast.

4. RADIOVISIOGRAPHY (RVG)

– It produces diagnostically useful images at low radiation.

– It provides an instantaneous image on a monitor, while reducing radiation exposure by 80%.

– *It has 3 components*

(i) *Radio* : Has sensitive intra-oral sensor.

(ii) *Visio* : Video monitor display processing unit.

(iii) *Graphy* : High resolution printers.

Advantages

– Reduction of radiation exposure.

– Instantaneous image and display.

– Control of contrast.

– Elimination of X-ray film.

– Ability to enlarge special areas.

– Potential for computer storage.

NON-RADIOGRAPHIC METHODS

– The main disadvantages of radiographic methods are,

– Radiation exposure

– No definitive interpretation

– Time consuming

– Due to morphologic variability of the root canal, apical foramen does not correspond to root tip.

– Possible distortion

– To overcome these disadvantages some electrical devices which can determine the working length have been invented.

1. ELECTRICAL RESISTANCE METHOD

– Working length is determined by comparing the electrical resistance of apical periodontal membrane with the gingiva surrounding the tooth and both should be similar.

Technique

– A probe such as a file is attached to the electronic instrument with a cord and is inserted into the root canal till it contacts the periodontal ligament.

– The second probe is attached to the gingival.

– When the file touches the soft tissues, the electrical resistance gauges of both periodontal ligament and gingiva should have the same reading.

– By measuring the depth of probe, one can determine the working length.

2. AUDIOMETRIC METHOD

– Has slight variation from the electronic method.

– In this method a variation in the principle of electrical resistance of comparative tissue uses frequency oscillation sound to indicate when a similarity to electrical resistance has occurred by a similar sound response.

Technique

– Introduce an instrument into the gingival sulcus and induce an electric current until a sound is produced.

– The same procedure is repeated by introducing the instrument into the root canal and length is determined when the same sound is produced.

– These gadgets are commonly called APEX LOCATORS.

APEX LOCATORS

– In many of these instruments, the event is signalled by a beep, flashing lights and digital reading.
– One electrode is attached to the chip and the other to the file and the patient forms the circuit.

Trade Names

Endo meter

Sonoexplorer

Neosone

Classification

1. First Generation

– Also known as 'resistance apex locators'.
– Measure opposition to the flow of direct current or resistance.

2. Second Generation

– Also known as 'Impedance apex locators'.
– Measure opposition to the flow of alternating current or impedance.

– *Disadvantage:* Root canal should be free from electroconductive materials to use this.

APEX FINDER

– This is a new instrument used to locate the apex, as well as the working length.
– Insert a fine plastic tapered shaft through a bevelled tube into the root canal.
– Resistance to withdrawal indicates that some barbs have engaged the apical region and the shaft is marked at this level of cusp tip.
– The distance between the barb and marker is determined.
– The barbs that are engaged with resistance will show apical inclination which will be in the opposite inclination of the other barbs.

MASTER APICAL FILE DETERMINATION

– Master Apical File (MAF) is defined as *the largest file that binds slightly at correct working length after straight line access.*
– It is determined of passively placing successively larger files until a size is reached that slightly binds at the tip.

CHAPTER 11

CLEANING AND SHAPING (BIOMECHANICAL PREPARATION) OF THE ROOT CANAL

CLEANING AND SHAPING

- Schilder defined the general objective of canal preparation as follows:
- Root canal system must be *cleaned and shaped, cleaned of their organic remnants and shaped to receive a three dimensional hermetic filling of the entire root canal space.*

AIMS OF ROOT CANAL PREPARATION

1. To reduce the bacterial load of the root canal.
2. To dissolute and debride the inflament and infected tissue.
3. To create a shape, which is suitable for obturation.

SCHILDER'S MECHANICAL OBJECTIVES OF ROOT CANAL PREPARATION (Fig. 11.1)

1. Develop a continuously tapering conical form in the root canal preparation.
2. Make the canal narrower apically, with the narrowest cross-sectional diameter at its terminus.
3. Make the preparation in multiple steps.
4. Never transport the foramen.
5. Keep the apical foramen as small as in practical.

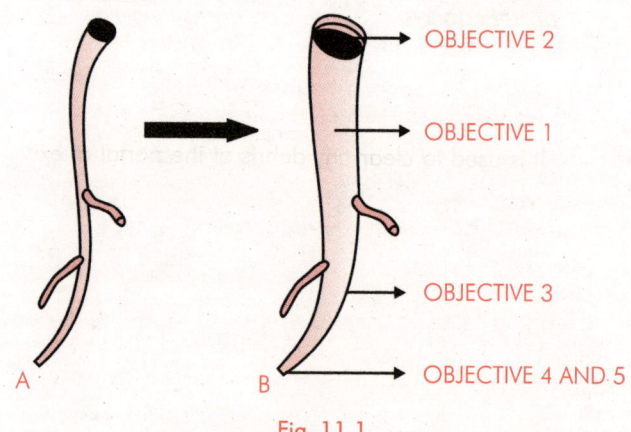

Fig. 11.1

The LOOK

- Schilder refers to 'the look' as the radiographic appearance of three-dimensional obturation, when all five mechanical objectives have been achieved.

MOTIONS OF CLEANING AND SHAPING

- There are six distinctive motion of files and reamers.

1. Follow

- Usually performs with files.
- They can be used during cleaning and shaping or any time an obstruction blocks the foramen.

Follow-Withdraw

- It is an in-and-out, passive motion that makes no attempt to shape the canal.
- File is the most useful instrument for this purpose.
- This motion is used when the foramen is reached, and the next step is to create the path from access cavity to foramen.

3. Cart

- Refers to the extension of a reamer to or near the radiographic terminus.
- Reamer should gently and randomly touch the dentinal walls and 'cart' away debris.

4. Carve

- Carving is for shaping.
- Reamers are best for carving.
- Instrument should not be pressed apically but simply touches the dentin and shape on withdraw.

5. Smooth / Circumferential

- Usually accomplished by files.
- If the above procedures are followed, smoothing is not required.

6. Patency

- Achieved with files or reamers.
- It is used to clear any debris at the portal of exit.

PURPOSE OF CLEANING AND SHAPING

- Cleaning and shaping is the basis for endodontic therapy.
- Cleaning is a combined chemical and mechanical process.
- Shaping is purely mechanical.
- Cleaning removes affected, infected antigenic, and substrate material from the canal system.
- Shaping enlarges the canals diameter and smoothens the walls as it removes crevices, fissures and irregularities from the canal, and facilitates obturation.

RULES MUST BE FOLLOWED DURING CLEANING AND SHAPING

1. Straight line access.
2. The length of the tooth should be correctly determined.
3. Instruments should be used in a sequence of sizes with periodic recapitulation, returning to smaller sizes to avoid blockage and ledging.

4. The instruments must be used as quarter to half turn in pull strokes.
5. Barbed broach should be used cautiously and only when the root canal is wide enough to permit their insertion and rotation without binding.
6. Should not force the instrument if it binds.
7. Clean, sterile instruments should be used.
8. Debris should not be forced through apical foramen.
9. Instrument should confine to root canal.
10. The apical portion of root canal 3–4 mm should be enlarged atleast 3 sizes greater than the first instrument that binds and until the walls are tapered without irregularities.

TECHNIQUES OF RADICULAR CAVITY PREPARATION

- There are two techniques present,
  1. Step-back preparation
  2. Step-down preparation

1. STEP - BACK PREPARATION

- Also called as *serial technique or telescopic preparation.*
- *Preparation starts at the apex with fine instruments and working one's way back up (or down) the canal with progressively larger instruments.*
- Designed to overcome instrument transportation in the apical third canal.

Technique

- *Mullaney* divided the preparation into two phases,
  1. *Phase I:* Apical preparation starting at the apical constriction.
  2. *Phase II:* Preparation of the remainder of the canal, gradually stepping back while increasing in size.

1. *Phase I: Apical Preparation*

- Apical portion of the canal is enlarged to atleast 25 to 30 sized instruments or the apical portion is enlarged using 1-2 sizes larger that the first file that binds.

2. *Phase II*

- To complete the instrumentation of remaining portion of root canal by successively using larger instruments and each larger instrument should be kept 1 mm shorter than previous instrument.

– The remainder of the root canal is prepared in a step back manner.

– Thus the preparation steps back up the canal 1 mm and one larger instrument at a time.

Advantages

1. Less likely to cause periapical trauma.

2. Facilitates removal of more debris.

3. Greater flare that results from instrumentation facilitates packing of gutta-percha by either lateral or vertical condensation.

4. One can obtain development of apical matrix or step which prevent overfilling of root canal.

5. Greater condensation pressure can be exerted which often fills lateral canals.

Objectives

– To keep the apical portion of preparation as small as possible, with an increasing taper throughout the remainder of the canal.

– In addition, the final apical preparation should be at or close to the original canal preparation.

– It creates a smooth flow and more tapered preparation from apical portion to coronal portion.

2. STEP DOWN TECHNIQUE (Crown Down Pressure less Technique)

– This involves cleaning and shaping of the canal from coronal third down to the apical third.

– Apical third is approached only after the coronal two-thirds preparations.

Technique

1. Coronal and Midroot Preparation

– Working length is determined.

– Coronal (16 mm) is prepared with H-files or Gates Glidden of sizes 15–40.

– Each larger file is inserted shorter than its predecessor.

2. Apical Preparation

– It involves enlargement of the apex by 2–3 sizes from the first file that binds apically.

3. To do stepback to connect apical and coronal taper.

Advantages

1. Elimination of debris and microorganisms from the more coronal parts of the root canal system there by preventing inoculation of apical tissues with contaminated debris.

2. Elimination of coronally placed interferences that might adversely influence instrumentation.

3. Early movement of large volumes of irrigant and lubricant to the apical part of the canal.

4. Facilitation of accurate working length determination as coronal curvature is eliminated early in the preparation.

Clinical Benefits

1. Easy removal of pulp stones.

2. Enhanced tactile feedback with instruments by removal of coronal interferences.

3. Enhanced apical movement of instruments into the canal.

4. Enhanced working length determination due to minimal tooth contact in the coronal third.

5. Increased space for irrigant penetration and debridement.

6. Rapid removal of pulp tissue located in the coronal third.

7. Straight line access to the root curves and canal junctions.

8. Enhanced coronal movement of debris.

9. Decreased deviation of instruments in canal curvatures.

10. Decreased canal blockages.

11. Minimization of instrument separation.

12. Predictable quality of canal cleaning and shaping.

13. Faster preparation.

Biological Benefits

1. Rapid removal of contaminated, infected tissue from the root canal.

2. Removal of tissue debris coronally thereby minimizing pushing of debris apically.

3. Reduction of postoperative pain.

4. Better dissolution of tissue with increased irrigant penetration.

5. Easy removal of smearlayer.

6. Enhanced disinfection of canal irregularities due to irrigant penetration.

RECAPITULATION

- Refers to repeated reintroduction and reapplication of instruments previously used throughout the cleaning and shaping process in order to create a well designed unclogged, smooth, evenly tapered unstepped root canals.
- The entire procedure is called **serial reaming** and filing and constant recapitulation.

EVALUATION CRITERIA FOR APICAL PREPARATION

- Three criteria are described.

1. Debridement

- Following preparation, the MAF tip is pressed against each wall on the outstroke. All walls should feel smooth.

2. Adequate taper

- The selected spreader or plugger passes easily to or within 1 mm of the working length with space left alongside for gutta-percha.

3. Apical preparation

- A seat or a stop or neither is identified by using a file smaller than the MAF at the working length.

CHAPTER 12

DISINFECTION OF THE ROOT CANAL

DISINFECTION

- It is the destruction of pathogenic microorganisms, presupposes adequate removal of pulp tissue and debris clearing and enlarging of the canal by biomechanical means and clearing of its contents by irrigation.

- The four factors either predispose the teeth to infection or counteract disinfection whether it may be of a wound or the root canal of a pulpless tooth, i.e. trauma, devitalized tissue, dead spaces and accumulation of exudate.

- Disinfection of the root canal is accomplished by intra canal medication.

- Microorganisms present in the canal can invade the periapical tissue and may not only give rise to pain but also destroy the periodontium including bone.

- The intracanal medication reduces or eliminates the microbial flora present in the root canal.

INTRACANAL MEDICAMENTS

Functions of Intracanal Medicaments

A. Primary functions

1. Antimicrobial activity
2. Antisepsis
3. Disinfection

B. Secondary functions

1. Hard tissue formation
2. Pain control
3. Exudation control
4. Resorption control

Requirements

- It should,

1. Be an effective germicide and fungicide.
2. Be nonirritating to the periapical tissue.
3. Remain stable in solution.
4. Have a prolonged antimicrobial effect.
5. Be active in the presence of blood, serum and protein derivatives of tissue.
6. Not interfere with repair of periapical tissues.
7. Not stain tooth structure.
8. Be capable of inactivation in a culture medium.
9. Have low surface tension.
10. Not induce a cell mediated immune response.

Classification

– May be classified arbitarily as,

A. Essential oils
B. Phenolic compounds
C. Halogens
D. Other material
E. Antibiotics

A. ESSENTIAL OILS

– These are weak disinfectants.

Eugenol

– Chemical essence of oil of clove and is related to phenol.
– Antiseptic and anodyne.
– Slightly more irritating than oil of clove.

B. PHENOLIC COMPOUNDS

1. Phenol

– A white crystalline substance which has a characteristic odour derived from coal tar.
– Liquefied phenol (carbolic acid) consists of 9 parts of phenol and 1 part water.
– Phenol is a protoplasm poison and produces necrosis of soft tissue.

2. Parachlorophenol

– A substitution product of phenol in which chlorine replaces one of the hydrogen atoms ($C_6 H_4 OCl$).
– On trituration with gum camphor these substances combine to form an oily liquid.
– Harrison and Madonia have recommended 1% aqueous solution of parachlorophenol.
– Penetrates deeper into the dentinal tubules than camphorated chlorophenol.

3. Formocresol

– This substance is a combination of formalin and cresol in the proportions of 1:2 or 1:1.
– It is a nonspecific bactericidal medicament most effective against aerobic and anaerobic organisms found in a root canal.

4. Glutaraldehyde

– S'Gravenmade and Dankert have recommended it in low concentration (2%).
– It is a strong disinfectant and fixative.
– This colourless oil is slightly soluble in water and thereby has a slightly acidic reaction.

5. Crestatin (Metacresylacetate)

– A clear, stable, oily liquid of low volatility.
– It has antiseptic and obtundant properties.

C. HALOGENS

1. Sodium hypochlorite

– Sometimes used as an intracanal medicament.
– Sodium hypochlorite vapours were bactericidal, whereas those of formocresol, aqueous parachlorophenol and camphorated chlorophenol were bacteriostatic.
– As the activity of sodium hypochlorite is intense but of short duration, the compound should preferably be applied to the root canal every other day.

2. Iodides

– Engstrom and Spangberg have recommended a 2% solution of iodine of potassium iodide as a root canal disinfectant.
– This compound consists of,
  – Iodine crystals: 2 parts
  – Potassium iodide: 4 parts
  – Distilled water: 94 parts
– Antibacterial effect is of short duration.

D. OTHER MATERIALS

1. Quaternary Ammonium

– The quats are compounds that lower the surface tension of solutions.
– 9-aminoacridine, an antiseptic but it may stain tooth structure.

2. Calcium Hydroxide

– It is best used as an intracanal medicament when one anticipates an excessive delay between appointments because it is efficacious as long as it remains within the root canal.

3. N2 (Sargentis Paste)

– A compound containing paraformaldehyde as its primary ingredient, contains eugenol and phenyl mercuric borate and at times additional ingredients including lead, corticosteriods, antibiotics and perfume.
– An intracanal medicament and sealer.
– Available as 'RC-2B'.

4. Antibiotics

- They should not be used routinely as an intra-canal medicament as they cause allergy, development of resistance to microorganisms, drug toxicity.

- PBSC (Polyantibiotic pastes) was used as an intracanal medicament.

- It is seldom used nowadays.

- PBSC consists of,

  - Penicillin—effective against gram positive.

  - Bacitracin—effective against penicillin resistant micro organisms.

  - Streptomycin—effective against gram-negative.

  - Caprolate sodium - effective against fungi.

FREQUENCY OF MEDICATION

- In accordance with general principles of root canal management disinfectant dressings should preferably be renewed in a week and not longer than 2 weeks.

- Because dressing become diluted by periapical exudate and are decomposed by interaction with the micro-organisms.

- Length of time for which the medicament remains effective depends on,

  1. Size of apical foramen

     - Wide apical foramen : washing of medicaments is quick. So they will not remain effective for long.

  2. Size of the dentinal tubules

     - Young teeth with little secondary dentin will allow greater diffusion of medicament.

     - So it will not remain effective longer in the canal for as long as older teeth.

3. Presence of Smear layer

- Smear layer initially delays the release of components and can have the effect of not allowing the medicaments to reach the regions of infection or inflammation in suitable therapeutic concentrations.

4. Presence of remnants of pulp tissue

- If pulp tissue is left in the canal, it will dissolve the medicaments and it will be rapidly cleared from the canal system.

5. Temporary sealing of the access cavity

- If the access cavity is not effectively sealed, then medicaments will not last long due to dissolution.

6. Medicament that is used

- The material should be preferably in the past form and have low solubility.

ELECTROSTERILIZATION

- It is a combined and simultaneous use of medicaments and direct electric current.

- The process of sterilization depends upon the passage of direct current through an electrolyte.

- A suitable Iridoplatinum electrode is selected which reaches the apex and fits the canal loosely.

- The canal is flooded with zinc iodide iodine solution.

- The electrode is then inserted and retracted in the root canal in order to eliminate air bubbles, and pump the solution to the apex.

- After the tooth electrode is adjusted, a hand electrode to be held in the hand and current is turned on gradually.

- The patient is instructed to signal the operator by raising the hand when there is tingling sensation.

- Amount of current tolerated by the patient is registered and duration of treatment is then calculated.

CHAPTER 13

TEMPORARY FILLING MATERIALS

DEFINITION

– *These are the materials used to seal the root canals to prevent from the leakage.*

REQUIREMENTS

– The material should,

1. Be impervious to fluids of the mouth and bacteria.
2. Hermetically seal the access cavity peripherally.
3. Not cause pressure on the dressing during insertion.
4. Set within a few minute after insertion.
5. Withstand the force of mastication.
6. Be easy to manipulate and to remove.
7. Harmonize with the colour of the tooth structure.

MATERIALS

1. CAVIT

– It is a moisture initiated, auto polymerized, premixed calcium sulfate-polyvinyl chloride acetate.

– **Composition:** Zincoxide, calcium sulfate, glycol-acetate, polyvinyl acetate, polyvinyl chloride, triethanolamine and red colouring.

– Thickness of at least 3.5 mm is necessary to prevent leakage.

Advantages

1. Superior sealing.
2. Ability to withstand thermal changes.
3. Easy to insertion.
4. Can also be used as retrograde filling material.

Disadvantages

– It was found that long periods between appointments predisposed the tooth to leakage.

2. INTERMEDIATE RESTORATIVE MATERIAL (IRM)

– It is a ZOE (Type III) based cement to which reinforcing particles are added to improve the strength and toughness of the set material.

– Its longevity can extend a year or longer.

– There is no evidence of leakage.

3. TERM

– It is a light activated particle filled composite resin for which there is no need of acid etching prior to placement.

– Main component is urethane dimethacrylate polymer.

ROOT CANAL SEALERS / CEMENTS

DEFINITION

– These are the cements which are used in adjunct to obturating material to seal the canal perfectly.

FUNCTIONS

1. Cementing the core material into the canal.
2. Filling of the discrepancies between the canal walls and core material.
3. Acting as a lubricant.
4. Bactericidal agent.
5. Acting as a marker for accessory canals, resorptive defects, root fractures and other spaces into which the main core material may not penetrate.

IDEAL PROPERTIES

– It should,

1. Provide an excellent seal when sets.
2. Produce adequate adhesion among the canal walls and the filling material.
3. Be radiopaque
4. Be nonstaining
5. Be dimensionally stable
6. Be easily mixed and introduced into canals.
7. Be easily removed if necessary.
8. Be insoluble in tissue fluids.
9. Be bactericidal or discourage bacterial growth.
10. Be nonirritating to periapical tissues.
11. Be slow setting, to ensure sufficient working time.

CLASSIFICATION

– Based on the composition,

A. Eugenol sealers

1. Grossman's sealer
2. Kerr root canal sealer
3. Wach's cement
4. Rickert's sealer
5. Tubli seal

B. Non-eugenol sealers

1. Chloropercha
2. Diaket
3. AH 26
4. Paraformaldehyde cement

C. Resorbable pastes with therapeutic values
- Zinc oxide eugenol paste + Iodoform + thymoliodide + camphorated phenol + paraformaldehyde.

1. GROSSMAN'S SEALER

- It is a nonstaining sealer which meets ideal requisites.

Composition
Powder

Zinc oxide	-	42%
Staybelite resin	-	27%
Bismuth subcarbonate	-	15%
Barium sulfate	-	15%
Sodium borate anhydrous	-	1%

Liquid
- Eugenol or oil of pigmenta leaf.
- Powder and liquid is mixed to creamy consistency.
- Different tests, to test for proper consistency are drop test and string test.

Drop Test
- The cement is gathered and the spatula is held edgewise.
- The cement should not drop off the spatula's edge in less than 10 to 12 seconds.

String Test
- The mixed cement should string out for at least 1 inch when the spatula is raised from the glass slab.

2. CHLOROPERCHA

Composition
Powder

Zinc oxide

Canada balsam

Rosin

Gutta-percha

Liquid

Chloroform

3. DIAKET

- It is a polyvinyl resin (polyketone).
- It consists of a fine, pure white powder and a viscous, honey coloured liquid.

Composition
Powder

Zinc oxide

Bismuth phosphate

Liquid

Polyvinyl resin

Advantages
- Good adhesion to teeth.
- Rapid set.
- High tensile strength.
- Resistance to permeability.

4. AH-26

- An epoxy resin containing a non toxic hardener.
- Radiopacity is imparted by bismuth oxide.

Advantages
- Strong adhesive properties.
- Provides good seal.

Disadvantages
- Staining of tooth structure.
- Insoluble in solvents.

5. RICKERT'S SEALER

- It is germicidal.

Composition
Powder

Zinc oxide

Precipitated silver

White resin

Thymol iodide

Liquid

Oil of cloves

Canada balsam

Advantages
1. Excellent lubricating property.
2. Excellent adhesion.
3. Adequate setting time.

Disadvantage
- Possibility of discoloration of tooth (due to silver).

6. TUBLISEAL

Composition

Zincoxide

Bismuth trioxide

Oleoresins

Thymol iodide

Oils

Modifiers

Advantages

1. Excellent lubricating property.
2. Does not stain the tooth.

Disadvantage

– Rapid setting

7. WACH'S SEALER

– It is germicidal.

Composition

Powder

Zinc Oxide	-	10 g
Calcium phosphate	-	2 g
Bismuth subnitrate	-	3.5 g
Heavy magnesium oxide	-	0.5 g

Liquid

Canada balsam	-	20 ml
Oil of clove	-	6 ml

Advantages

– Low tissue irritation
– Adequate setting time
– Limited lubricating qualities

CHAPTER 15

OBTURATION OF THE ROOT CANAL

– *Obturation:* It is the final phase of root canal therapy, refers to filling the entire root canal completely and densely with a non-irritating, air-tight sealing agent.

OBJECTIVES

1. To prevent percolation and microleakage of periapical exudate into the root canal space.
2. To prevent reinfection.
3. To create a favourable biologic environment for the process of tissue healing to take place.

APPROPRIATE TIME FOR OBTURATION (OR WHEN TO OBTURATE)

– Root canal should be obturated when,
1. Tooth is asymptomatic-no tenderness and pain.
2. The canal is dry
3. There is no sinus tract
4. There is no foul odor
5. Successive negative culture is obtained.
6. The temporary filling is intact.

OBTURATING MATERIALS OR ROOT CANAL FILING MATERIALS

REQUIREMENTS FOR AN IDEAL ROOT CANAL FILLING MATERIAL

– It should,
   – Be easily introduced
   – Be liquid or semisolid and should become solid
   – Seal laterally and apically
   – Be impervious to moisture
   – Not shrink
   – Be bacteriostatic
   – Not stain tooth
   – Not irritate periapical tissues
   – Be easily removed
   – Be sterile or sterilizable
   – Be radiopaque
   – They are the bulk that will fill the canal space
   – They may or may not be used in conjunction with sealer.

CLASSIFICATION OF OBTURATING MATERIALS

1. Pastes

- Chloropercha
- Calcium hydroxide
- N_2

2. Solids

a.	*Semirigid Flexible*	Silvercones
b.	*Rigid*	Vitallium implants
c.	*Plastic*	Gutta-percha
		Epoxy resin acrylate
d.	*Cements*	Zinc oxide eugenol

1. GUTTA-PERCHA : (GP) (Fig. 15.1 A and B)

- Most widely used and accepted root canal filling material.
- GP is a hydrocarbon resembling a rubber in origin.
- Pure GP is not used.

Composition

Zinc oxide	-	66 % (filled)
Gutta-percha	-	20% (Matrix)
Heavy metal surfaces	-	11% (radiopacifier)
Waxes or resins	-	3% (plasticizer)

- GP is manufactured in two different shapes,

1. Standardized

- The standardized sizes coordinate with the ISO sizes of the root canal file.
- They are used primarily as the main core material for obturation.

2. Nonstandardized

- They are more tapered from the tip or point to the top.
- These are usually designated as extra fine, fine-fine, medium-fine, fine-medium, medium, medium-large, large and extra large.
- These are used as secondary and auxillary cones.
- GP may come in either pellet form or in cannulas for the injectable thermoplastic obturation techniques.
- It is available in heatable syringes for thermo-mechanical techniques.

- Guttapercha cones have become available containing an iodoform component called medicated guttapercha, an this enhances the anti microbial properties.

Advantages

1. As it is plastic, it adapts and seals better with irregularities and contour of canal.
2. It is least toxic or inert.
3. Tissue tolerant or nonallergic.
4. Radiopaque.
5. It will not discolour the tooth structure.
6. It does not shrink after insertion unless it is plasticised by a solvent / heat.
7. It does not encourage bacterial growth.
8. It can be easily sterilized and easily removed from root canal when necessary.

Disadvantages

1. It lacks rigidity so difficult to place in narrow canals and canals with extreme curvature.
2. Lacks adhesive quality hence used with a sealer.
3. Can become brittle with age.
4. It can be easily displaced by pressure.

Technique to rejuvenate the aged brittle cone

- By momentary immersion in hot tap water (55°C) followed by instant cooling in cold tap water.

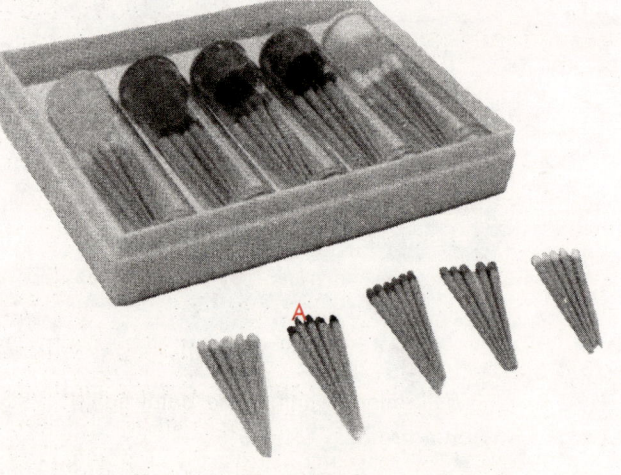

Fig. 15.1 A and B

2. SILVER CONES

- Are usually used in fine, tortuous canals as a solid core.
- May also as a retro-grade root canal filling.

Advantages

1. Made of pure silver.
2. When extreme curvatures are present, it can be conveniently used.

Disadvantages

1. Non adaptability
2. Corrosion
3. Difficulty in removal for retreatment and for restorative reasons.
4. Post space preparation while trying to remove a portion of silver point it may disturb the apical seal or cause lateral perforation.

MASTER CONE SELECTION

- There are 4 methods to determine the proper fit of master cone,
  1. Visual test
  2. Tactile test
  3. Radiograph
  4. Patient response

1. Visual test

- Grasp the measured point at a position with in 1 mm short of the prepared length of the canal with cotton pliers.
- Then the point is carried into the canal until the cotton pliers touch the external reference point of the tooth.
- If the working length of the tooth is correct and the point goes completely to position, the visual test has been passed unless the point can be pushed this position.
- This can be determined by grasping 1 mm further back on the point and attempting to push it apically.

2. Tactile test

- It determines whether the point tightly fits the canal or not.
- In the event the apical 3–4 mm of the canal have been prepared with near parallel walls (in contrast to a continous taper), some degree of force should be required to seat the point and once it is in position, a pulling force should be there to dislodge it. This is known as `TUG BACK'.
- If tugback is present tactile test is passed.

3. Patient response

- Patient's who are not anesthesitized during a treatment of non-vital pulp or at the second appointment of vital pulp may feel the GP penetrating the foramen.
- Adjustments can be made until it is completely comfortable.
- This is a good test when the position of the foramen cannot be determined accurately by radiograph or by tactile sensation.

4. Radiograph Test

- After visual and tactile test its position must be checked by the radiograph.
- The film must show the point extending to within 1 mm from the tip of the preparation.

OBTURATION TECHNIQUES FOR GUTTA-PERCHA

1. Single cone technique.
2. Lateral condensation technique
3. Vertical condensation technique or warm gutta-percha technique.
4. Combination of lateral and vertical condensation techniques.
5. Inverted cone method.
6. Rolled cone technique.
7. Sectional method.
8. Chemically plasticized gutta-percha technique.
9. Compaction (McSpadden technique).
10. Thermoplasticized injection moulded method.
   - We have described only lateral and vertical condensation techniques in detail.

1. LATERAL CONDENSATION TECHNIQUE

Significance

- It is a preferred technique for most of the canals as most teeth present wide canals or flares that cannot be densely filled with the single cone technique.

Technique (Fig. 15.2 A to D)

- This is a procedure where additional auxillary cones are inserted and condensed laterally around the primary cone.
- Tapered preparation is necessary.

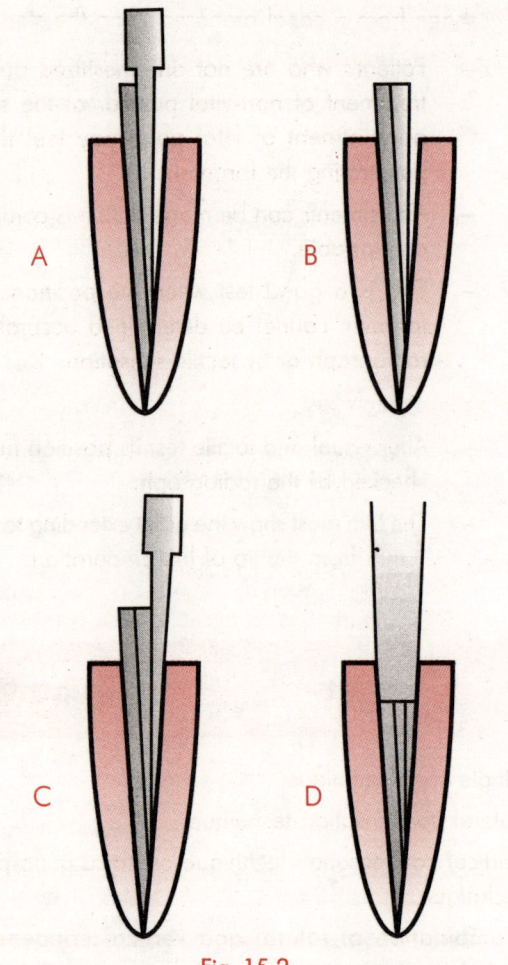

Fig. 15.2

Selection of master cone

– GP cone is inserted to the working length and should fit snugly and resist to removal or 'tug back'.

– A radiograph is taken to determine the apical and lateral fit of the primary cone.

– Cone is fitted in canal short of 1mm from the apex.

– Once the primary cone is accurately fitted in the root canal, it is removed to dry the canal.

– Walls are coated with thin layer of cement.

– Now the selected master cone is inserted and condensed with spreader.

– If gap is present then accessory cone is inserted and condensed.

– The process continues till the canal is filled completely.

– Cementing is not necessary for accessory canals.

– After verifying the canal by radiograph the buttend of GP in the pulp chamber is cut-off with a hot instrument.

– The chamber is cleaned and temporary restoration is placed in the access cavity.

2. VERTICAL CONDENSATION OR WARM GUTTA-PERCHA TECHNIQUE

– Introduced by SCHILDER.

– This technique is especially used with 'Step Back Technique'.

Indications

1. Method is specifically indicated when maximum condensation is desired.

2. They are used when reaching of conventional master cone to the apical portion of canal is impossible, as when there is ledge formation, perforation or unusual canal curvature.

3. This method can be used when other kind of treatment fail.

Advantages

1. Excellent seal of the canal apically, laterally.

2. Obturation of lateral and accessory canal.

Disadvantages

1. Complicated
2. Difficulty in length control
3. Risk of vertical root fracture
4. Overfilling of gutta-percha

Technique (15.3 A to F)

– In this method, the flow property of GP to heat is utilized.

– Master cone is selected based on working length.

– The canal wall is coated with a thin layer of root canal cement.

– The selected cone is coated with cement.

– The coronal (butt) end of the cone is cut-off with a hot instrument.

– A heat carrier (plugger) is heated and carried into the canal vertically and this causes the flow of gutta-percha.

– This procedure is repeated until the canal is three dimensionally filled.

– The maximum temperature is 80° C in vertical condensation and temperature at apical region is 40–42° C.

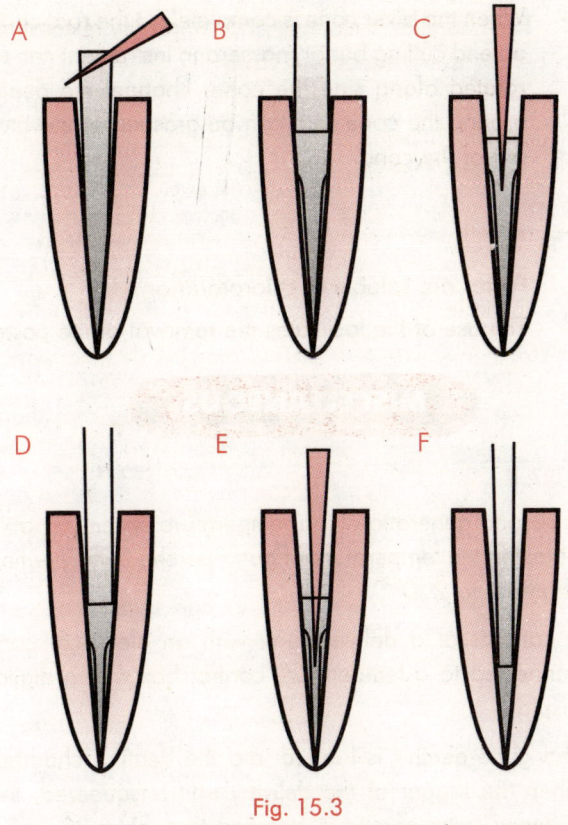

Fig. 15.3

METAL CORE OBTURATION

– It includes obturating the root canal with a silver cone, a sectioned silver cone, stainless steel (instrument blade) or amalgam.

1. SILVER CONE METHOD

Significance

– Use is restricted to teeth with fine, tortuous canals that cannot be filled properly with gutta-percha.

Technique

– Select a cone corresponding in size to the largest instrument used in the preparation of the canal.

– Sterilize the cone by alcohol flaming three times or by passing it through on open flame two or three times.

– Insert the cone in the canal using silver cone pliers or Stieglitz forceps, and press it apically.

– The cone should fit snugly and should bind at the apical foramen.

– A canal instrumented for silver cone obturation should have tapered converging walls differing in

shape from a canal prepared using the step back technique.

– Take a radiograph to check the fit of the cone in the canal.

– If it protrudes beyond the apex, cut-off the excess at the tip. So the final fit will terminate at 0.5 mm short of the root apex.

– If the silver cone is too short, select another that fits or reprepare the canal so the selected cone seats properly.

– Coat the canal with cement and insert the sterilized silver cone with slight pressure to the measured length.

– Take another radiograph to ensure that the filling is properly positioned.

– Laterally condense secondary gutta-percha cones around the primary silver cone.

– Wipe the walls, clean with chloroform or alcohol and fill the crown with zinc phosphate cement.

2. SECTIONAL OR SPLIT CONE METHOD

Significance

– Designed for a tooth whose restoration may require a post and core.

Technique

– The method consists of fitting the cone snugly as described earlier.

– The cone is notched approx. 6 mm from the apical tip it is sterilized and it is cemented in the root canal.

– The wedged cemented cone is rotated until it breaks at the notch, and the free end is removed to leave enough space for preparation of a post.

3. STAINLESS STEEL METHOD

Significance

– Can be used to fill fine, tortuous canals.

Technique

– Because steel files are much more rigid than silver cones, they can be inserted into a canal with greater ease.

– Once the file has been cemented, its handle must be cut-off with a high speed bur, 3 or 4 mm below the occlusal surface to allow space for a restoration.

REMOVAL OF ROOT CANAL FILLINGS

1. GUTTA-PERCHA

Objective

– To remove it without forcing the filling material into the periapical tissue.

Technique

– Remove the GP from the chamber by searing it with a heated excavator, or grind it out with a slowly resolving round bur.

– Flood the pulp chamber with chloroform or xylol to soften the GP.

– Insert a no. 25 or 30 reamer or file into the canal along side the GP and remove the softened filling piece by piece.

– Repeat the process of softening the filling and instrumenting pieces out of the canal until all the GP has been removed.

– If an instrument binds excessively withdraw it carefully to avoid breakage, deposit another a few drops of solvent to soften the GP and continue the procedure.

– As the apex is approached, insert and rotate a heated instrument so its tip is embedded in the remaining GP. Allow it to cool and withdraw the remaining filling from the canal.

– A radiograph is taken to determine whether the GP has been completely removed from the canal.

2. SILVER CONES

– A silver cone is not removed as easily as a GP filling unless the butt end extends into the pulp chamber.

– In such cases chloroform or xylol is used to soften the cement and GP surrounding the butt end of the silver cone.

– An explorer tip can be used to free the silver cone of GP and cement around the canal orifice.

– First, flood the pulp chamber with chloroform to dissolve the cement.

– Grasp the projecting section of silver cone with a pair of narrow beak pliers (Stieglitz) and remove it from the canal.

– Be careful not to severe the butt end of the silver cone during this procedure.

– When the silver cone is completely in the root canal an end cutting bur or masserann instrument can be rotated along side the cone, channel the dentin around the cone so it can be grasped or elevated out of the canal.

3. PASTES

– Pastes are soluble in chloroform or xylol.

– The use of file facilitates the removal of the paste.

MISCELLANEOUS

OBTURA II

– A second generation high temperature system capable of taking the temperature of gutta-percha in the heating chamber to 200°C.

– It consists of a delivery unit with an electrical cord connected to a temperature control box with a digital display.

– The gutta-percha is loaded into the heating chamber when the trigger of the delivery unit is squeezed, the softened gutta-percha is extruded through a 20 or 23 gauge.

Advantages

1. Well adaptation to the prepared canal.
2. Used for back filling canals after establishing an apical plug.
3. Used for filling large and irregular canals.

THERMAFIL

– It is a patented endodontic obturator consisting of a flexible central carrier, sized and tapered to match variable tapered files.

– The central carrier is uniformly coated with a layer of a refined and tested a-phased guttapercha.

Advantages

– Significantly less strained during delivery and compaction.

– Easy flowing of GP into canal irregularities.

– Allows simple, fast, predictable filling of root canal.

– Especially used for small or very curved canals.

Disadvantages

– No apical stop or definitive apical constriction to prevent the GP extension beyond the root canal.

UNDER FILLING OF ROOT CANAL

Causes

- Natural barrier in the canal.

- A ledge created during preparation.

- Insufficient flaring.

- Poorly adapted master cone.

- Inadequate condensation pressure.

Treatment

- Removal and retreatment is preferred.

OVER FILLING OF ROOT CANAL

Causes

- Sequela of overinstrumentation through the apical foramen.

- Uncontrolled condensation forces extrude materials.

- Other causes are inflammatory resorption and incomplete development of the root.

- Extruded obturation material causes issue damage and inflammation.

Treatment

- Apical surgery may be required to remove the material from apical tissues and place a retrograde material.

CHAPTER 16

RESTORATION OF THE ENDODONTICALLY TREATED TEETH

- Restorations for endodontically treated teeth are designed to protect the remaining tooth structure from fracture and to replace the missing tooth structure.
- The final restoration includes the combination of 1. Dowel, 2. Core, and 3. Coronal restoration.
- Not every endodontically treated tooth needs a crown or a dowel; some need all three components and some need only an access seal for the coronal restoration.
- The final configuration of the restored tooth includes the following (Fig. 16.1).
  1. Residual tooth structure and its periodontal attachment apparatus.
  2. Dowel material
  3. Core material
  4. Definitive coronal restoration

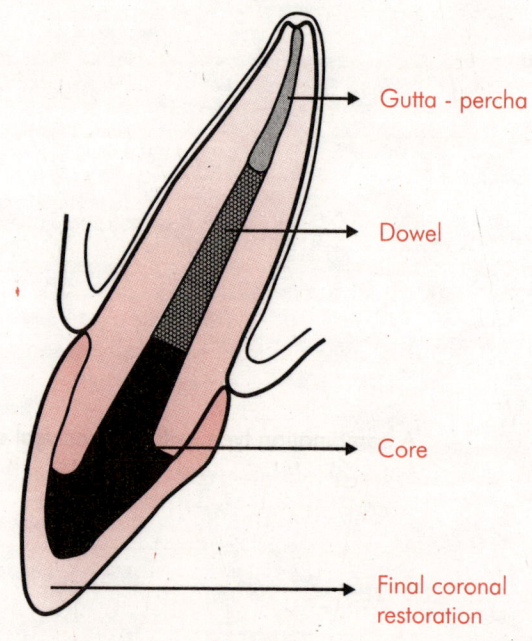

Fig. 16.1

1. DOWEL (POST)

- *The Dowel is a post or other relatively rigid, restorative material placed in the root of a nonvital tooth.*
- *Provides retention for the core and coronal restorations and must be designed to minimize the potential for root fracture from functional forces.*

Ideal Properties

- Dowels should provide,
1. Maximum protection of the root.
2. Adequate retention with in the root.

3. Maximum retention of the core and crown.

4. Maximum protection of the crown margin cement seal.

5. Pleasing esthetics if indicated.

6. High radiographic visibility.

7. Retrievability.

8. Biocompatibility.

Materials

– Include alloys of gold, stainless steel, titanium and dental amalgam.

Classification

– Based on the type of fabrication,

1. Custom cast posts

1. Tapered smooth
2. Parallel serrated

2. Prefabricated posts

– Prefabricated root canal posts are classified into three main types according to the general shape of their root portion,

i. *Parallel-sided*

– Cylindrical in shape with rounded corners.
– Has same diameter from one end to another.

ii. *Taper type*

– The sides are tapered from one end to other.

iii. *Parallel tapered type*

– A combination type, with the occlusal one-half to two-thirds being parallel sided and the apical portion being tapered.

– Prefabricated posts are also classified according to the surface texture,

i. *Smooth surface posts*

– Used in a cemented technique procedure.
– The post channel is larger in diameter than the post.

ii. *Serrated surface posts*

– Used in cemented technique procedure.

iii. *Threaded surface posts*

– Used with a screw in procedure.
– Post channel is slightly narrower in diameter than the post.

2. CORE

– *The core is a restorative material placed in the coronal area of a tooth which replaces carious,* *fractured or missing coronal structure and retains the final crown.*

– The core is anchored to the tooth by extending into the coronal portion of the root canal or through the endodontic dowel.

– The attachment between tooth, dowel, and core are mechanical or both, because of the core and dowel are usually fabricated of different materials.

Ideal Properties

– The core materials should have,

1. High compressive strength.
2. Dimensional stability.
3. Ease of manipulation.
4. Short setting time (for cement).
5. An ability to bond to both tooth and dowel.

CORE MATERIALS

– *Include cast metal or ceramic, amalgam, composite resin and glass ionomer resin (sometimes).*

A. Cast Core

– A cast metal dowel and core is a traditional way to restore endodontically treated teeth.

– The core is an integral extension of the dowel and the cast core does not depend on mechanical means for retention to the dowel.

– This type of construction avoids dislodgment of the core and crown from the dowel and root when minimal tooth structure remains.

Advantages

1. Non-corrosive final restoration.
2. Increased stiffness.
3. Decreased dentin deformation.

Disadvantages

1. High rate of root fracture
2. Not economic
3. Technique sensitive fabrication
4. Require two appointments

B. Amalgam Core

– Has high rate of clinical success.

Advantages

1. High strength
2. Improved marginal seal
3. Easy manipulation
4. Rapid setting time

Disadvantages

1. Potential for corrosion.
2. Discoloration of the gingiva and dentin.
3. Not eco friendly.

C. Composite Resin Core

- To get optimum composite resin core function,
1. There should be more than 2 mm of sound tooth structure should remain at the margin.
2. The composite resin core and the bonding agent must be compatible.

Advantages

1. Ease of manipulation
2. Very rapid set
3. High compressive strength

Disadvantages

1. Polymerization shrinkage
2. Micro leakage

D. Glass Ionomer Core

Advantages

1. Good adhesion
2. Anticariogenic property

Disadvantages

1. Limited to small restorations
2. Brittle
3. Low retention
4. High solubility

- Glass ionomer core is indicated in posterior teeth in which,
1. A bulk of core material is possible.
2. Significant sound dentin remains.
3. Additional retention is available with pins or dentin preparations.
4. Moisture control is assured.
5. Caries control is indicated.

E. Resin-modified glass ionomer Core

- It is a combination of glass ionomer and composite resin technologies. They exhibit properties of both materials.
- They exhibit minimal microleakage.

3. CORONAL RESTORATION

- This is the final component of the endodontic reconstruction.

Significance

1. Re-establishes function
2. Restores esthetics
3. Isolation of the dentin and endodontic fill materials from microleakage.
4. Distributes functional forces.

- The coronal restoration for endodontically treated intact anterior teeth consists of sealing the lingual access cavity. Posterior teeth need coronal coverage to protect against fracture from occlusal forces, regardless of the amount of remaining tooth structure.

- The final coronal restoration provides added security to the tooth by consolidating the remaining cusps and prepared tooth structure and by creating a ferrule effect.

FERRULE

- It is a metal band that encircles the external dimension of the residual tooth, similar to the metal bands around a barrel or a shovel handle.

- It is formed by the walls of the crown or cast telescopic coping encasing the gingival 1 to 2 mm of the axial walls of the preparation above the crown margin.

Significance

1. Increases the fracture resistance of the tooth.
2. Increases the retention and resistance of the restoration.

Requirements of a Ferrule

1. Should have a minimum of 1 to 2 mm dentin axial wall height.
2. Should have parallel axial walls.
3. Must totally encircle the tooth.
4. Must be on the sound tooth structure.
5. Must not invade the attachment apparatus of the tooth.

CHAPTER 17

SINGLE-VISIT ENDODONTICS

ADVANTAGES

1. Immediate familiarity with the internal anatomy facilities obturation.
2. No risk of bacterial leakage beyond the temporary coronal seal between the appointments.
3. Reduction of clinic time.
4. No additional appointments.
5. Economic.

DISADVANTAGES

1. Difficult apical access in flared-up canals.
2. Fatigue to the dentist with extended operating time.
3. Patient fatigue with extended chair side time.
4. No opportunity to place an intracanal disinfectant.

OLIET'S CRITERIA FOR CASE SELECTION

1. Positive patient acceptance.
2. Sufficient available time to complete the procedure properly.
3. Absence of acute symptoms requiring drainage via the canal and of persistent continuous flow of exudate or blood.
4. Absence of anatomical obstacles (calcified canals, fine tortuous canals, bifurcated or accessory canals) and procedural difficulties (ledge formation, blockage, perforations, inadequate fills).

INDICATIONS

1. Uncomplicated vital teeth.
2. Fractured anterior or bicuspid teeth where esthetics is a concern and temporary post and crown are required.
3. Patients who are physically unable to return for the completion.
4. Patients with heart valve damage or prosthetic implants who require repeated regimens of prophylactic antibiotics.
5. Necrotic, uncomplicated teeth with sinus draining tracts.
6. Patients who require sedation.

CONTRAINDICATIONS

1. Painful, necrotic tooth with no sinus tract for drainage.
2. Teeth with severe anatomic anomalies.
3. Asymptomatic nonvital molars with periodical radiolucencies and no sirus tract.
4. Patients with acute apical periodontitis.
5. Most retreatments.

CHAPTER 18

PULPAL THERAPY

PULPOTOMY

Definition

– It is defined as complete removal of cornal portion of dental pulp followed by a placement of suitable dressing or medicament that will promote healing and preserve vitality of tooth.

Indications

1. Vital tooth with healthy periodontium.
2. A restorable tooth.
3. Absence of spontaneous pain.
4. Atleast 2/3 of root length should be present.
5. During pulpotomy procedure haemorrhage at amputation site should be pale red and easily controllable.

ContraIndications

1. Spontaneous pain (especially at night)
2. Swelling
3. Presence of fistula
4. Tender on percussion
5. Pathologic mobility
6. External root resorption
7. Internal root resorption
8. Periapical or inter radicular radiolucency
9. Profuse haemorrhage from amputated radicular stumps
10. Pus or exudate at exposure site
11. Presence of pulp calcifications

Material used

1. Formocresol
2. Glutaraldehyde

1. Formocresol

Buckley's formula

– *Formaldehyde 19%* : This binds with cellular proteins and helps in fixation of tissues.

– *Tricresol 35%* : Increase solubility and permeability of cell wall membrane.

– *Glycerine (25%) + water (21%)* : It acts as emulsifier and prevents conversion of formaldehyde into paraformaldehyde.

2. Glutaraldehyde (Introduced by Kopel)

– This is dialdehyde compound. It has super fixative properties, self limiting penetration and low toxicity.

Procedure

- Radiographic interpretation.
- Administration of local anaesthesia.
- Rubber dam application.
- Initial penetration with round bur followed by use of 169 L bur to remove roof of pulp chamber.
- Following removal of roof, coronal pulp contents are removed using long shank spoon excavators.
- The walls of coronal pulp chamber are defined.
- Following removal of coronal pulp contents the root orifices become evident (amputation site).
- The haemorrhage from pulp stumps is controlled using pressure condensation or with help of adrenalin soaked pallets.
- Cotton pellet is impregnated with formocresol.
- The pellet is placed over amputation site. The recommended time being 5 min while recent studies advocate 1 min application of same.
- A mix of formocresolised zinc oxide eugenol is lightly condensed over amputation site followed by a hard setting cement (zinc polycarboxylate) followed by silver amalgam restoration.
- As this is a pulp treated tooth a stainless steel crown is recommended.

CVEK type pulpotomy / Shallow pulpotomy

- Administration of local anesthesia and rubberdam isolation.
- With a spoon excavator remove granulation tissue from the exposure site.
- Remove pulp tissue from the pulp proper to a depth of 1 to 2 mm with a water cooled, round diamond stone.
- Visualize the removal, layer by layer.
- Irrigate with a coolant water spray.
- After preparing the pulp tissue, bleeding is controlled by placing a cotton pellet moistened with saline.
- Wash the wound with saline.
- Apply the calcium hydroxide over the wound and cover all exposed adjacent dentin.
- An intermediate base of hard setting zinc phosphate cement or glass ionomer cement is placed.
- Restoration with composite resin.

MTA (Mineral Trioxide Aggregate)

- This is an alternative to calcium hydroxide.

- The technique for managing a traumatic pulp exposure using MTA is in many ways similar to that used with calcium hydroxide but with some minor modifications.
- Tooth is anaesthetized and isolated with rubber dam.
- Site is disinfected using sodium hypochlorite solution.
- A shallow pulpotomy is done.
- Removal of pulp tissue to a depth of at least 2 mm.
- Bleeding is allowed to stop.
- Some moisture is required for the proper curing of the material.
- Mixture of MTA powder and liquid is placed on the wound surface and gently tapped with moist cotton pellet.
- Entire access into the pulp should be filled in a similar manner with small amounts of MTA.
- MTA when exposed to saliva will allow it to cure.
- A minimum of 6 hours is required for a material to adequately set.
- The tooth can then be restored with a definite restoration.

DEVITALISATION PULPOTOMY
(Pulp Mummification Procedure)

- This is a two stage procedure.
- Paraformaldehyde is used to fix the pulpal tissue.

Materials used

- Hobsons paste - contains paraformaldehyde, lignocaine, carmine, carbovax and propylene glycol.

  Mummifying agent

  - Beachwood creosote
  - Hobson's paste

Procedure

- Administration of local anesthesia.
- Initial access preparation
- Superficial layer of coronal pulp content excavation.
- Mummifying agent (Hobson's paste or Beachwood Cresote) is placed on to which a thin mix of zinc oxide eugenol is lightly condensed.
- The patient is recalled after a week during which period the mummifying procedure occurs and a routine pulpotomy is carried out.

Indications

- In cases of non-negotiable radicular canals or in cases where the patient is uncooperative.

LASER PULPOTOMY

- Nd : YAG LASER has been used for pulpotomy in primary teeth with a high degree of success.
- Not very popular as it is expensive.

ELECTROSURGICAL PULPOTOMY

- Electrocarty procedure carbonises and heat that is generated denatures the pulp and bacterial contamination.
- After the surgical amputation of coronal pulp, pulp stumps are cartriged through this method.
- This is followed by the obturation of coronal pulp chamber with zinc oxide eugenol over which a layer of hard setting restoration is placed, over which a stainless steel crown is recommended.

PULPECTOMY

- *It is a complete removal of coronal and radicular pulp and replacing the same with a suitable obturating material.*

Indications

1. In all cases of irreversible pulp disease.
2. In cases of acute pulpitis resulting from infection, injury or operative trauma.
3. In case of carious or mechanical exposure it is the treatment of choice.
4. In other cases, intentional extirpation is required for restorative and fixed prosthetic procedures.

Procedure

- Administration of local anaesthesia.
- Rubberdam application.
- Access cavity preparation.
- Roof of pulp chamber is removed followed by extirpation of radicular pulp using barbed broaches.
- Following pulp extirpation, biomechanical preparation is carried out using suitable reamers and files.
- Radicular morphology of primary molars is characterisatic termed as *ribbon shaped* because the canals are narrower mesiodistally and broader buccolingually. Hence, instrumentation may be difficult. In case of difficulty in negotiating canals one should not make an attempt to forcefully negotiate the instrument apically because of chances of perforation of root.

- Irrigation is carried out using H_2O_2 or sodium hypochlorite.
- Canals are dried using paper points after which a thin mix of zinc oxide eugenol or formocresolised ZOE is used to obturate canals and coronal chamber.
- Gutta-percha and silver points are contraindicated in primary dentition because they are nonresorbable.
- Following placement of obturating material a hard setting cement is condensed over the same followed by a silver amalgam restoration.
- As this is a pulp treated tooth, a stainless steel crown is recommended.

Other recommended materials for Root Canal Obturation in Primary Dentition

1. *Walkhoff Paste:* Contains parachlorophenol camphor and menthol.
2. *KRI Paste:* Contains Iodoform, camphor, para-chlorophenol and menthol.
3. *Misto Paste:* Contains zinc oxide, iodoform, thymol, chlorphenol, camphor.

APEXIFICATION

- Pulpal therapy for young permanent teeth.
- *It is a method which is intended to induce further development of root apex of an immaturely developed permanent tooth by formation of osteodentin and cementum.*

Indications

1. Long standing fracture of crown involving pulp.
2. Long standing caries exposure.

Contraindications

1. All vertical and most horizontal root fractures.
2. Replacement resorption (ankylosis).
3. Very short roots.

Aim

- To obtain normal narrowing of canal and also an apical closure against which an obturation can be achieved.

Procedure

1. Radiographic interpretation to access the radiographic length and working length.
2. Working length should be maintained 1.5–2 mm short of existing radiographic length.

3. Administration of local anesthesia.

4. Application of rubberdam.

5. Pulp extirpation followed by biomechanical preparation.

6. The young permanent dentition has characteristic broad canal with a wide opened apex and hence called as 'Blunder buss canals'.

7. H_2O_2 is contraindicated as an irrigating agent because of its effervescent nature and as any debris can be pushed apically, hence irrigation is limitated to use of sodium hypochlorite and normal saline.

8. Canal is obturated with a mix of calcium hydroxide and CMCP (Camphorated Para-mono-chlorophenol).

9. The access opening is filled with a hard setting cement.

10. The patient is recalled periodicallly for further radiographic examination to determine the presence of root closure.

11. Once the narrowing and root enclosure is achieved the existing root canal obturated material is removed and a routine root canal therapy is carried out.

– A better approach to apexification may be one in which a combination procedure,

1. Use calcium hydroxide for a short period of time about 2 weeks to assist in disinfection of the root canal.

2. Place MTA (Mineral Trioxide Aggregate) in the apical part of the canal to serve as an apical plug that promotes apical repair.

– After checking that the MTA has cured, complete the root canal treatment with gutta-percha and a bonded resin restoration extending below the cervical level of the tooth to strengthen the root's resistance to fracture.

APEXOGENESIS

Definition

– It is defined as, physiological root end development and formation.

– The procedure is used to initiate a full apical closure.

Indications

1. Immature tooth with incomplete root formation.

2. Damage to the coronal pulp but with a healthy radicular pulp.

Contraindications

1. Avulsed and replanted a severely luxated tooth.

2. Severe crown root fracture that requires intraradicular retention for restoration.

3. Tooth with an unfavourable horizontal root fracture.

4. Carious tooth that is unrestorable.

CHAPTER 19

SURGICAL ENDODONTICS

OBJECTIVE

– As in all endodontic procedures the objective of periapical surgery is to ensure the placement of a proper seal between the periodontium and the root canal foramina. When this seal cannot be achieved satisfactorily by working through the canal system (orthograde system), a surgical procedure permits visual and manipulative control of the area and placement of the seal (retrograde filling) through the surgical site.

– The better the seal, the better the endodontic prognosis of the tooth; this feature accounts for the high percentage of healing in surgically treated teeth.

INDICATIONS

1. Any condition or obstruction that prevents direct access to the apical third of the canal. For Ex: 1. Anatomic conditions like calcifications, curvatures, bifurcations, dens in dente and pulp stone, etc. and 2. Iatrogenic conditions like ledging, blockage from debris, broken instruments, old root canal fillings and cemented posts.

2. Iatrogenic or resorptive perforation that can not be treated with calcium hydroxide.

3. Periradicular disease associated with a foreign body.

4. Incomplete apexogenesis with blunderbuss canals or other apices that do not respond to apexification procedures and are inadequately sealed with an orthograde filling.

5. Abscess formation necessitating incision and drainage.

6. Horizontally fractured root tip with periradicular disease.

7. Periodontal lesions with furcation involvement that do not respond to periodontal treatment thus necessitating radisectomy.

8. Replantation of avulsed teeth.

9. Intentional extraction and replantation.

10. Necessity for diagnostic biopsy.

11. Predictable failure.

CONTRAINDICATIONS

A. General

1. Medcially compromised or brittle patient (i.e. a patient with an active systemic disease such as uncontrolled diabetes, TB, syphilis, nephritis, blood dyscrasias, osteoradionecrosis or in any other medical condition in which the health of the patient restricts surgical intervention.

2. Emotionally distressed patient, i.e a patient unable psychologically to withstand or cope up with any surgical procedure.

3. Limitations in the surgical still and experience of the operator.

B. Local

1. Localized acute inflammation (in this condition, emergency procedure such as incision and drainage or trephination may be indicated, elective periapical surgery should be avoided).

2. Anatomic considerations (procedures that penetrate the mandibular canal, maxillary sinus, mental foramen, floor of the nares or that severe the greater palitatine blood vessel should be avoided whenever possible).

3. Inaccessible surgical sites.

4. Teeth with poor prognosis.

CLASSIFICATION OF ENDODONTIC SURGICAL PROCEDURES

A. Surgical Drainage

1. Incision and drainage

2. Cortical trephination (Fistulative surgery)

B. Periradicular Surgery

1. Curettage

2. Biopsy

3. Root end resection

4. Root end preparation and filling

5. Corrective surgery

 i. Perforation repair

 ii. Root resection

 iii. Hemisection

C. Replacement Surgery

– Extraction / Replantation

D. Implant Surgery

1. Endodontic implants.

2. Root form osseointegrated implants.

RETROGRADE FILLING

– A retrograde filling is placed in the apically resected root when the canal is poorly sealed from the surrounding tissue.

– The technique used for resection and retrograde filling depends on the accessibility of the root tip in the operative site, the presence of hazardous anatomic structures surrounding the surgical site. The configuration, location and accessibility of the apical foramina to be used.

– The root is bevelled, to achieve the access needed to fill all the foramina present on the resected root surface.

Materials Used

– Zinc and zinc free amalgam-widely used

– ZOE cements

– Cavit

– Polycarboxylate cement

– Glass ionomer cement

– Composite fillings

– Zinc phosphate cement

– Silver cones

– Gold foil

Apical Seal

– The filling at the interface of the canal and periapical tissue should seal the root canal from the surrounding tissue.

Technique

– The cavity in the bevelled surface of the root is prepared for a retrograde filling with small, round burs followed by inverted cone burs.

– The ideal preparation has the smallest exposed surface at the apex while encompassing all foramina and extends about 2 mm inside the root canal.

1. Debride the operative site, wipe and dry the root tip and isolate the root tip with sterile cotton pellets to prevent any seepage into the cavity and to collect any excess amalgam particles that fall into the wound during packing and condensation.

2. Place a varnish over the prepared cavity. Pack the amalgam into the cavity using a retrofilling amalgam carrier or a plastic instrument and condense amalgam with a retrofill amalgam plugger.

3. Wipe and adapt the margins of amalgam to dentin with a moist cotton pellet.

4. Remove all the cotton pellets surrounding the root apex, cautiously to prevent amalgam particles trapped in the cotton from falling into the surrounding tissue.

5. Irrigate the wound with sterile saline or anesthetic solution and aspirate the solution thoroughly to debride the wound site.

6. Examine the root tip, filling and surrounding tissue, both visually and radiographically to that the canals have been properly sealed.

RADISECTOMY/ROOT RESECTION

Definition

–   Denotes the removal of one or more roots of a molar.

Indications

–   When endodontic treatment of one root is technically impossible or when such treatment has failed.
–   When untreatable furcation involvement is present and removal of the root will facilitate oral hygiene in that area.
–   When extensive loss of bone has occurred around one root of an upper molar.
–   When a fractured root of an upper molar is present.
–   When a root has been perforated and cannot be treated endodontically.
–   When a root has been destroyed by extensive decay.

Contraindications

–   When loss of bone involves more than one root and the remaining root would have inadequate support.
–   When the bridge span is long and the abutment tooth would lend inadequate support.
–   When the roots are fused.

Technique of Root Resection (Fig. 19.1)

–   Administration of local anesthesia.
–   Probe the area to determine the extent and outline of alveolar bone destruction around the root to be removed.
–   Elevate the mucoperiosteal flap.
–   With the contra angle handpiece and cross cut bur severe the root where it joins the crown and remove the root.
–   With a stone or diamond point smooth the resected root stumps and contour the tooth.
–   Scale and plane the root surface area.
–   Clean the area and replace the flap and suture.
–   Cover it with a periodontal pack.
–   Remove the pack and suture after 1 week.

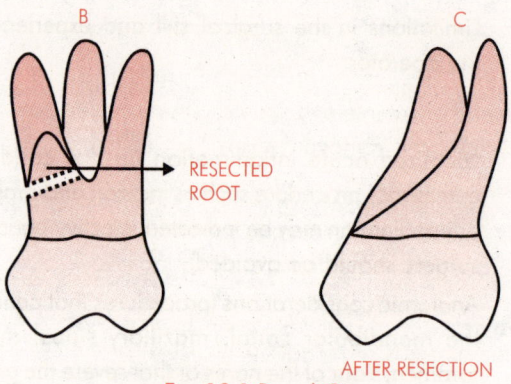

Fig. 19.1 B and C

HEMISECTION

Definition

–   Procedure in which one root and its corresponding crown portion is cut and removed.

Indications

–   When the periodontal involvement of one root is severe.
–   When loss of bone is extensive in the furcation area.
–   When caries involves much of the roots.

Contraindications

–   Similar to radisectomy.

Technique (Fig. 19.2)

–   It involves the same technique as that is used for root resection.
–   In this procedure, half of the crown is removed alone with one of roots of mandibular molar.
–   The retained mesial and distal halves serves as abutment for prosthesis or restoration.

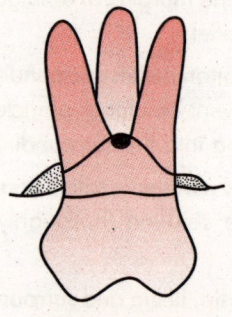

BEFORE RESECTION

Fig. 19.1 A

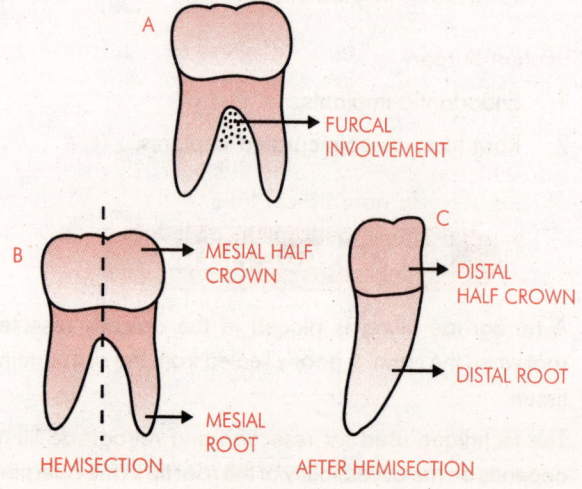

Fig. 19.2 A to C

BICUSPIDIZATION / BISECTION

– Molar is cut into two separate mesial and distal portion without the removal of any part of the root or crown (Fig. 19.3).

– It is performed when the mandibular molars exhibit proper anatomic features and stability.

– Molar with divergent roots and bone loss restricted to furcal areas are ideal for bicuspidization.

– The tunnel like effect of the furcation involvement is eliminated by creating two separate teeth from single molar.

– The portion of the teeth will require crowns.

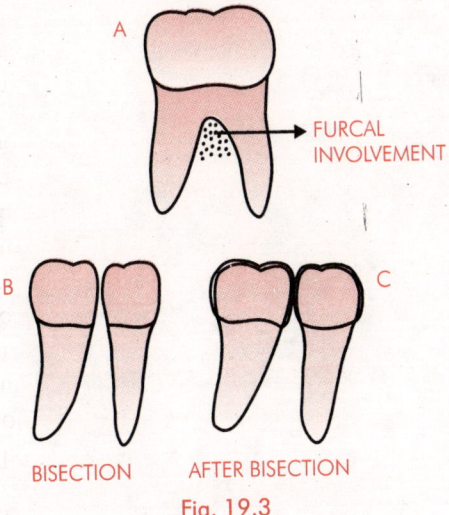

Fig. 19.3

APICOECTOMY

– Apicoetomy is the removal of the root tip.

Indications

1. When the anatomy of the canal system has not been conductive to nonsurgical treatment.
2. When iatrogenic perforation or ledges prevent apical sealing.
3. When the root tip is resorbed or fractured.
4. When a retrograde filling must be placed in an apex because of an unremovable obstruction exists in the canal.

Procedure (Fig. 19.4)

– Radiograph is taken to determine the level at which the root should be amputated.

– Design the mucoperiosteal flap.

– Now the mucoperiosteal flap is raised make an opening into the periapical.

– Bony defect using a surgical bur or chisel.

– Extend the opening in the labial plate to obtain good access to the limits of the defect.

– Then with a fissured cylindrical bur amputate the root at the appropriate level.

– Apical foramen is sealed either by retrograde filling or sealing the gutta-percha in the canal.

– Control haemorrhage within the defect by crushing bleeding points in bone by pressure or by cotton pledgets dipped in epinephrine.

– Suture the mucoperiosteal flap and maintain firm pressure over the area for 10 minutes.

– Obtain an immediate postoperative radiograph to check the level of root amputation and future comparison.

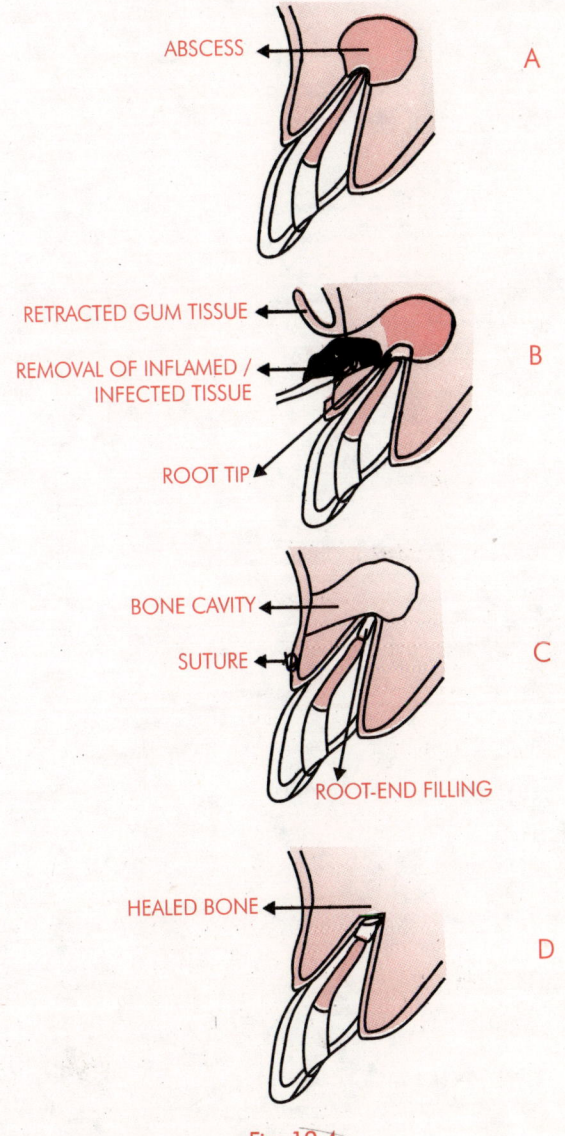

Fig. 19.4

Section III

Dental Biomaterials

CHAPTER 01

DENTAL AMALGAM

Dentists have more than a century of experience using amalgam as a direct filling material. Dental amalgam has a much longer service record, than most drugs and biomaterials in use today and except for gold, all other dental restorative materials. There is more information about dental amalgam than about any other dental restorative material presently used, yet concerns are raised periodically about the safety of dental amalgam relative to one of its ingredients-elemental mercury.

DEFINITION

- *Amalgam* is an alloy of mercury with another metal or metals.
- *Dental amalgam* is produced by mixing liquid mercury with solid particles of an alloy of silver, tin, copper and some times zinc, palladium, indium and selenium. This combination of solid metals is called *Amalgam alloy*.
- The reaction between mercury and alloy follows mixing is termed an *amalgamation* reaction. It results in the formation of a hard restorative material of silver-grey appearance.

APPLICATIONS

- *It is the strongest and most widely used filling material.*
- It is used in /as,
    1. Class I and II cavities on the posterior teeth.
    2. Class V cavities where esthetics are not considered.
    3. Core build-up for crown preparation in a grossly destructed tooth.
    4. Retrograde root canal filling.
    5. Preparation of dies.
    6. Combination with retentive pins to restore a crown in which one or two walls of cavity are missing.
    7. Restoration of disto-facial cusps of canine.
    8. The patients where moisture control is difficult.

ADVANTAGES

1. Easy to manipulate.
2. Least technique sensitive.
3. Self sealing property.
4. Good strength.
5. Long lasting.
6. Economic.
7. Good wear resistance.

8. Applicable in a broad range of clinical situations

9. Less chair side time required.

10. Direct restorative material.

11. Easy to repair.

12. Durable.

DISADVANTAGES

1. Cannot be used in esthetic zones.

2. More brittle and less tough.

3. Do not bond to the tooth structure.

4. Mercury toxicity.

5. Galvanic action.

6. Prone to tarnish and corrosion.

7. Marginal breakdown.

8. Microleakage.

9. Delayed expansion and resultant pulpitis.

10. Some destruction of sound tooth structure.

CLASSIFICATION

I. Based on size of alloy particle

1. Microcut

2. Macrocut

II. Based on shape of alloy particle

1. Lathecut

2. Spherical

3. Spheroidal / Admixed (Spherical with irregular surface)

III. Based on number of alloying metals

1. Binary: Two metals—silver, tin.

2. Ternary: Three metals—silver, tin, copper.

3. Quaternary: Four metals—silver, tin, copper, indium.

IV. Based on noble-metal content

1. Non noble metal alloys.

2. Noble metal alloys.

V. Based on copper content

1. **Low copper/conventional/traditional alloys:** Contain less than 6% of copper.

2. **High copper alloys:** Contain more than 6% of copper.

These are classified into,

i. *Admixed / Dispersed / Blended alloys*
   It is a mixture of spherical eutectic high copper alloy and lathecut low copper alloy.

ii. *Single / Unicomposition alloys*

VI. Based on zinc content

1. *Zinc containing alloys*
   Contain more than 0.01% of zinc.

2. *Zinc free alloys*
   Contain less than 0.01% of zinc.

COMPOSITION

– According to *ADA specification no.1,*

Silver	- 69.4%
Tin	- 26.2%
Copper	- 3.6%
Zinc	- 0.8%

ROLE OF MAJOR COMPONENTS IN AMALGAM

1. Silver

   – Major element

   – Whitens the alloys

   – Decreases the creep

   – Increases the strength

   – Increases the setting expansion

   – Reduces tarnish and corrosion

2. Tin

   – Controls the reaction between silver and mercury.

   – Reduces strength and hardness of the amalgam.

   – Reduces tarnish resistance of the amalgam.

3. Copper

   – Increases strength and hardness.

   – Increases setting expansion.

   – Decreases the brittleness of the alloy.

4. Zinc

   – Acts as a *scavenger or deoxidizer:* Prevents the oxidation of silver, copper and tin during manufacture of alloy powder.

   – Adds plasticity to the mix.

   – Zinc less alloys are more brittle.

   – Zinc causes delayed expansion if its content is > 0.01%.

5. Platinum and Palladium

– Increases the hardness and whitens the alloy.

6. Mercury

– Necessary for the reaction to form plastic mass.

MANUFACTURING OF ALLOY

1. Lathe-cut powder

– The metal ingredients are heated and protected from oxidation until melted, then poured into a mold to form an ingot.

– Lathe-cut alloys are normally subjected to two heat treating procedures.

– The first is a **homogenization** heat treatment, normally carried out on the alloy ingot before lathe cutting and designed to produce homogenous grains in which the $Ag_3Sn(\gamma)$ intermetallic compound predominates. Homogenization ensures that each filing has similar composition and properties. The heat treatment involves heating to about 420°C for several hours. The resulting alloy contains relatively larger grains of γ–phase material.

– The second is **heat treatment** which is carried out after lathe-cutting.

– This is a lower temperature treatment typically involving heating the alloy powder to approximately 100°C for about 1 hour. This treatment is called as **'alloy ageing'** ; it is to remove residual stresses introduced during cutting and ensures that the alloy remains stable during future storage.

2. Spherical powder

– Manufactured by **atomization** process.

– All the desired elements are melted together. The liquid alloy is then sprayed, under high pressure of an inert gas, through a fine crack in a crucible into a large chamber. The droplets of alloy solidify as they falldown. The produced particles are either spherical or spheriodal in nature.

3. Particle size

– The average particle size of amalgam is 15–35 microns.

– Average small particle size alloys have high strength and produce rapid hardening.

4. Comparison of alloy-powder particles

– Lathe-cut and admixed alloys require more condensation pressure and tend to resist condensation better than spherical alloys.

– Spherical alloy amalgams are more plastic.

– Spherical alloy requires less mercury than lathe-cut alloys.

5. Admixed alloys

– These alloy powder particles contain both lathe-cut and spherical alloy particles.

– Contain 30 to 55 wt% spherical high-copper powder.

DIFFERENCES BETWEEN *LOW COPPER* AND *HIGH COPPER* ALLOYS

Low Copper Alloys	High Copper Alloys
1. Less compressive strength (presence of γ_2 phase).	1. High compressive strength.
2. Less corrosion resistance.	2. High corrosion resistance.
3. Less marginal integrity.	3. High marginal integrity.
4. High creep: 0.8–8%.	4. Low creep : 0–1%.

DIFFERENCES BETWEEN *LATHE-CUT* AND *SPHERICAL* ALLOYS

Lathe-Cut Alloys	Spherical Alloys
1. Particles are irregular in shape.	1. Particles are in spherical shape.
2. Manufactured by milling an annealed ingot of alloy.	2. Manufactured by atomization of molten alloy.
3. Less plastic and resists condensation pressure.	3. More plastic.
4. More mercury required hence has inferior properties.	4. Requires less mercury hence has better properties.

ADVANTAGES AND DISADVANTAGES OF *ADMIXED* AND *SPHERICAL* HIGH COPPER AMALGAMS

Admixed High Copper Amalgam	Spherical High Copper Amalgam
Advantages	*Advantages*
1. Longer working time.	1. Sets faster.
2. Less dimensional change.	2. Lower residual mercury.
3. Displacement of matrix.	3. Lower creep.
	4. Faster finishing.
	5. Higher early strength.
	6. Low condensation pressure.
Disadvantages	*Disadvantages*
1. Slower set.	1. Less working time.
2. High residual mercury.	2. Greater dimensional change.
3. Higher creep.	
4. Less early strength.	
5. Harder to finish.	

SETTING REACTIONS AND STRUCTURE (AMALGAMATION PROCESS)

Phases in amalgam alloys and set dental amalgam	Stoichiometric formula
γ (gamma)	Ag_3Sn
γ_1	Ag_2Hg_3
γ_2	$Sn_{7-8}Hg$
ε (epsilon)	Cu_3Sn
η (eta)	Cu_6Sn_5
Silver–copper eutectic	$AgCu$

γ_1 - *noble phase*, γ_2 - *weakest phase*.

A. Low copper alloys

- Silver and tin can form an intermetallic compound of formula $Ag_3Sn(\gamma)$ which contains 73.15% silver and 26.85% Tin.

- The reaction is,

$$Ag_3Sn + Hg \rightarrow Ag_2Hg_3 + Sn_{7-8}Hg + \underset{(unreacted)}{Ag_3Sn}$$
$$\quad \gamma \qquad\qquad \gamma_1 \qquad\quad \gamma_2 \qquad\quad \gamma$$

- **Structure of set material:** A core of unreacted γ and a matrix of the γ_1 and γ_2 compounds.

- The percentages are γ_1 - 54 to 56%; γ_2 - 11 to 13%; γ - 27 to 35% by volume.

- Mercury has limited solubility for silver (0.035 wt%) and tin (0.6 wt%).

- Because the solubility of silver in mercury is much lower than that of tin, the γ_1 phase precipitates first and the γ_2 phase precipitates later.

- γ_1 has body-centred cubic structure and γ_2 has hexagonal structure.

- The more unconsumed $Ag-Sr$ particles that are retained in the final structure, the stronger the amalgam.

- γ_2 phase is least stable to corrosion environment and suffer corrosion attack especially at 'crevices' of the restorations.

B. High-Copper Admixed Alloys

- It has silver-copper eutectic alloy (71.9 wt% silver and 28.1 wt% Copper).

- **Main feature:** The set structure is essentially free of γ_2 phase.

- The reactions are,

(1)
$$\underset{(\gamma)}{Ag_3Sn} + \underset{(eutectic)}{Ag-Cu} + Hg$$
$$\downarrow$$
$$\underset{(\gamma_1)}{Ag_2Hg_3} + \underset{(\gamma_2)}{Sn_{7-8}Hg} + \underset{(\gamma)}{Ag_3Sn} + \underset{(eutectic)}{Ag-Cu}$$

(2)
$$\underset{(\gamma_2)}{Sn_{7-8}Hg} + \underset{(eutectic)}{Ag-Cu} \longrightarrow \underset{(\eta)}{Cu_6Sn_5} + \underset{(\gamma_1)}{Ag_2Hg_3}$$

- **Set material:** Consists of a core of Ag_3Sn and $Ag-Cu$ surrounded by a halo of Cu_6Sn_5 and a matrix of γ_1.

C. High-Copper Unicomposition Alloys

- **Main feature:** The set structure is free of γ_2 phase.
- The reaction is,

$$Ag_3Sn + Cu_3Sn + Hg \rightarrow Ag_2Hg_3 + Cu_6Sn_5$$
$$\quad(\gamma)\qquad(\epsilon)\qquad\qquad(\gamma_1)\qquad(\eta)$$

- **Set material:** Consists of a core of Ag_3Sn and and Cu_6Sn_5 is present in the γ_1 matrix rather than as a halo.

PROPERTIES OF AMALGAM

- **ADA Specification no: 1 for Amalgam Alloys** lists three physical properties as a measure of amalgam quality: *Creep, compressive strength and dimensional change.*
- According to ADA, when a cylindrical specimen is 7 days old, a 36 Mpa stress is applied in a environment. The maximum allowable creep is 3%. The minimum allowable compressive strength 1 hour after setting, when a cylindrical specimen is compressed at a rate of 0.25 mm/min is 80 Mpa. The dimensional change between 5 min and 24 hrs. must fall within the range of 20 μm/cm.

1. Creep

- *Creep is the time-dependent strain or deformation that is produced by a stress.*
- Creep can cause an amalgam restoration to extend out of the cavity preparation, there by increasing its susceptibility to marginal breakdown.
- Creep values of low-copper amalgams: 0.8–8% and of high-copper amalgams: < 0.1%.
- Creep rates increase with higher γ_1 and γ_2 volume fractions.
- Creep also increases with high mercury / alloy ratio and low condensation pressure.

2. Compressive Strength

- Set amalgam has a very weak tensile and a very high compressive strength.
- The following factors affect the strength of the amalgam,

  #### 1. Temperature
  It loses 50% of its room temperature strength when its temperature is elevated to 600°C (as when hot coffee flows over it).

  #### 2. Trituration
  Under-trituration and over-triturartion decreases the strength.

  #### 3. Mercury
  Higher the residual mercury, lower the strength.

  #### 4. Condensation
  Greater the condensation pressure, higher the strength.

  #### 5. Porosity
  It results from under-trituration, under-condensation, irregularly shaped particles of the alloy powder, insertion of too large increments into the cavity, delayed insertion.

  #### 6. Gamma 2 Phase
  Its reduction or the prevention of its formation can definitely increase the strength.

3. Dimensional change

- During setting, amalgam undergoes three distinct dimensional changes, i.e.
- **Stage 1: Initial contraction:** Results from the absorption of the mercury into the interparticular spaces of the alloy powder.
- **Stage 2: Expansion:** Due to the formation and growth of the matrix crystals.
- **Stage 3: Limited, delayed contraction of the mass:** Results from the absorption of unreacted mercury.
- The following are the factors affect the dimensional change,

  #### 1. Constituents
  The more the basic gamma-phase, the more the expansion.

  Greater traces of tin produce lesser expansion.

  #### 2. Mercury
  More mercury produces a more prolonged second stage of amalgamation (expansion).

  #### 3. Particle Size
  Smaller the particle size, the less the expansion.

  #### 4. Trituration
  Good trituration causes no apparent expansion.

  #### 5. Condensation
  Higher condensation pressure induces more contraction.

  #### 6. Contamination with moisture
  If it contaminate, causes delayed expansion.

4. Corrosion

- The order of corrosion resistance of the different stages of amalgamation are,

$$\underset{\substack{(\gamma_1)\\ \text{(Most resistant)}}}{Ag_2Hg_3} > \underset{(\gamma)}{Ag_3Sn} > Ag-Cu > \underset{(\epsilon)}{Cu_3Sn} >$$

$$\underset{(\eta)}{Cu_6Sn_5} > \underset{(\gamma_2)}{Sn_{7-8}Hg}\ \text{(Least resistant)}$$

1. Low-Cu system

- In the low-copper amalgam system, the most corrodable phase is the γ_2 phase.
- Corrosion results in the formation of tin oxychloride from the tin in the γ_2 phase and also liberates mercury.

$$Sn_{7-8}Hg + \frac{1}{2}O_2 + H_2O + Cl^- \rightarrow Sn_4(OH)_6 Cl_2 + Hg$$

2. High-Cu System

- Cu_6Sn_5 (η) is the least resistant phase.
- The corrosion product is $CuCl_2 . 3Cu(OH)_2$.

$$Cu_6Sn_5 + \frac{1}{2}O_2 + H_2O + Cl^- \rightarrow CuCl_2 . 3Cu(OH)_2 + SnO$$

5. Delayed Expansion / Secondary Expansion

- Defined as *the gradual expansion of a zinc containing amalgam over weeks to months which is associated with hydrogen gas development caused by contamination of the plastic mass with moisture during its manipulation in a cavity preparation.*
- The expansion usually starts after 3 to 5 days and may continue for months, reaching values greater than 400 μm(4%).

Complications

- Protrusion of the restoration out of the cavity.
- Increased microleakage space around the restoration.
- Restoration perforation.
- Blister formation on the restoration surface.
- Increased flow and creep.
- Pulpal pressure pain.

TECHNICAL CONSIDERATIONS

- The following steps are involved in the building up of an amalgam restoration.

1. Choice of the Alloy and Mercury

- Select an alloy certified by the ADA.
- High-copper amalgam is recommended because of its superior clinical performance.
- There is no decision in the choice of mercury except that it should follow the USP specifications.
- Alloys are available in powder, tablet and pre-proportioned forms.
- Most operators prefer diposable capsules.

2. Proportioning of the alloy and mercury

- Two techniques are available for the purpose of proportioning.

1. High-mercury technique

- Also called as *increasing dryness technique*.
- The initial amalgam mix contains a little or more mercury than needed for the powder (52–53% Hg) producing a very plastic mix.
- It is necessary to continue squeezing the mercury out of the mix increments being introduced during build-up of the restoration so that each increment will be dryer than the previous one.

2. Minimum mercury technique

- Also called as *1:1 technique or 'Eame's technique' or 'No-squeeze cloth technique'*.
- It is more popular technique.
- The initial amalgam mix contains equal amounts of mercury and powder alloy.
- With this techniques one can assume that 50% or less mercury will be in the final restoration.
- Proportioning of the alloy and mercury should be done by weight.

3. Trituration

- Defined as *the process of mixing the amalgam alloy particles with mercury in an amalgamator.*

Objectives

1. To achieve a workable mass of amalgam in a minimum time.
2. To remove oxides from the surface of powder particles.
3. To pulverize the pellets into particles that can be easily wetted by the mercury.
4. To reduce particle size so as to increase the surface area of the alloy particles per unit volume.
5. To dissolve the particles or part of the particles of the powder in mercury, which initiate the formations of the matrix crystals.
6. To keep the amount of γ_1 or $\gamma_1 - \gamma_2$ matrix crystals as minimal as possible.

Methods of Trituration

- The two methods of trituration are,

1. Hand Trituration

- Alloy and mercury are triturated by hand with a mortar and pestle: its use is diminishing now a days.

2. Mechanical Trituration

- Used universally.

– Has a metal or plastic capsule to contain the powder and mercury which serves as a mortar.

– A cylindrical metal or plastic piston of smaller diameter than the capsule is inserted into the capsule and this serves as the pestle.

– The *three* basic movements of mechanical triturators are,

   i. The mixing arm carrying a capsule moves back and forth in a straight line at varying speeds.

   ii. The mixing arm travels back and forth in a figure of 8 at varying speeds.

   iii. The mixing arm travels in a centrifugal fashion.

Normal Mix

– Appears shiny and separates in a single mass from the capsule.

– Has maximum strength.

– Carved surface retains its lustre after polishing.

– Mix may be warm (not hot) when it is removed from the capsule.

Under-triturated mix

– Appears dull and crumbly.

– Mix is rough and grainy.

– Susceptable to tarnish after carving.

– Less strength.

Over-triturated mix

– Appears soapy and tends to stick to the inside of the capsule.

– Decreased working time.

– Results in higher contraction of amalgam.

– Increased creep.

4. Mulling

– It is a continuation of trituration.

– *It is done to improve the homogenity of the mass and to assure a consistent mix.*

– There are two ways to accomplish the mulling, i.e.

   i. The mix is enveloped in a dry piece of rubber dam and vigorously rubbed between the index finger and thumb or the thumb of one hand and palm of another hand. This process should not exceed 2 to 5 sec.

   ii. After trituration pestle is removed from the capsule and the mix in triturated in the pestle free capsule for 2 to 3 seconds. In addition to fulfilling the objectives of mulling, this process delivers the mix in one single coherent and consistent mass.

5. Condensation

– Defined as *the process of compaction of the alloy into the prepared cavity to attain greatest possible density with adequate mercury present to ensure maximum continuity of the noble phase Ag_2Hg_3 between the remaining alloy particles.*

1. Objectives

1. To adapt amalgam intimately to the prepared walls and margins.

2. To produce a uniform and viod-free restoration as possible.

3. To minimize the residual mercury content.

4. It brings the strongest phase of amalgam close together, thereby increasing the strength of the restoration.

– Condensation should be done immediately after trituration.

– Condensation can be done by the hand or mechanical condensers.

– It is shown that mechanical condensation is superior to hand condensation.

– Condensers are available in different shapes and sizes, i.e. round, parallelogram, diamond, etc. and as well as in various angulations to facilitate access.

– The face or nib of the condenser is inversely proportional to the square of its surface area.

– *Condensation pressure : 66.7 N.*

2. Condensation of Non-Spherical alloy

– Amalgam should be inserted in small increments and condensed with small condensers, to eliminate voids, to bind the increments together and to facilitate the filling of minor details of the prepared cavity.

– Once the surface of the preparation is reached, larger condensers should be used to avoid undue pressure on the enamel at the cavo surface.

– Condensation forces should be applied at 45° to walls and floors, i.e. bisecting line angles and trisecting point angles.

– Further increments are condensed at 90° to the previous portion to avoid shear force that may displace the already condensed amalgam.

– *Amalgam should be condensed from its center to periphery to avoid overlapping or bridging of voids at critical areas.*

– Excess mercury or splashy amalgam which appears on the surface should be excavated and discarded before inserting another increment.

3. Condensation of spherical alloy

– Here, increments are taken in such a way so as to fill the entire cavity or a large part of the cavity.

– Largest condenser is used to prevent the lateral escape of the spherical particles during condensation pressure toward the cavity floor.

4. Blotting mix

– After completely filling the prepared cavity and covering the cavosurface anatomy, an over dried amalgam mix (made by squeezing off mercury in squeezing cloth) is condensed heavily over the restoration using the largest condensers possible for the involved tooth. This mix is called the blotting mix.

– It serves to blot excess mercury from the critical marginal and surface area of the restoration and to adapt amalgam more intimately to the cavosurface anatomy.

– The mix is excavated and discarded after its use.

5. Delayed condensation

– It results in a mix with increased residual mercury, less strength, higher creep, decreased plasticity and the mix does not adapt well to the cavity walls.

– Higher concentrations of mercury is located around the margins of the restorartions.

6. Burnishing or Surfacing

– *It is the process of rubbing usually performed to make a surface shiny or lustrous.*

– Immediately, after discarding the blotting mix, a large rounded burnisher is used for burnishing.

– Burnishing proceeds from the amalgam surface to the tooth surface on the occlusal and other conspicuous portions of the restoration.

– Inaccessible areas, such as the proximal portion of the restoration are burnished with a beaver tail burnisher and / or sprately burnisher or T-burnisher.

Objectives

1. As a continuation of condensation to reduce the voids.
2. To bring out excess mercury to the surface.
3. To adapt the amalgam further to cavosurface anatomy.
4. Condition the surface amalgam to the carving step.

Precarve burnishing

– It is a form of condensation done to improve the benefits of condensation.

– It produces a denser amalgam at the margins of occlusal preparations restored with high-copper amalgam and initiates carving.

Postcarve burnishing

– Done to improve smoothness and to produce a Satin (not shiny) appearance.

– To improve marginal integrity of high copper amalgams.

– Produces denser amalgam at the margins of occlusal preparation restored with low-copper amalgam.

7. Carving

– Defined as *the anatomical sculpturing of the amalgam material.*

Objectives

1. To produce a restoration with no underhangs.
2. To produce a restoration with the proper physio-logical contours.
3. To produce a restoration with minimal flash.
4. To produce a restoration with functional, non-intefering occlusal anatomy.
5. To produce a restoration with adequate, compatible marginal ridges.
6. To produce a restoration with physiologically compatible embrasures.

– Carving can be achieved by Hollenbeck carvers, Ward's carvers, Diamond carvers, Cleiod, Discoid carvers, etc.

– Under carving leaves thin portions of amalgam (subjected to fracture) on the unprepared tooth surface. Such margins give the appearance that the amalgam has expanded beyond the preparation. *The thin portion of amalgam extending beyond the margin is referred to as `flash'.*

MERCURY TOXICITY

– OSHA has set a Threshold Limit Value (TLV) of 0.05 mg/m^3 as the maximum amount of mercury vapour allowed in the work place.

– The lowest dose of mercury that elicits a toxic reaction is 3 to 7 µg/kg body weight.

– The dosage of mercury to cause death is 4000 µg/kg body weight.

– The maximum allowable level of mercury in the blood is 3 µg/kg.

– Free mercury should not be sprayed or exposed to the atmosphere.

– Mercury hazard can arise during trituration, condensation, finishing and polishing of the restoration and also during the removal of old restoration at high speed.

– Skin contact with mercury should be avoided as it can be absorbed by the skin.

– Dentists and dental assistants are having the high risk of mercury intoxication.

– Mercury vapour can be inhaled.

Effects of Mercury Toxicity

1. CNS disturbances: Tremors, headache, depression, insomnia.
2. Excessive salivation.
3. Glossitis, stomatitis.
4. Dark opaque line on the free gingival margin.

Precautions

– Air contamination is managed by proper ventilation.

– Mercury from the carpets is removed by sprinkling the sulphur (sulphur reacts with mercury to form cinnabar which can be easily disposed).

– Excess mercury removed during condensation, mulling, trituration is stored in well sealed jars.

– Adequate use of water or coolant during polishing will minimize the inhalation of mercury vapour.

– Skin contacted with mercury should be thoroughly washed with soap and water.

– Excess mercury should not be thrown into sinks.

– The alloy mercury capsules should have a tightly fitting cap to avoid leakage.

– The excess amalgam spilled on the floor is picked and stored in well sealed containers.

BONDED AMALGAM

– It is a newly introduced concept.

– Amalgam bonding systems are used to seal underlying tooth structure and bond amalgam to enamel and dentin.

– Amalgam is strongly hydrophobic whereas enamel and dentin are hydrophilic. Therefore, the bonding system is modified with a wetting agent which has the capacity to wet both hydrophobic and hydrophilic surfaces.

– The frequently used bonding system is 4-META (4 Methyloxy Ethyl Trimellitic Anhydride).

– The bonding system is applied in thicker layers (10 to 50 µm) to improve micromechanical bonding.

Indication

– Indicated when weakened tooth structure remains and bonding may improve the overall resistance form of the restored tooth.

Advantages

1. Dentin sealing
2. Improved resistance form

Disadvantages

– Poor micromechanical bonding at the interface of amalgam with the bonding system.

GALLIUM ALLOYS

– These are developed to overcome the toxic effects of the mercury.

– In this, gallium is used as the liquid instead of mercury and then it is triturated with a silver, tin, copper alloy powder in the same fashion as dental amalgam.

Gallium Amalgam

– It is a product formed by the reaction of an alloy powder (silver, tin, copper) with a gallium-based liquid alloy (gallium, indium, tin).

Composition

Powder

Silver	-	50%
Tin	-	25.7%
Copper	-	15%
Palladium	-	9%
Trace elements	-	0.3%

Liquid

Gallium	-	65%
Indium	-	18.95%
Tin	-	16%
Trace elements	-	0.5%

– Indium and tin are added to the gallium liquid to decrease its melting temperature.

Structure

– The structure of set alloy consists of a reaction zone of $CuGa_2$ and $PdGa_5$, surrounded by the unreacted zone, which consists of a matrix of Ag_9In_4 and islands of Ag_9Ga_3 and beta-tin particles.

Properties

– Measured at 24 hours.

1.	Compressive strength	-	383 Mpa
2.	Tensile strength	-	57 Mpa
3.	Creep	-	0.17%
4.	Dimensional change	-	16 µm/cm

CHAPTER 02

DENTAL CEMENTS

- Cements are widely used in dentistry for a variety of applications, i.e. for lining, luting, restorative purposes, etc.

Classification

I. Cements-based on Phosphoric acid

1. Zinc phosphate cements.
2. Silicophosphate cements.
3. Copper phosphate cements

II. Cements-based on organometallic chelate compounds

1. Zinc oxide eugenol cements.
2. Ortho-ethoxybenzoic acid (EBA) cements.
3. Calcium hydroxide cements.

III. Cements-based on polyalkenoic acids

1. Polycarboxylate cements.
2. Glass ionomer/polyalkenoate cements.

ZINC PHOSPHATE CEMENT

- *Oldest of the luting cements.*
- It is the traditional crown and bridge cement used for alloy restorations.

COMPOSITION AND SETTING

Powder

ZnO	:	90.2%
MgO	:	8.2%
SiO_2	:	1.4%
Bi_2O_3	:	0.1%
Miscellaneous	:	0.1%

(BaO, Ba_2SO_4, CaO)

Liquid

- Phosphoric acid (free acid) - 38.2%.
- Phosphoric acid (combined with Al and Zn)-16.2%.

Al	-	2.5%
Zn	-	7.1%
H_2O	-	36.0%

- Water controls the ionization of the acid, which in turn influences the rate of the liquid-powder (acid–base) reaction.
- The set cement is a cored structure consisting primarily of unreacted zinc oxide particles embedded in a cohesive amorphous matrix of zinc aluminophosphate.

MANIPULATION

1. *Powder / Liquid Ratio:* 1.4 g powder to 0.5 ml liquid.
2. *Mixing:* The cement is mixed over a large area of the cooled slab to dissipate the heat of the reaction (exothermic reaction).
3. *Mixing Time :* 60–90 sec.
4. *Setting Time:* According to ADA Specification no: 96, it is 2.5–8 min.

PROPERTIES

1. *Consistency and film thickness*
   Luting 25 μm (max).
2. *Strength*
   i. Compressive strength: 96–133 Mpa
   ii. Tensile Strength: 3.1–4.5 Mpa
3. *Retention*
   Bonding occurs by mechanical interlocking at interfaces, not by chemical interactions.
4. *Biological*
   Pulp response is *moderate* as compared with *silicate cement*.
   The pH of the cement two minutes after the start of the mixing is 2.14. The pH then increases rapidly to 5.5 at 24 hour.

APPLICATIONS

1. For luting permanent metal restorations.
2. As a base.
3. For the cementation of orthodontic brackets.

ADVANTAGES

1. Easy manipulation.
2. Sharp setting.
3. Adequate strength after setting.

DISADVANTAGES

1. Pulp irritation.
2. No antibacterial action.
3. Brittleness
4. No adhesion property.
5. Solubility in oral fluids.

SILICO PHOSPHATE CEMENT

- This is a hybrid of zinc phosphate and silicate materials.
- They are supplied as powder and liquid.

- Powder is a mixture of zinc oxide and aluminosilicate glass.
- Liquid is an aqueous solution of phosphoric acid containing buffers.
- The set cement contains a matrix of zinc and aluminium phosphates enclosing unreacted cores of zinc oxide and glass particles.
- It has anticariogenic property.
- Used primarily as luting cements for porcelain crowns because of their extra translucency at the margins.
- Used as temporary filling materials also.

COPPER CEMENT

- Not widely used nowadays.
- They are closely related to the zinc phosphate cements.
- Supplied as powder and liquid.
- Powder is a mixture of zinc oxide and black copper oxide.
- Liquid is an aqueous solution of phosphoric acid.
- It possess bactericidal effect due to the copper.
- They can be used in primary teeth where complete excavation of caries is not possible.
- Used for cementation of splints and orthodontic appliances.

ZINC OXIDE EUGENOL CEMENT

- It is the least irritant among all dental materials (pH is 7 at the time of placement).

COMPOSITION AND SETTING

Powder

ZnO	-	69.0%
White rosin	-	29.3%
Zinc stearate	-	1.0%
Zinc acetate	-	0.7%

Liquid

Eugenol	-	85.0%
Olive oil	-	15.0%

- The setting of ZOE cements is a chelation reaction in which an *amorphous zinc eugenolate* is formed.
- The set material consists of a matrix of amorphous zinc eugenolate that binds the unreacted zinc oxide particles together.

TYPES OF ZOE

– According to ADA Specification no. 30,

Type I	:	Temporary cementation.
Type II	:	Long-term cementation of fixed prosthesis.
Type III	:	Temporary fillings, thermal insulating bases.
Type IV	:	Intermediate restorations.

ADVANTAGES OF ZOE

1. Bland and obtundent effect on pulp.
2. Good sealing ability.
3. Resistance to marginal penetration.

DISADVANTAGES OF ZOE

1. Low strength and abrasion resistance.
2. Solubility in oral fluids.
3. Little anticariogenic action.

MODIFICATIONS OF ZOE

– Two compositional changes have been used to increase the strength of the cement for luting purposes.

1. Polymer reinforced ZOE

– Contains 80% zinc oxide and 20% polymethyl methacrylate in the powder and eugenol in the liquid.

– Can be used for final cementation of fixed prosthesis, cement bases, cavity liners and provisional restorations. Ex : IRM (Type III).

Advantages

1. Minimal biologic effects.
2. Good sealing property.
3. Adequate strength for final cementation.

Disadvantages

1. Higher solubility.
2. Hydrolytic instability.
3. Possible discoloration.

2. EBA - Alumina - reinforced ZOE

– Contains 70% zinc oxide and 30% alumina by weight in the powder.

– The liquid contains 62.5% ortho EBA by weight and 37.5% eugenol by weight.

– It is stronger than reinforced ZOE.

– Has lower solubility.

– Forms a suitable cavity lining for amalgam due to their adequate strength and resistance.

– Primarily used as luting agent.

Advantages

1. Easy manipulation.
2. Long working time.
3. Good flow.
4. Low irritation to pulp.

Disadvantages

1. Critical proportioning.
2. Hydrolytic instability.
3. Poor retention.

MANIPULATION

– Supplied as a powder and liquid or as two pastes.

Mixing time :	30 to 60 sec
Setting Time :	4 to 10 min
	(ADA Specification No. 30)

PROPERTIES

1. *Film thickness*

   For permanent cementation: 25 μm (max).

   For temporary cementation : 40 μm (max).

2. *Strength*

   Compressive strength: 35 Mpa.

3. *Retention*

   By mechanical retention.

4. *Biological*

   Pulp response is *mild* when compared to *silicate cement*.

APPLICATIONS

1. Cement bases
2. Lining of deep cavities
3. As obtundent
4. Temporary cementation
5. Permanent cementation
6. Provisional restorations
7. Endodontic sealers

CALCIUM HYDROXIDE

COMPOSITION AND SETTING: (BASE)

– It is supplied as two pastes system,

1. *Paste I*

Calcium hydroxide	-	50%
Zinc oxide	-	10%
Zinc stearate	-	0.5%
Ethyltoluene sulphonamide	-	39.5%

2. *Paste - II*

Glycol salicylate — 40%

Titanium dioxide

Calcium sulphate

Calcium tungstate

- The setting reaction occurs between calcium hydroxide and salicylate and yields calcium disalicylate.

pH

- Above 12.
- The high pH of calcium hydroxide leads to extreme cytotoxicity of bacteria and there by it is bactiricidal.

COMPOSITION AND SETTING (LINER)

- Calcium hydroxide, used as a cavity liner is suspended in a solvent carrier with a thickening agent.
- When it is placed on the pulpal floor, the solvent evaporates and leaves a thin film of calcium hydroxide.
- It can neutralize acids that migrate toward the pulp and in the process, induce the formation of reparative dentin.

APPLICATIONS

1. Pulp capping procedures.
2. Reparative dentin formation.
3. Liners.
4. Root canal sealer.
5. Low strength base.
6. Perforation repairs.

ADVANTAGES

1. Easy manipulation.
2. Rapid setting in thin layers.
3. Good sealing property.
4. Beneficial effects on carious dentin and exposed pulp.

DISADVANTAGES

1. Low strength.
2. Plastic deformation.
3. Moisture sensitivity.
4. Soluble in acidic conditions.

ZINC POLYCARBOXYLATE CEMENT

- It is also called as *Zinc Poly Acrylate Cement*.
- *It is the first cement system that developed an adhesive bond to tooth structure.*

COMPOSITION AND SETTING

Powder

Zinc Oxide (Mainly)

Magnesium oxide

Stannous fluoride (Small quantities)

Liquid

- An aqueous solution of polyacrylic acid or a copolymer of acrylic acid with other carboxylic acids, such as itaconic acid.
- The acid concentration varies from 32 to 42% by weight.
- The set cement is a zinc polyacrylate ionic gel matrix that unites unreacted zinc oxide particles.

MANIPULATION

1. *Powder / Liquid Ratio*

   1.5 parts of powder to 3 parts of liquid by weight.

2. *Mixing*

   The powder is rapidly incorporated into the liquid in large quantities.

   - If good bonding to tooth structure is to be achieved, the cement must be adapted against the tooth surface before it looses its glossy appearance.
   - The glossy appearance indicates a sufficient amount of free carboxylic acid groups on the surface of the mixture that are vital for bonding to tooth structure.

3. *Mixing Time:* 30–60 sec

4. *Setting Time:* 6–9 min (ADA Specification No. 96)

PROPERTIES

1. *Consistency and Film thickness :* 25–48 µm.

2. *Strength*

   Compressive strength : 57–99 MPa

   Tensile Strength : 3.6–6.3 MPa

3. *Bonding to Tooth Structure*

   - It bonds chemically to the tooth structure.
   - The polyacrylic acid is believed to react with calcium ions via carboxyl groups on the surface of enamel or dentin. *Thus, the bond strength to enamel is greater than that to dentin.*

4. *Biological*

   - Pulp response is *mild* when compared with *silicate cement.*

- The pH of zinc polycarboxylate cement is higher than that of a zinc phosphate cement.
- Its mild irritation is due to that, the larger size of the poly acrylic acid molecule compared with phosphoric acid molecule may limit its diffusion through the dentinal tubules.

APPLICATIONS

1. Primarily for luting permanent alloy restorations and as bases.
2. Also used for cementation of orthodontic bands.

ADVANTAGES

1. Adhesion to tooth structure
2. Less irritation
3. Easy manipulation
4. Strength
5. Film thickness properties

DISADVANTAGES

1. Critical proportioning
2. Lower compressive strength
3. Requires clean surface

GLASS IONOMER CEMENT

- It is "an aqueous based material that hardens following an acid–base reaction between fluoroalumino silicate glass powder and a polyacrylic acid solution" also referred to as conventional GIC.

SYNONYMS

1. Poly alkenoate cement
2. ASPA (Alumino Silicate Polyacrylic Acid)

TYPES

Type I	:	for luting
Type II	:	for restorations
Type III	:	liners and bases

COMPOSITION AND SETTING

Powder

- It is an acid soluble calcium fluoroaluminosilicate glass.

Silica	-	41.9%
Alumina	-	28.6%
Aluminium fluoride	-	1.6%
Calcium fluoride	-	15.7%
Sodium fluoride	-	9.3%
Aluminium phosphate	-	3.8%

- *Lanthanum, strontium, barium* or *zinc oxide* are added to provide radiopacity.

Liquid

- Earlier, the liquids for GIC were aqueous solutions of polyacrylic acid in a concentration of about 40 to 50%. The liquid was quite viscous and tends to gel over time.
- In most of the current cements liquid contains,
  - Polyacrylic acid in the form of copolymer with itaconic, maleic or tricarboxylic acids.
  - Tartaric acid
  - Water
- On mixing the powder and liquid, the acid slowly degrades the outer layers of the glass particles releasing Ca^{2+} and Al^{3+} ions.
- During the early stages of setting, Ca^{2+} is released more rapidly and is primarily responsible for reacting with the poly acid to form a reaction product. Al^{3+} is released more slowly and becomes involved in setting at a later stage, often referred to as a secondary reaction stage.
- The set cement consists of an agglomeration of unreacted powder particles surrounded by a silica gel in an amorphous matrix of hydrated calcium and aluminium polysalts.
- Water serves as the reaction medium initially and then slowly hydrates the cross linked matrix, thereby yielding a stable gel structure that is stronger and less susceptible to moisture.
- If freshly mixed cements are exposed to ambient air without any protective covering, the surface will craze and crack as a result of desiccation.
- Any contamination by water that occurs at this stage can cause dissolution of the matrix forming cations and anions in the surrounding areas.
- Therefore conventional GIC must be protected against desiccation and water changes in the structure during placements.

MANIPULATION

1. **P/L Ratio :** Manufacturer's recommendation to be followed.

2. *Mixing :* It is done on the paper pad with an agate or lastic spatula. Metal spatula is not used because it corrodes the formed matrix.

3. *Mixing time :* 45 to 60 sec.

4. *Setting Time :* According to ADA specification No. 96, it is 2.5 to 6.0 min.

PROPERTIES

1. *Film thickness*

   Luting : 15 μm

   Restorative : 50 μm

2. *Strength*

   Compressive strength : 93–226 Mpa

   Tensile strength : 4.2–5.3 Mpa

3. *Mechanism of Adhesion*

   - The mechanism has not been clearly identified.

   - It primarily involves chelation of carboxyl groups of the poly acids with the calcium in the apatite of the enamel and dentin.

   - The bond strength to enamel is always higher than that to dentin because of the greater inorganic content of enamel and its greater homogenicity.

4. *Biological*

   - Pulp response is *mild* to *moderate*.

   - They elicit a greater pulp reaction than ZOE but generally less than that from zinc phosphate cement.

5. *Anticariogenic*

   - They release fluoride in amounts comparable to those released initially from silicate cement and continue to do so over an extended period.

   - In addition, due to its adhesive effect they have the potential for reducing infiltration of oral fluids at the cement tooth interface, there by preventing secondary caries.

APPLICATIONS

1. Anterior esthetic restorative material for class III cavities.

2. For eroded areas and class V restorations.

3. Luting agents.

4. Liners and bases.

5. Orthodontic bracket adhesives.

6. Pit and fissure sealants.

7. Intermediate resotrations.

ADVANTAGES

1. Esthetics.

2. Low thermal conductivity.

3. No galvanic reaction.

4. Direct restoration.

5. Minimal removal of sound tooth structure.

DISADVANTAGES

1. Technique sensitive.

2. Moisture sensitive.

MODIFICATIONS OF GIC

1. Metal reinforced GIC .

2. Resin modified GIC (Hybrid Ionomer).

3. Compomer.

1. METAL REINFORCED GIC

They were introduced to improve the strength, fracture toughness and resistance to wear.

Types

1. *Silver alloy admixed / miracle mix*

   Spherical amalgam alloy powder is mixed with type - II GIC powder.

2. *Cermet*

   Prepared by fusing glass powder to silver particles through sintering.

Properties

- Nearly same as conventional GIC.

- Metallic fillers have little or no influence on the mechanical properties of restorative glass ionomers.

- They release appreciable amount of fluoride initially, but the magnitude decreases substantially overtime.

Applications

1. Restoration of small class I cavities as an alternative to amalgam or composites.

2. For core build-up of grossly destructed teeth (not be used wherever the cement will constitute greater than 40% of the total core building).

2. RESIN MODIFIED GIC (RMGIC)

Also called as *Hybrid Ionomer*.

Developed to overcome the moisture sensitivity and low early strength of GIC'S.

Composition and Setting Reactions

Powder

- Ion leachable fluoroaluminosilicate glass particles.
- Initiatos for light curing and / or chemical curing.

Liquid

- Water and polyacrylic acid or polyacrylic acid modified with methacrylate and hydroxyethyl methacrylate (HEMA) monomers.
- The initial setting reaction of the material occurs by the polymerization of methacrylate groups. The slow acid–base reaction will ultimately be responsible for the unique maturing process and the final strength.

Advantages

1. Improved translucency.
2. Fluoride release at the same level as conventional GIC .
3. Higher tensile strength.
4. Higher bond strength to tooth structure.

Disadvantages

1. Polymerization shrinkage
2. Microleakages

Applications

1. Liners and bases
2. Fissure sealants
3. Core buildups
4. Restoratives
5. Adhesives for orthodontic brackets
6. Repair materials for damaged amalgam cores or cusps
7. Retrograde root filling materials
8. Cervical lesions
9. Sandwich technique
10. Root caries
11. High caries risk patients

3. COMPOMER

Also known as *poly acid modified composites*.

Developed to get the properties of fluoride releasing capability of conventional GIC and the durability of composites.

Composition and Setting Reaction

1. Single Component System

- Provides as a one paste, light curable material for restorative applications.

- It consists of silicate glass particles, sodium fluoride and polyacid—modified monomer without any water.
- Setting is initiated by photopolymerization of the acidic monomer that yields a rigid material.
- During the service life of the restoration, the set material begins to absorb water in the saliva that contributes the acid–base reaction between the acidic functional groups with in the matrix and silicate glass particles. This reaction eventually sustains fluoride release.
- Because of the absence of water in the formulation the cement mixture is *not self adhesive like conventional GIC and hybrid GIC.*

2. *Two Component System*

- Consists of powder and liquid or of two pastes.
- Used for luting applications.
- The powder is composed of strontium aluminium fluorosilicate, metallic oxides and chemically activated and / or light activated initiators.
- The liquid contains polymerizable methacrylate / carboxylic acid monomers, multifunctional acrylate monomers and water.
- The pastes have same ingredients as powder and liquid.
- Because of the presence of water in the liquid, these materials are self adhesive and an acid base reaction starts at the time of mixing.

Advantages

1. High bond strength
2. High compressive strength
3. High flexural strength
4. Low solubility
5. Sustained fluoride release

Disadvantages

1. Less fluoride release.
2. Physical properties inferior to composites.

Applications

1. Class I and II restorations in children.
2. Cervical lesions.
3. Cementation of cast alloy crowns and bridges, porcelain fused to metal crowns and bridges, gold cast inlays and onlays.
4. Orthodontic bonding.

CHAPTER 03

AGENTS FOR PULP PROTECTION

- Cavity varnishes are natural gums, such as copals, resins, or synthetic resins dissolved in an organic solvent, such as acetone, chloroform or ether.
- They form a coating on the tooth by evaporation of the solvent.
- *Varnishes are applied on all the surfaces of the cavity preparation including the margins·*
- Minimum of two layers of varnish is applied to attain a uniform and continuous coating. When the first layer dries, small pinholes develop. A second or third application fills in most of these voids and thereby producing a more continuous coating.
- *Varnish is not indicated for adhesive materials, such as GIC and resin based composite·*

Uses

1. Reduces microleakage around the margins of newly placed amalgam restorations thereby reducing post-operative sensitivity.
2. Prevent penetration of corrosion products of amalgams into the dentinal tubules thereby reducing the tooth discoloration.
3. Reduces the passage of irritants into the dentinal tubules from the overlying restoration or base.
4. Used as a surface coating over certain restorations to protect them from dehydration or contact with oral fluids.
5. Applied on the metallic restorations as a temporary protection in cases of galvanic shock.

Properties

- Varnishes neither possess mechanical strength nor provide thermal insulation because of inadequate film thickness.
- Contact angles of varnishes on dentin range from 53 to 106 degrees.

CAVITY LINERS

- *Liners are applied only onto the pulpal floor.*

Composition

- Liners are suspensions of calcium hydroxide in an organic liquid such as methyl ethyl ketone or ethyl alcohol or in an aqueous solution of methyl cellulose. On evaporation of the volatile solvent, the liner forms a thin film on the prepared tooth surface.

Properties

– Liners neither possess mechanical strength nor provide any significant thermal insulation.

– Calcium hydroxide liners are soluble and should not be applied at the margins of restorations.

Uses

1. To provide a barrier against the passage of irritants from cements or other restorative materials.

2. To reduce the sensitivity of freshly cut dentin.

3. To accelerate the formation of reparative dentin (due to the presence of calcium hydroxide).

Other Liners

1. Type III glass ionomer.

2. Type IV ZOE.

CEMENT BASES

Cement base

– It is a *material used in the cavity preparation to restore internal outline form and to provide chemical and thermal insulation.*

Intermediary Base

– It is a *material used in the cavity preparation to act as a protective barrier between dentin and the restorative material or to provide some therapeutic benefit to the tooth.*

Classification of Cement Bases

I. *Low Strength Bases*

– Have minimum strength and low rigidity.

– Main function is to act as a barrier to irritating chemicals and to provide therapeutic benefit to the pulp.

Ex: Calcium hydroxide , ZOE.

II. *High Strength Bases*

– Used to provide thermal protection for the pulp and mechanical support for a restoration.

Ex: Zinc phosphate, Zinc polycarboxylate, Glass ionomer, Hybrid ionomer, Compomer, Polymer reinforced ZOE.

Functions

1. To prevent thermal shock.

2. To prevent galvanic shock.

3. To prevent chemical irritation.

4. To support forces of condensation.

5. To support the restoration under masticatory load.

6. To provide therapeutic action.

Thickness of the Base: *0.5 to 0.75 mm*

Clinical Considerations

– The selection of a base depends to an extent by the design of the cavity, the type of restorative material used and the proximity of the pulp relative to the cavity wall.

1. *For amalgam restorations*

   Calcium hydroxide or ZOE.

2. *For direct filling gold*

   Zinc phosphate , Zinc polycarboxylate or GIC.

3. *For resin based composites*

   Calcium hydroxide, GIC.

Principles of Intermediary Basing

1. Do not apply the intermediary base material on margins or surrounding walls but confine it to pulpal and axial walls only.

2. Confine the intermediary base material to the deepest part of the pulpal floor and or the axial walls.

3. Apply in minimal thickness to fulfill the objectives.

4. Therapeutic bases are always very weak so they should be covered with a stronger and more durable base.

Effective Depth

– It is the *area of minimum thickness of sound dentin separating the pulpal tissues from the carious lesion or the thickness of the dentin bridge between the floor of the cavity and the roof of the pulp chamber.*

– The lesser the effective depth, the nearer the irritating ingredients to the pulp, so the more destructive the pulpal reaction will be.

	Effective depth	Reaction on Pulp–Dentin organ
1.	≥ 2 mm	Healthy reparative reaction.
2.	0.8 to 2 mm	Unhealthy reparative reaction.
3.	< 0.3 to 0.8 mm	Pulpal destruction.

Determination of effective depth

– Radiographic method is the most reliable method.

Procedure

On the radiograph, measure the dentin bridge at its deepest portion and the thickness of any clinically measurable anatomical landmark of the tooth. Ex. enamel thickness at the periphery of the preparation on the tooth measure the same anatomical mark. Then follow the following equation.

$$\frac{\text{Effective depth in the radiograph}}{\text{Enamel thickness in the radiograph}} = \frac{\text{Actual effective depth}}{\text{Actual enamel thickness}}$$

$$\text{Actual effective depth} = \frac{\text{Effective in radiograph} \times \text{Actual enamel thickness}}{\text{Enamel thickness in the radiograph}}$$

Disadvantage

– Radiograph is a two dimensional measure rather than three dimensional.

CHAPTER 04

DENTAL INVESTMENTS AND DIE MATERIALS

DENTAL INVESTMENTS

- Investment is defined as a ceramic material that is suitable for forming a mold into which a metal or alloy is cast. The operation of forming the mold is described as *investing*.

IDEAL PROPERTIES

- It should,
  1. Be easily manipulated.
  2. Have sufficient strength at room temperature.
  3. Have stability at higher temperatures.
  4. Have sufficient expansion.
  5. Have beneficial casting temperatures.
  6. Be adequately porous.
  7. Have smooth surface.
  8. Be inexpensive.

COMPOSITION

- In general an investment is a mixture of three distinct types of materials, i.e.

  1. **Refractory material**
     - Usually a form of silicon oxide such as quartz, tridymite or cristoballite or a mixture of these.
     - The purposes are to act as a material that can withstand high temperatures and to regulate the thermal expansion.

  2. **Binder material**
     - It sets and bind together the particles of refractory substance.
     - The common binder used for dental casting gold alloy is α – calcium sulfate hemihydrate.

  3. **Other chemicals**
     - Other chemicals such as sodium chloride, boric acid, potassium sulfate, graphite, copper powder or magnesium oxide are often added in small quantities to modify various physical properties.

Types

- There are three types of investment materials, i.e.
  1. *Gypsum bonded investments.*
  2. *Phosphate bonded investments.*
  3. *Ethyl silica bonded investments.*
- They all contain silica as the refractory material, but the type of binder used is different.

1. GYPSUM BONDED INVESTMENTS

Classification

– According to ADA specification no: 2,

Type I : *Inlay thermal, for casting inlays and crowns.*

Type II : *Inlay hygroscopic, for casting inlays and crowns.*

Type III : *Partial denture, thermal.*

Uses

– Limited to gold castings and other low fusing alloys.

2. PHOSPHATE BONDED INVESTMENTS

– Supplied as a powder containing silica, primary ammonium phosphate ($NH_4H_2PO_4$) and Magnesium oxide (MgO).

– The setting reaction in aqueous solution is,

$$NH_4H_2PO_4 + MgO \longrightarrow NH_4MgPO_4 + H_2O$$

Classification

– According to ADA specification no. 42,

Type I : *For inlays, crowns and other fixed restorations.*

Type II : *For partial dentures and other cast removable restorations.*

Uses

– Used for high fusing alloys (i.e. palladium and base metal alloys) with porcelain.

3. ETHYL SILICA BONDED INVESTMENTS

– Used for high fusing alloys.

Disadvantages

– Gives off flammable components during processing.

– Expensive.

DIE, CAST AND MODEL MATERIALS

DIE: Defined as a *reproduction of a prepared tooth made from a gypsum product, epoxy resin, a metal or a refractory material.*

CAST: Deifned as a *reproduction of the shape and features of a surface made from an impression of the surface.*

MODEL: Defined as a *positive full-scale replica of teeth, soft tissues and restored structures used as a diagnostic aid for construction of orthodontic and prosthetic appliances.*

– Dental stones plaster, electroformed silver and copper, epoxy resin and casting investment are some of the materials used to make casts or dies from dental impressions.

– Impressions in agar or alginate hydrocolloid can be used only with a gypsum material such as plaster, stone or casting investment.

– Compound impressions can be used to produce dies of plaster stone or electroformed copper.

– Various rubber impression materials can be used to prepare gypsum, electroformed or epoxy dies.

1. DENTAL STONES

– The most commonly used die materials are type IV (dental stone, high strength) and type V (dental stone, high strength, high expansion) improved stones.

– Type IV stones have a setting expansion of 0.1% or less and type V has 0.3% in accordance with ADA specification no. 25.

– The greater expansion is useful for compensation of the relatively large solidification shrinkage of base metal alloys.

Advantages

1. Relatively inexpensive.
2. Easy to use.
3. Compatible with all impression materials.
4. Good strength.

Disadvantages

1. Brittle.
2. Susceptibility to abrasion of edges and occlusal surface.

2. ELECTROFORMING

– Also known as *electroplating or electrodeposition*.

– Electroforming is a process by which a thin coating of metal is deposited on the impression.

– Metals used for electroforming are copper and silver; plating can be done for individual tooth impression, full arch impression; plating is done on compound impression; (usually copper plated) polysulphide impression (usually silver plated) and silicone impression.

– Hydrocolloid impressions are extremely difficult to electroplate and the process is not feasable for dental use.

Components

1. *Cathode:* The impression to be coated.

2. *Anode:* The metal to be deposited, i.e. copper or silver.

3. *Anode holder* and *cathode holder*.

4. *Electrolyte:* The solution through which the electric current is passed.

5. *Ammeter:* Registers the current in milliamperes.

6. *Plating tank:* Made of glass or rubber with well fitting cover to prevent evaporation.

Procedure

1. Wash and dry the impression.

2. Attach the impression to the cathode holder with an insulated wire.

3. *Metallizing* the impression to make it to conduct electricity. In this process a thin layer of metal such as silver powder is deposited on the surface of the impression material. The metallizing agents are bronzing powder, aqueous suspensions of silver powder and powdered graphite.

4. The surface of the copper ring or impression tray is covered by wax, 2 mm beyond the impression margin to avoid the plating of ring or the tray.

5. With a dropper, the impression is filled with the electrolyte without air bubbles.

6. The electrode is attached to the cathode and the impression is immersed in the electrolyte bath.

7. The direct current is applied for approximately 10 hr.

8. The current is disconnected. The impression is washed, then the die is completed by pouring dental stone. When the stone hardens, the impression is removed and the die is trimmed.

Advantages

1. Excellent abrasion resistance.

2. Moderately high strength.

3. Dimensional accuracy.

Disadvantages

1. Difficult to trim.

2. Health hazard from silver bath.

3. Not compatible with all impression materials.

3. EPOXY RESINS

– They are most effective with rubber impression materials.

Advantages

Tougher and more abrasion resistant than die materials.

Disadvantages

1. Slight shrinkage.

2. Viscous.

3. More setting time (may take up to 24 hrs).

4. DIVESTMENT

– It is a *die stone investment combination*.

– This is a combination of die material and investing medium.

– A gypsum bonded material called divestment is mixed with a colloidal silica liquid. A die is prepared from the mix and a wax pattern is constructed on it. Then the wax pattern together with die is invested in divestment.

Advantages

1. Possibility of distortion of wax pattern during removal from the die or during setting of the investment is minimized.

2. Highly accurate technique for conventional gold alloys especially for extra coronal preparations.

Disadvantages

Not recommended for high fusing alloys.

Ex: metal ceramic alloys (as it is a gypsum bonded material).

5. DIVESTMENT PHOSPHATE OR DVP

– This is a phosphate bonded investment that is used in the same manner as divestment.

– Suitable for high fusing alloys.

CHAPTER 05

DENTAL CASTING PROCEDURES

- *Casting* can be defined as *The act of forming an object in a mould*.
- The casting procedure is used to make dental restorations such as inlays, onlays, crowns, bridges and removable partial dentures.
- The steps involved in the casting procedure are,
    1. Tooth /teeth preparation
    2. Die preparation
    3. Waxing
    4. Spruing
    5. Casting ringlining
    6. Investing
    7. Burnout
    8. Casting process
    9. Cleaning and finishing of the casting

1. TOOTH/TEETH PREPARATION

- The tooth/teeth are prepared by the dentist to receive a cast restoration.

2. DIE PREPARATION

- A die is prepared from die stone or the impression is electroformed. A die spacer is coated or painted over the die which provides space for the luting cement.

3. WAXING/FORMATION OF THE WAX PATTERN

- There are two fundamental ways to prepare a wax pattern for a dental restoration.
- They are,
    I. Direct wax pattern
    II. Indirect wax pattern

I. Direct wax pattern

- In this direct method, the pattern is prepared on the tooth in the mouth.
- This method can only be used for small inlay restorations.

Technique

- Type I inlay wax is used.
- It is heated sufficiently to have adequate flow and plasticity under compression to reproduce all the details of the prepared cavity.
- Over heating of the wax should be avoided to prevent tissue damage, discomfort to the patient and difficulty in compression of the over heated wax.
- The heating and annealing of the wax is accomplished in a dry-heat oven.

-- Wax may be annealed in water that is at a proper temperature and the storage for longer periods should be avoided under these conditions.

- Prolonged heating of the wax in water, especially at high temperatures, may result in a crymply mass.

- Ample time for cooling (from the working temperature to mouth temperature) should be allowed.

- Adequate compression of the wax is required for forming direct wax patterns.

- Carving instruments should be sufficiently warmed as desirable to soften, but not melt, the wax as the marginal adaptation and contour are developed and to minimize the formation of stresses in the wax.

II. Indirect wax pattern

- In this method, a model (die) of the tooth is first made, and then the pattern is made on the die.

- This method is used for all types of restorations.

Technique

- A metal or stone die is used in indirect method, which is the positive replica of a portion of the surrounding tooth structure and the cavity preparation.

- Type II inlay wax is used.

- The advantage of the indirect method is, it makes the property of flow less critical, because pattern may be removed at a lower temperature and with greater ease from the die.

- A lubricant is applied to the die to release the wax pattern from the die (In the mouth saliva or dentinal fluid acts as lubricant). Excess seperator should be avoided as it results in the inaccuracies in the wax pattern and poor surface of the cast alloy.

- The wax may be adapted to the die either by the flowing of small melted increments from a spatula to build-up the desired contour or by the compression method as in direct method.

- The metal die is warmed throughout to near body temperature, so that the wax solidifies more evenly throughout its mass, resulting in better adaptation.

- The die can be warmed by placing it under an electric lamp or on an electric heating pad that is at a suitable temperature.

- The wax pattern is carved with a warm instrument, to minimize the formation of stresses in the wax.

4. SPRUING

I. Definition: Sprue is defined as *The mold channel through which molten metal or ceramic flows into the mold cavity.*

II. Purpose of spuruing

1. To form a mount for the wax pattern.

2. To create a channel for the elimination of wax during burn out.

3. To form a channel for the flowing-in of molten alloy during casting.

4. To compensate for alloy shrinkage during solidification procedure.

III. Sprue size and design

- Large inlays require sprues that are 14-gauge (4 to 5 mm long) and small inlays require 16-gauge (3 to 4 mm long) sprues.

- Large crowns require 10-gauge sprues and small crowns require 12-gauge sprues with an average sprue length of 4 to 5 mm.

IV. Types / selection of sprue materials

- Several types of materials are used for sprues, depending on the type of restoration being cast.

- For small inlays, a hollow-metal sprue may be used.

- Round wax is a commonly used sprue material for many restorations of all sizes.

- Plastic sprues have also been used for casting.

V. Sprue diameter

- The sprue former should have a diameter that is approximately the same size as the thickest area of the wax pattern.

- Attaching a large sprue former to a thin delicate pattern could cause distortion.

- If the sprue former diameter is too small than the molten metal in this area will solidify before the casting itself and localized shrinkage porosity develops.

- The Y-sprue design is often used on MOD inlay restorations.

VI. Sprue location

- The ideal area for the spure former is the point of greatest bulk in the pattern to avoid distorting thin areas of wax during attachment to the pattern and to permit complete flow of the alloy into the mold cavity.

VII. Sprue direction

- The sprue should be directed toward the margins such that it minimizes the turbulence of the flow of the molten metal and favours the fine margins of the wax pattern.

- To get a satisfactory casting it is attached at a 45 degree angle to the proximal area.

VIII. Sprue length

- The wax pattern should be positioned approximately 6 mm from the end of the casting ring.

- If it is less than 6 mm of space, there is not enough thickness of investment to keep the molten alloy from breaking through.

- If is is more than 6 mm of space, the alloy will solidify before the escape of entrapped air, resulting in rounded margins, incomplete casting, mold fracture, etc.

IX. Sprue attachment

- Once the sprue is attached to the restoration the other end of the sprue is attached to a sprue base usually made of hard rubber.

- As with the attachment of the sprue to the restoration, the base-sprue attachment should avoid sharp corners to ensure smooth non turbulent flow of the **metal** into the pattern during casting.

- A reservoir should be **added** to a sprue network to prevent localized shrinkage porosity. When the molten alloy fills the heated casting ring the pattern area should solidify first and the reservoir last. Because of its large mass of alloy and position in the heat center of the ring, the resevoir remains molten to furnish liquid alloy into the mold as it solidifies

5. CASTING RING LINING

Purposes

1. Allows for mould expansion.
2. Reduces the heat loss (as it is a thermal insulator) when the ring is transferred from the furnace to the casting.
3. Permits the easy removal of the investment after casting.

Types of Ring liners

I. Asbestos ring liners

Use has been discontinued due to its health hazards.

II. Non-asbestos ring liners

1. Alumino silicate ceramic liner
2. Cellulose (paper) liner

Placement

- The ceramic paper liner is cut to fit the inside of the metal ring and is held in place with the finger.

- The ring with the liner is then dipped into water until the liner is completely wet and water is dripping from it.

- After the liner has been soaked, it should not be touched because this reduces the cushioning effect, which is needed for the lateral expansion of the investment.

- The liner is 3 mm short of the top and bottom of the ring to lock in the investment during burn out and casting.

6. INVESTING

- Investing is the process by which the sprued wax pattern is embedded in a material called an investment.

- Gypsum and phoshate bonded investment materials are the two types of materials used for this purpose.

- A casting ring is added to contain the investment while the investment material is poured carefully around the pattern.

Procedure

- A wetting agent is applied on the wax pattern to reduce air bubbles.

- Place the casting ring into the crucible former so that the wax pattern is located near the centre of the ring.

- Mix the investment in a vaccum mixer and vibrate.

- Some investment is applied on the wax pattern with a brush to reduce the trapping of air bubbles.

- The ring is reseated on the crucible former and placed on the vibrator and gradually filled with the remaining investment mix. Allow it to set for 1 hour.

7. BURNOUT

- *Burnout is the process of heating an invested mold to eliminate the embedded wax or plastic pattern.*

Purpose

1. To eliminate the wax (pattern) from the mould.
2. To expand the mould (thermal expansion).

Procedure

- Separate the crucible former from the ring; if a metallic sprue former is used it should be removed before burnout.

- Burnout is started when the mould is wet.
- The heating should be gradual. Rapid heating produces steam which causes the walls of the mould cavity to flake and also causes cracks in the investment due to uneven expansion.
- The ring is placed in a burnout furnace and heated gradually to 400°C in 20 min. Maintain it for 30 min. In the next 30 min raise the temperature to 700°C and again maintain it for 30 min.
- The casting should be completed as soon as the ring is ready. If casting is delayed the ring cools and the investment contracts and the crown becomes smaller.

8. CASTING PROCESS

- It involves the process of melting the casting alloy and forcing the molten alloy into the mold by using casting machines.

I. Melting of the Alloy

- There are two methods of alloy melting, i.e.
  - i. Torch melting
  - ii. Electrical melting

i. Torch Melting

- Most common method of melting.
- Used for melting of gold alloys.
- The natural gas / air is used by using a torch.

ii. Electrical melting

- It includes electric resistane melting which uses a furnace with a carbon or ceramic crucible.
- Can be used for all types of alloys.

II. Casting Machines

1. Casting Crucible

- It is a refractory device which is that part of the casting machine, upon which the alloy is seated.
- There are four types of casting crucibles are available, i.e. clay, carbon, quartz and zirconia - alumina.
- Clay crucibles are used for crown and bridge alloys.
- Carbon crucibles are used for both crown and bridge alloys and also for higher fusing gold based metal ceramic alloys.
- Crucibles made from alumna, quartz or silica are recommended for high fusing alloys of any type.

2. Types of Casting Machines

i. Centrifugal force type

- Available as spring driven or motor driven.
- It rapidly spins the mold, crucible and molten alloy in a circle. Casting occurs when the spinning starts suddenly.
- The advantages are simplicity of design and operation with the opportunity to cast both large and small castings on the same machine.

ii. Vacuum / Air pressure type

- Either compressed air or gases like carbon dioxide or nitrogen can be used to force the molten metal into the mould.
- The crucible and casting ring are stationary and only the molten metal moves.
- Used to make small casting.

III. Casting Procedure

- When the alloy is molten, it has a mirror like appearance like a ball of mercury.
- The hot casting ring is then shifted from the burnout furnace to the casting machine.
- Place the ring in the casting cradle so that the sprue hole adjoins the crucible.
- Sprinkle flux powder over the molten metal to reduce the oxides and increase its fluidity for casting.
- Release the arm and allow it to rotate till it comes to rest. This create centrifugal force which forces the metal into the mold cavity.

9. CLEANING AND FINISHING OF THE CASTING

1. Quenching

- It is done for gold alloys.
- After the casting has solidified, the ring is removed and quenched in water.

Advantages

1. The alloy is left in an annealed (softened) condition for burnishing, polishing and similar procedures.
2. The investment becomes soft and granular, and is easily removed.

2. Recovery of casting

- The investment is removed and the casting is recovered.

3. Pickling

- *It is a process of removal of surface films which consists of heating the discolored casting in an acid.*

– The acids used are 50% hydrochloric acid and sulphuric acid.

– The disadvantages of HCl are corrosion health hazard fumes.

4. Polishing

– Minimum polishing is required if all the procedures from the wax pattern to casting are followed meticulously.

CASTING DEFECTS

– The casting defects are classified into,

1. Distortion
2. Surface roughness and irregularities
3. Porosity
4. Incomplete or missing detail

1. Distortion

– Distortion of the casting is due to the distortion of the wax pattern.

– It is minimized by the proper manipulation of wax and handling of the pattern.

2. Surface Roughness

– It is usually be traced to,

1. Air bubbles on wax pattern which can be avoided by proper mixing of investment and application of wetting agent.
2. Too rapid heating cracks the investment resulting in fins which can be avoided by heating the ring gradually to 700°C.
3. Higher w/p ratio gives rougher casting which can be avoided by using correct w/p ratio.
4. Composition of investment: Proportion of quartz and binder influences the surface texture of casting.

3. Porosity

– Porosity may internal or external.

– Porosities are classified as,

1. *Solidification defects*

i. Localized shrinkage porosity

ii. Microporosity

2. *Trapped gases*

i. Pin hole porosity

ii. Gas inclusions

iii. Subsurface porosity

3. *Residual air*

i. *Localized shrinkage porosity*

– Caused by premature termination of the flow of molten metal during solidification.

– Generally occurs near the sprue casting junction.

– Can be avoided by using sprue of correct thickness, attaching sprue to thickest portion of wax pattern and placing a reservoir close to the wax pattern.

Suck-back porosity

– Often occurs at an occluso axial line angle or inciso axial line angle that is not well rounded.

– The entering metal impinges on to the mold surface at this point and creates a higher localized mold temperature in this region known as a hot spot.

– Suck back porosity can be eliminated by flaring the point of sprue attachment and reducing the mold - melt temperature differential, i.e. lowering the casting temperature by about 300°C.

ii. *Microporosity*

– It results in small irregular voids.

– It occurs from rapid solidification if the mold or casting temperature is too low.

– It can be reduced by increasing the melting temperature of the metal and mould temperature.

iii. *Pin hole porosity*

– Results from the entrapment of gas during solidification.

– Many metals dissolve or occlude gases while they are molten. On solidification, the absorbed gases are expelled and thus pinhole porosity results.

– It can be minimized by premelting the gold alloy on a graphite crucible or a graphite block if the alloy has been used before.

iv. *Gas inclusion porosity*

– It is also results from the entrapment of gas during solidification and are usually much larger than pin hole porosities.

– These porosities are caused by gas occluded from a poorly adjusted torch flame or by use of the mixing or oxidizing zones of the flame rather than the reducing zone.

– It can be avoided by correctly adjusting and positioning the torch flame during melting.

v. *Sub surface porosity*

– They may be caused by the simultaneous nucleation of solid grains and gas bubbles at the first moment that the alloy freezes at the mold walls.

– Can be diminished by controlling the rate at which the molten metal enters the mold.

vi. *Entrapped-air porosity / Back pressure porosity*

– It produces large concave depressions which are caused by the inability of the air in the mold to escape through the pores in the investment or by the pressure gradient that displaces the air pocket toward the end of the investment via the molten sprue and button.

– It is frequently found in a 'pocket' at the cavity surface of a crown on mesio occlusal distal casting.

– It can be eliminated by proper burnout, an adequate mold and casting temperature, a sufficiently high casting pressure and proper P/L ratio.

4. Incomplete Casting

– It is due to the molten alloy that has been prevented from completely filling the mold.

– The causes are,
  – Use of insufficient alloy
  – High viscosity of the alloy
  – Premature solidification of alloy
  – Insufficient venting of the mold
  – Low casting pressure

CHAPTER 06

DENTAL CERAMICS

CERAMIC

– Defined as *an inorganic compound with nonmetallic properties typically composed of metallic (or semimetallic) and nonmetallic elements* (Ex: Al_2O_3, CaO and Si_3N^4).

DENTAL CERAMIC

– Defined as *an inorganic compound with nonmetallic properties typically consisting of oxygen and one or more metallic or semimetallic elements* (Ex. Aluminium, calcium, lithium, magnesium, potassium, silicon, sodium, tin, titanium and zirconium) *that is formulated to produce the whole or part of a ceramic based dental prosthesis.*

CLASSIFICATION

I. *According to their use or indications*

1. Anterior
2. Posterior
3. Crowns
4. Veneers
5. Post and cores
6. FPD's
7. Stain ceramic
8. Glaze ceramic

II. *According to composition*

1. Pure alumina
2. Pure zirconia
3. Silica glass
4. Leucite-based glass-ceramic
5. Lithi-based glass ceramic

III. *According to processing method*

1. Sintering
2. Partial sintering
3. Glass infiltration
4. CAD-CAM
5. Copy milling

IV. *According to firing temperature*

1. Ultra-low fusing: < 850°C
2. Low-fusing: 850-1100°C
3. Medium-fusing: 1101–1300°C
4. High-fusing: > 1300°C

V. *According to microstructure*

1. Glass
2. Crystalline
3. Crystal-containing glass

VI. According to translucency

1. Opaque
2. Translucent
3. Transparent

APPLICATIONS

1. Ceramics for metal crowns and FPD's.
2. All-ceramic crowns, inlays, onlays and veneers.
3. Ceramic denture teeth.

COMPOSITION

- SiO_2, Al_2O_3, CaO, Na_2O, K_2O, B_2O_3, ZnO, ZrO_2 others like barium oxide, tin oxide, lithium oxide, etc.

PROCESSING

1. Sintering / Firing

- The process of heating closely packed particles to a specified temperature (below the melting point of the main component) to densify and strengthen a structure as a result of bonding, diffusion and flow phenomena.
- It can be done either by *temperature control alone* (the furnace temperature is raised at constant rate until a specified temperature is reached) or *by controlled temperature and a specified time* (the temperature is raised at a given rate until certain levels are reached, after which the temperature is maintained for a measured period until the desired reactions are completed).

2. Glazing

Natural glaze/Auto glazed/Self-glazed

A vitrified layer that forms on the surface of a dental ceramic containing glass phase when the ceramic is heated to a glazing temperature for a specified time.

Over glaze

The surface coating of glass formed by fusing a thin layer of glass powder that matures at a lower temperature than that associated with the ceramic substrate.

Over glazing should be avoided.

Disadvantages

1. Gives unnatural shiny appearance.
2. Causes loss of contour.
3. Causes shade modification.

Advantages of Glazing

1. Reduces crack propagation.
2. Increases strength.

CERAMIC MATERIALS

1. DICOR

- It is commercially available (castable ceramic).
- It was developed by corning glass works.
- Dicor is a castable glass that is formed into an inlay, facial veneer, or full-crown restoration by a lost-wax casting process similar to that employed for metals.
- Dicor glass-ceramic contains about 55 vol % of tetra silicic fluoromica crystals.

Advantages

1. Ease of fabrication.
2. Improved esthetics.
3. Minimal processing shrinkage.
4. Good marginal fit.
5. Moderately high flexural strength.
6. Low thermal expansion.
7. Minimal abrasiveness.

Disadvantages

1. Limited use in low-stress areas.
2. Inability to colour internally.
3. Decreased translucency.

Dicor MGC

- It is Dicor-Machinable glass ceramic.
- Dicor MGC is a higher quality product provided as CAD-CAM blanks or ingots.
- It contains 70 vol% tetra silicic fluormica platelets.
- Mechanical properties are similar to Dicor but has less translucency.

2. IN-CERAM

- It is supplied in three forms, i.e.

1. In-ceram spinell,
2. In ceram alumina, and
3. In-ceram zirconia.

1. In-Ceram Spinell (ICS)

- It consists of glass-infiltrated magnesium spinel ($MgAl_2O_4$).
- It is indicated for use as anterior single-unit inlays, onlays, crowns and veneers.
- Has greater translucency but lower strength and toughness than other types.

2. *In-Ceram Alumina (ICA)*

   – It consists of 70 wt% alumina infiltrated with 30 wt% sodium lanthanum glass.

   – It is indicated for anterior and posterior crowns and anterior three-unit FPD's.

   – Its advantages are moderately high flexural strength and fracture toughness, metal free structure, ability to be used successfully with conventional luting agents.

   – The disadvantages are poor marginal fit, high degree of opacity, inability to be elicited, technique sensitivity.

3. *In-Ceram Zirconia (ICZ)*

   – It contains approx. 30wt% zirconia, and 70wt% alumina.

   – It is indicated for posterior crowns and FPD's.

   – It is the strongest and toughest of the three types.

   – Its disadvantages are same as ICA.

4. ALUMINOUS PORCELAIN

   – Earlier, conventional ceramics are of low strength.

   – To compensate the strength, aluminous porcelain is developed which is similar to that of conventional porcelain but with increased alumina content (40–50%).

   – Alumina is used to build core over which conventional body and enamel porcelain are condensed and fired.

   Advantages

   1. Decreased crack formation.
   2. Increased strength than that of conventional porcelains.
   3. Less expensive than metal ceramic.
   4. Increased esthetics.

Section IV

Pre-Clinical
Operative Work Area

CHAPTER 01

PRE - CLINICAL OPERATIVE WORK AREA

1. PHANTOM HEAD

– Instead of a patient, there will be a phantom head (Fig. 1.1), which simulates the natural environment existing in a patiet to give the student, a prelude (introduction) of the working conditions in a clinical environment.

– A phantom head has provisions for attaching an upper arch and a lower arch. It also has a rubber face mask to give the student an idea about the limited access in the oral cavity.

– Phantom head can be tilted in an up and downward directions and in sides to permit the easy access and good visibility.

– The height of the phantom head can be adjusted depending on the need.

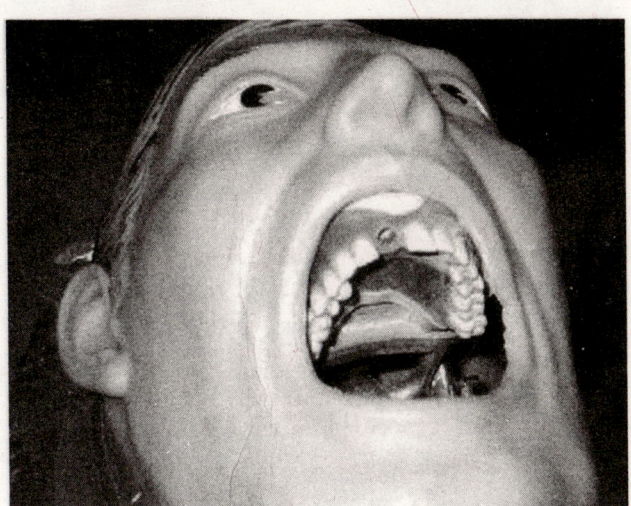

Fig. 1.1

2. TYPE OF TEETH USED

– Most of the colleges use readymade acrylic teeth (typhodont teeth) mounted on an acrylic base specially made for the preclinical student training (Fig. 1.2). (Natural teeth are also used).

– The acrylic base has a nut on the filting surface that can be fixed to the screw in the phantom head.

– The individual teeth are attached to the base either with individual screws or a friction grip.

– The advantages of Typhodant teeth are: (1) available in proportionate sizes, (2) standardized occlusion is achieved.

– The advantages of natural teeth are: (1) get the feeling of cutting enamel and dentin, (2) economical.

– The disadvantages are no proper occlusion as they are obtaining from various sources.

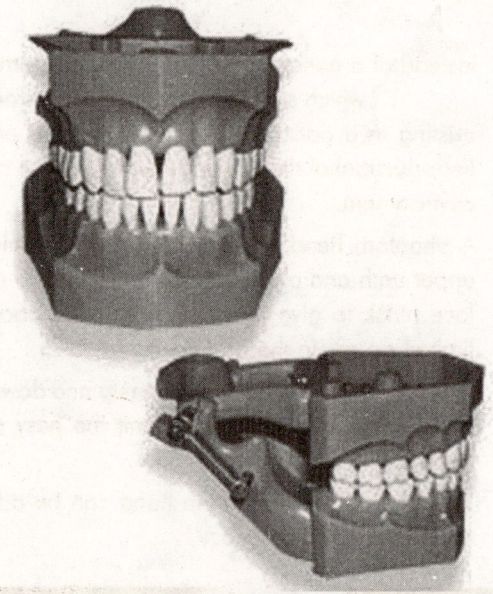

Fig. 1.2

3. LIGHTING

– Each phantom head will have one operating focus light with flexible arm.

– It should be directed to the operating area with a distance of 18 inches.

4. INSTRUMENTS ARRANGEMENT

– A clean set of instruments should be arranged in a proper sequence on the operating tray.

– If the tray is not available, the instruments should be arranged on the work table over a clean green cloth.

– Instruments should be arranged in the probable working order.

– After using every instrument, it should be returned to its alloted place, this type of working principles improves the operator's efficiency.

5. MAINTAINANCE OF STERILITY

– Sterility may not be needed for preclinical working area, but absolute cleanliness is mandatory.

– The student should be dressed in clean and should always wear a clean lab coat.

– Nails should be pared with well groomed hair and should give a neat and clean appearance.

6. TYPE OF CAVITIES PREPARED IN THE PRECLINICAL TRAINING

– During the preclinical training, cavities are prepared on noncarious teeth. In these cavities, the outline form is not affected by the extent of caries.

– The depth and the width of the cavity are kept at minimum.

– In short, ideal cavities are prepared by the student.

– The idea of preclinical training is only to obtain hand control and precision.

– When a student knows what features are expected in an ideal cavity (Figs 1.3–1.5) then he will be able to incorporate those features in the cavity.

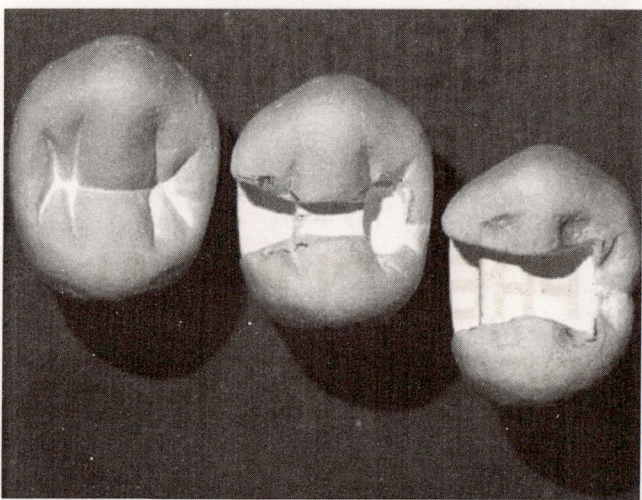

Fig. 1.3

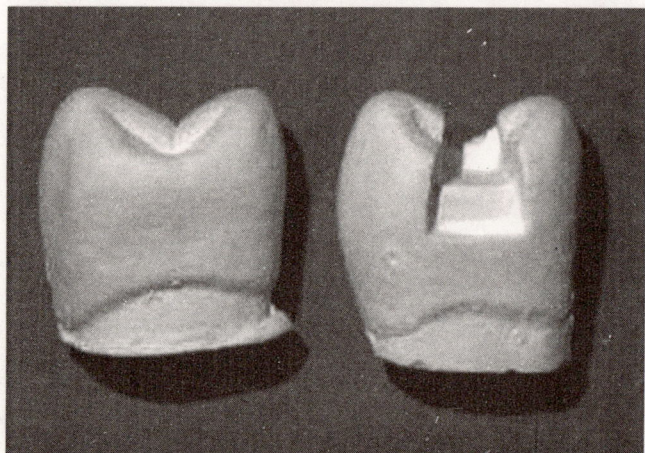

Fig. 1.4

7. PRELIMINARY CONSIDERATIONS AT THE WORK AREA

1. Adjustment of the phantom head at the proper position (at elbow level of the operator).

2. Adjustment of the operating stool for confortable seating at the correct operating position depending on the tooth to be worked upon (see the detail in Section V).

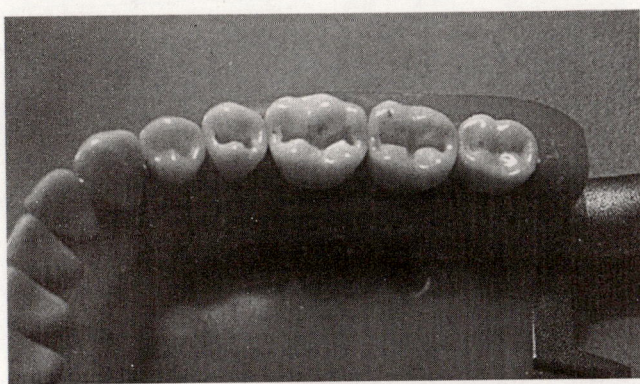

Fig. 1.5

3. Check the handpiece for the appropriate bur having been fixed firmly.

4. Arrangement of hand instruments in the proper order (Fig. 1.6).

5. Decision about the outline of the cavity and having a clear mental picture of the extent of the cavity.

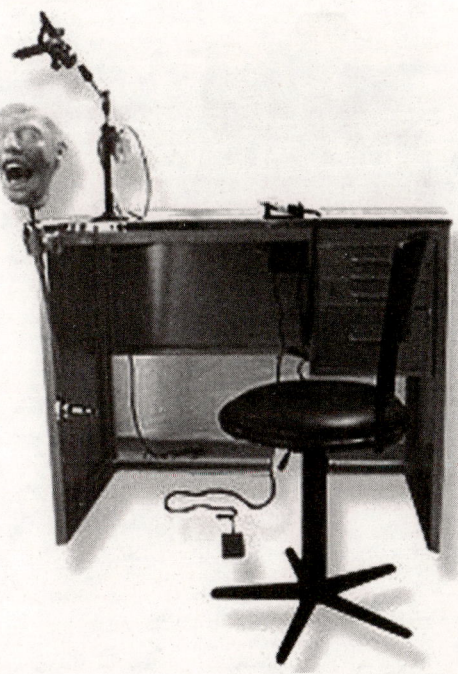

Fig. 1.6

Section V

Foundation to Clinical Dentistry

INFECTION CONTROL IN DENTISTRY

Dental staff and patients may be exposed to a wide variety of disease causing microorganisms that may be transmitted in the dental clinic. Diseases such as Hepatitis, HIV infection, Herpes, Tuberculosis have been joined by new diseases such as severe acute respiratory syndrome (SARS). The Microbiology subject in 2nd year BDS will provide you with the necessary foundation to understand the organisms that cause disease and introduce you to some of the diseases of concern for dentistry. The step - by - step procedures in the following sections will guide you through instrument processing, surface and equipment disinfection and personal protective wear. As new diseases evolve, dental healthcare professionals must adopt the newest and most effective infection-control techniques to prevent transmission in the dental setting.

MODES OF DISEASE TRANSMISSION

– These are four primary modes of diseases transmission in dentistry, i.e.

1. **Direct Contact**
   – Touching or contact with the patient's blood or other body fluids.

2. **Indirect Contact**
   – Touching or contact with a contaminated suface or instrument.

3. **Droplet Infection**
   – An infection that occurs through mucosal surfaces of the eyes, nose or mouth.

4. **Parenteral Transmission**
   – 'Parenteral' means through the skin.
   – Infection can occur though needlestick injuries, human bites, cuts, abrasions or any break in the skin.

DISEASE TRANSMISSION IN THE DENTAL OFFICE

– It can occur in a variety of ways, such as,
   1. 'Parenteral'.
   2. Dental team to patient.
   3. Dental office to community.
   4. Community to dental office to patient.

REGULATORY BODIES

– *OSHA:* Occupational Safety and Health Act was passed by U.S. Congress in 1970.

– *SOPS :* Standard Operating Procedures is a term used in former OSHA regulations.

REGULATIONS OF OSHA

1. Provision for hepatitis B vaccination.

2. Universal precautions such as,
   - Careful handling of sharp instruments.
   - Use of devices to reduce contamination risks (High volume suction, Rubberdam and Protective sharp containers).

3. Personal protective equipment: Gloves, Mask, Gown.

4. House keeping is term related to clean-up instruments, operatory equipment, floors, walls and management of waste, sterilization procedures.

5. Implement engineering controls to reduce the production of contaminated spatter, mist, aerosol. Ex : Rubberdam, High volume suction.

6. Implementation of work practice controls to minimize the splashing, spatter or contact of bare hands with contaminated surfaces. Ex: When using the brush to scrub instruments hold the instruments well down in the sink and brush away from yourself.

7. Never contact telephones, switches, door handles with soiled gloves.

8. Safe handling of needles.

9. Provision of proper washing facilities–washing hands after removing gloves.

10. Maintenance of proper sterilization of instruments.

11. Removal of blood contaminated waste properly and disposed thoroughly.

12. Provision of laundering of protective garments used for universal precautions.

INFECTION CONTROL PRACTICES

I. HANDWASHING

PURPOSES

1. Removes surface dirt and transient bacteria.

2. Dissolves the normal greasy film on the skin.

3. Rinses and removes all loosened debris and micro-organisms.

4. Provides disinfection with a long - acting antisetpic.

INDICATIONS

1. Before and after treating each pateint (before glove placement and after glove removal).

2. Before regloving (after removing gloves that are torn, cut or punctured).

3. After bare handed touching inanimate objects that may be contaminated with blood or saliva.

4. When hands are visibly soiled.

5. Before leaving the treatment room.

TYPES

1. Routine Handwash

   Materials: Water and nonantimicrobial soap (plain soap).

   Purpose: To remove soil and transient microorganisms.

   Procedure

   1. Wet the hands, apply soap (avoid hot water).

   2. Rub the hands together for at least 15 seconds ; cover all surfaces of fingers, hands and wrists.

   3. Rinse under running water.

   4. Dry thoroughly with disposable towels.

   5. Turn-off the tap with the towel.

2. Antiseptic Handwash

   Materials: Water and antimicrobial liquid soap (Ex: chlorhexidine, iodine and iodophors, triclosan, etc.).

   Purpose: To remove or destroy transient microorganisms and reduce resident flora.

   Procedure

   1. Remove watch and jewelery from hands.

   2. Tie the hair back securely.

   3. Wear protective eyewear and face mask before handwashing to prevent contamination of washed hands that are ready for gloving.

   4. Use cool water.

   5. Apply hands, wrists and forearms quickly with liquid antimicrobial soap.

   6. Rub all surfaces vigorously.

   7. Rinse thoroughly, running the water from finger tips down the hands, keep water running.

   8. Repeat two more times (one lathering for 3 min. is less effective than are 3 short latherings and 3 rinses in 30 sec. The latherings serve to loosen the debris and microorganisms and the rinsings wash them away).

   9. Use paper towels for drying and taking care not to recontaminate.

3. Antiseptic Hand Rub

Materials: Alcohol-based hand rub (contains 60 - 95% ethanol or isopronol).

Purpose: To remove or destroy transient microorganisms and reduce resident flora.

Procedure

1. Decontaminate the hands with an alcohol-based hand rub.

2. Apply the product (follow manufacturer's directions for amount to use) to the palm of one hand and rub hands together.

3. Rub the hands vigorously, covering all surfaces of fingers and hands, until the hands are dry.

4. Surgical Antisepsis / Surgical Scrub

Materials: Water and antimicrobial liquid soap.

Purpose

1. To remove or destroy transient microorganisms.

2. To reduce resident flora with a persistent or prolonged effect that inhibits proliferation or survival of microorgansims.

Procedure

1. Remove all jewellery.

2. Cover your hair and wear the protective eye-wear and face mask before performing a surgical scrub.

3. Under running water, use the orange stick to clean under your nails. Discard the stick and rinse your hands without touching the fancet or inside of the sink.

4. Wet the hands and forearms up to the elbows with warm water and then dispense about 5 ml of antimicrobial soap into cupped hands.

5. Use the surgical scrub brush to scrub the hands and forearms for seven minutes.

6. Rinse thoroughly with warm water, keep your hands up and above waist level. (This allows the water to run toward the elbows, keeping hands, clean).

7. Dispense another 5 ml of antimicrobial soap and repeat the scrub.

8. Wash for an additional seven minutes without using a brush. Rinse, so that the contaminated water runs down the arms and off the elbows.

9. Dry the hands and arms with a sterile towel, use a patting motion and continue up the forearms.

10. Keep your hands above your waist before wearing your sterile gown.

II. PERSONAL PROTECTIVE EQUIPMENT (PPE)

- It include protective clothing, protective masks, protective eye wear and gloves.

- Because dental team members are likely to come in contact with blood and saliva, they must wear PPE whenever they are performing procedures that may produce splash, spatter, acrosol or other contact with body fluids.

- We must also wear appropriate PPE when performing other clinical activities such as processing dental radiographs, handling dentures and other prosthetic appliances or contaminated equipment and surfaces.

1. PROTECTIVE CLOTHING

Purpose: To protect the skin and underclothing from exposure to saliva, blood, aerosol and other contaminated materials.

Types: Include smocks, pants, skirts, laboratory coats, surgical scrubs (hospital operating room clothing), scrub (surgical) hats and shoe covers.

Requirements

1. Should be made of fluid-resistant material.

2. Clothing should have long sleeves and a high neckline to minimize the amount of uncovered skin.

3. The design of the sleeve should allow the cuff to be tucked inside the band of the glove.

4. Protective clothing must cover dental personnel at least to the knees when seated.

5. Buttons, zippers and other ornamentation (which may harbour pathogens) should be kept to a minimum.

2. PROTECTIVE MASKS

- Worn over the nose and mouth.

Purpose: To protect from inhaling infectious organisms spread by the aerosol spray of the handpiece or air–water syringe and by accidental splashes.

Types:

1. *Dome shaped* - move prefer for lengthy procedures because, confirms (molds) more effectively to the face and creates an air space between the mask and the wearer (Fig. 1.1).

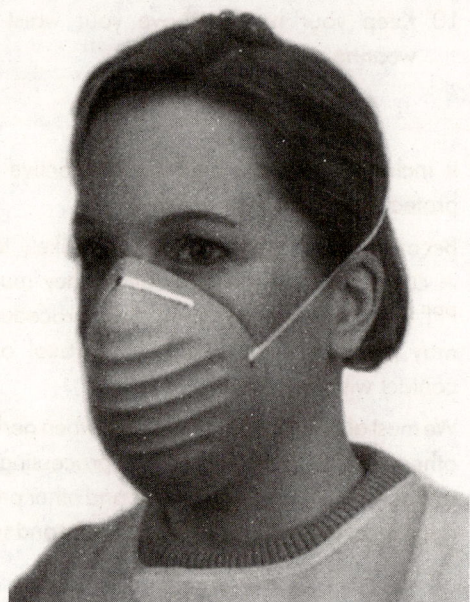

Fig. 1.1

2. *Flat type* (Fig. 1.2)

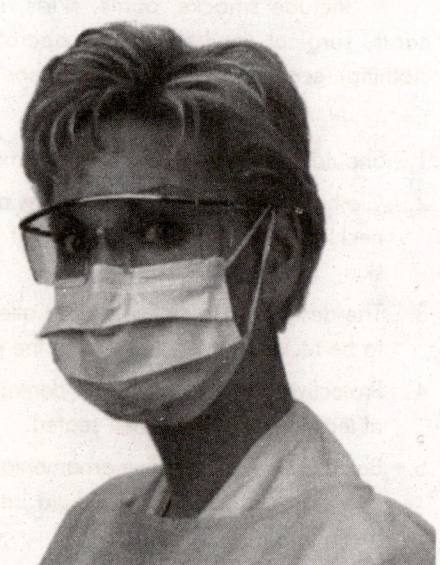

Fig. 1.2

Guidelines for the use of masks

– Masks should,
1. Be changed for every patient.
2. Be handled by touching only the side edges to avoid contact with the more heavily contaminated body of the mask.
3. Confirm to the shape of the face.
4. Not contact the mouth when being worn because the moisture generated will decrease the mask filtration efficiency.
5. A damp or wet mask is not an effective mask.

Characteristics:

– Face mask should,
1. Not contact with the wearer's nostrils or lips.
2. Have a high bacterial filtration efficiency rate.
3. Fit snugly around the entire edges of the mask.
4. Not fog eyewear.
5. Be convenient to put on and remove.
6. Be made of material that does not irritate skin or induce allergic reaction.
7. Not collapse during wear or when wet.

Materials used

– Various materials are used, i.e. gauze and other cloth, plastic foam, fiberglass, synthetic fiber mat and paper.

3. PROTECTIVE EYE WEAR

Purpose

– To protect the eyes,
1. Against damage from aerosolized pathogens.
2. From flying debris such as scrap amalgam and tooth fragments.
3. From the injury by splattered solutions and caustic chemicals.
– Eyewear should hve both front and side protection (solid side shields).

Types

1. *Glasses with protective side shields* (Fig. 1.3)

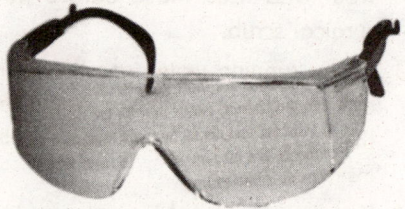

Fig. 1.3

2. *Clear face shields* (Fig. 1.4)

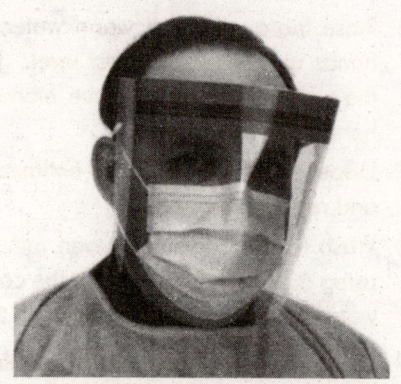

Fig. 1.4

Patient Eyewear

– Patients should be provided with protective eyewear because they also may be subject to eye damage from,

1. Handpiece spatter.
2. Spilled or splashed dental materials.
3. Airborn bits of acrylic or tooth fragments.

4. GLOVES AND GLOVING

– Wearing gloves is a standard practice to protect both the patient and the dentist from cross-contamination.

Types of Gloves

1. Examination / Treatment Gloves

– Usually made of latex or vinyl.
– Are inexpensive and are available in a range of sizes from extra small to extra large and fit either hand.
– Are nonsterile and serve strictly as a protective barrier for the wearer.
– Gloves are effective only when they are intact (not damaged, torn, ripped or punctured). If gloves are damaged during treatment, change them immediately and wash your hands before regloving.

2. Sterile Surgical Gloves

– They are the type used in hospital operating rooms.
– Should wear for invasive procedures involving the cutting of bone or significant amounts of blood or saliva such as oral surgery or periodontal treatment.
– Sterile gloves are supplied in prepackaged units to maintain sterility before use.
– They are provided in specific sizes and are fitted to the left or right hand.

3. Utility Gloves

– They are not used for direct patient care.
– They should wear,
  1. When the treatment room is cleaned and disinfected between patients.
  2. While contaminated instruments are being cleaned or handled.
  3. For surface cleaning and disinfecting.
– They may be washed, disinfected or sterilized and reused.

4. Non-latex containing gloves

– Occasionally, health care providers or patients may experience serious allergic reactions to latex.
– The person who is sensitive to latex can substitute with gloves made from other non-latex containing materials such as vinyl, nitrile.

Guidelines for the use of gloves

1. All gloves used in patient care must be discarded after a single use.
2. Replace torn or damaged gloves immediately.
3. Do not wear jewellery under gloves.
4. Change gloves frequently (i.e. if the procedure is long, change gloves about once in each hour).
5. Remove contaminated gloves before leaving the chairside during patient care and replace them with new gloves before returning to patient care.
6. Wash hands after glove removal and before regloving.

Wearing of gloves

1. Thoroughly wash and dry your hands.
2. Hold one glove at the cuff, place your opposite hand inside the glove and pull it onto your hand. Repeat with a new glove for your other hand.

Removal of Gloves

1. Use left hand fingers to pinch right glove near edge to fold back (Fig. 1.5).

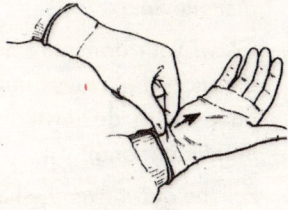

Fig. 1.5

2. Fold edge back without contact with clean inside surface (Fig. 1.6).

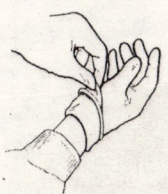

Fig. 1.6

3. Use right hand fingers to contact outside of left glove at the wrist to invert and remove (Fig. 1.7).

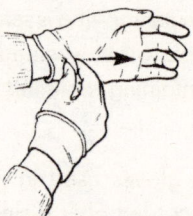

Fig. 1.7

4. Bunch the glove into the palm (Fig. 1.8).

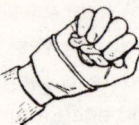

Fig. 1.8

5. With ungloved left hand, grasp inner non-contaminated portion of the right glove to peel it off, enclosing other glove as it is inverted (Fig. 1.9).

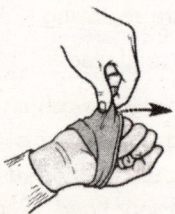

Fig. 1.9

Performing Sterile Gloving

1. The glove package should already be opened before the surgical scrub. Be sure to touch only the inside of the package at this point (Because the open glove pack is a sterile field).

2. Glove your dominant hand first (applying the second glove is more difficult and you have more dexterity (ability) with your dominant hand).

3. Pull the glove over the hand, touching only the folded cuff (because you need to touch only the inside of the glove) (Fig. 1.10).

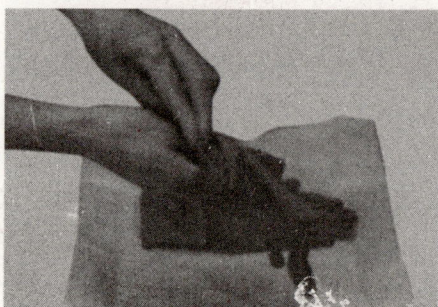

Fig. 1.10

4. With your dominant hand gloved, slide your fingers under the cuff of the other glove (you can only touch the sterile portion of the glove with your dominant hand) (Fig. 1.11).

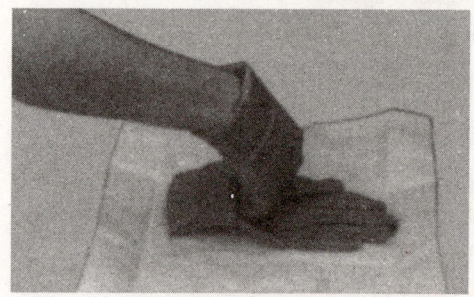

Fig. 1.11

5. Pull the glove up over your other hand (Fig. 1.12).

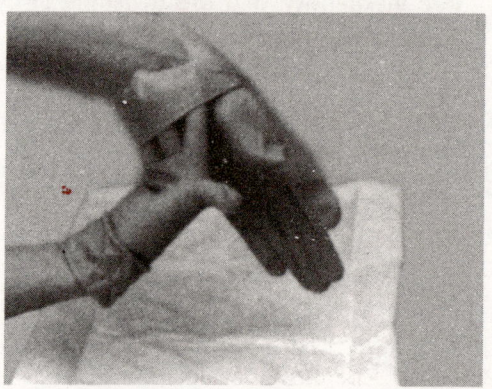

Fig. 1.12

6. Unroll the cuf from your gloves (Fig. 1.13).

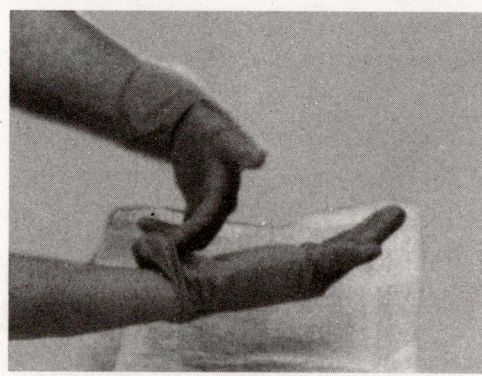

Fig. 1.13

WEARING PPE: Wear in the reverse order of what you change most frequently during the day, i.e.

1. Gloves—most oftenly changed.
2. Protective mask and eyewear—less often.
3. Protective clothing—least often.

–   So, first wear the protective clothing, then protective mask, eye wear and lastly the gloves (Figs 1.14–1.17).

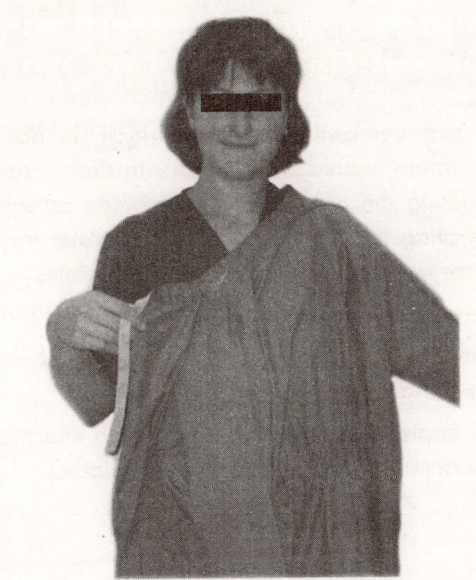

Fig. 1.14

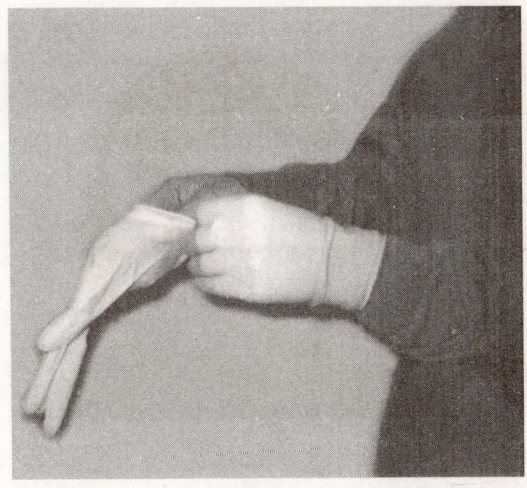

Fig. 1.17

REMOVAL OF PPE: Done in a manner to prevent contaminating hands, clothing, skin and mucous membranes, i.e. first remove gloves, then eye wear and mask and lastly protective clothing (Figs 1.18–1.20).

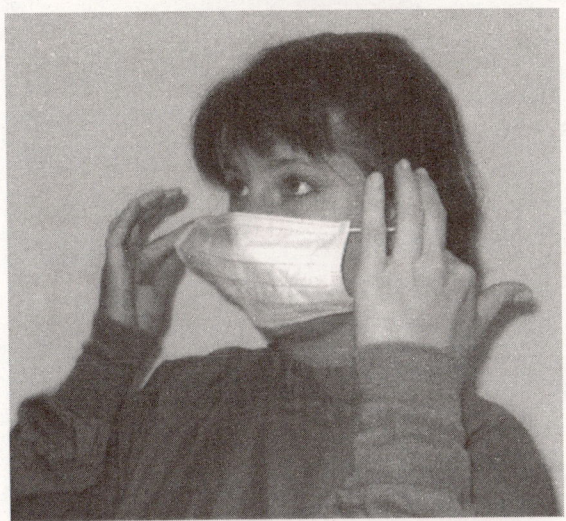

Fig. 1.15

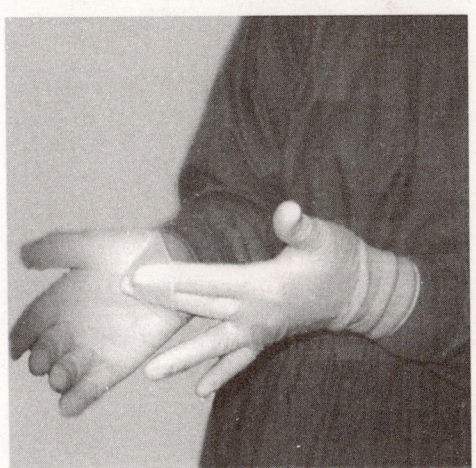

Fig. 1.18

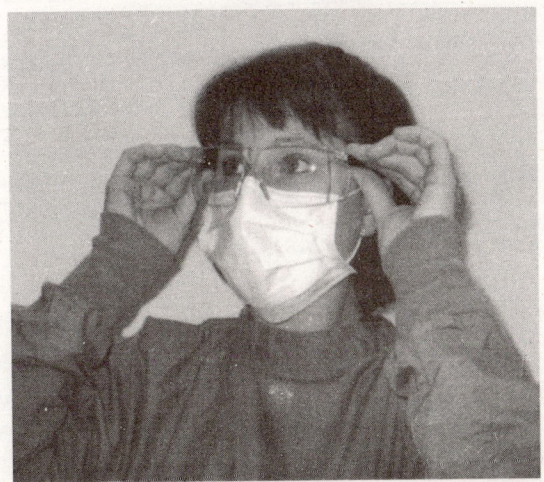

Fig. 1.16

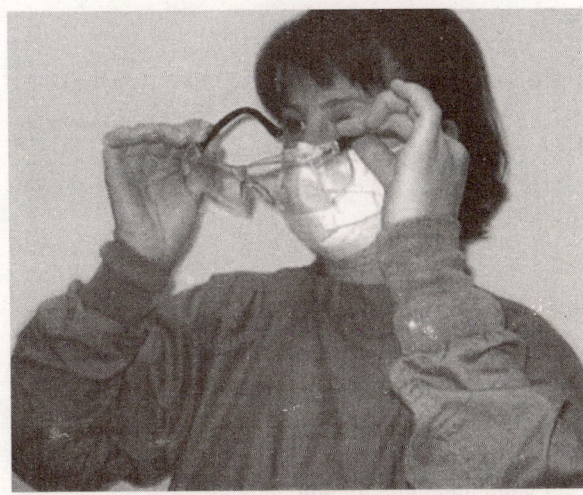

Fig. 1.19

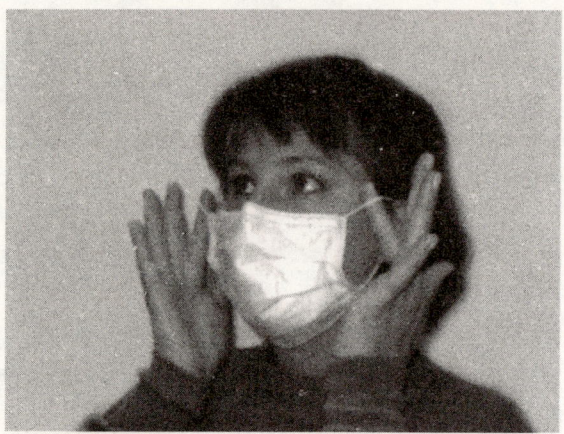

Fig. 1.20

DISINFECTION OF SURFACES AND EQUIPMENT IN THE DENTAL OFFICE

– The surfaces and equipment which do not permit sterilization should be treated with disinfectant prior to seating the patient and in between patients. Ex : Operating light handles, chair controls, tray arms, release levers and three way syringe handles.

– Detergent solutions assist in removing dried blood.

– Alcohol, 90% isopropyl or 70% ethyl alcohol aids in solubilizing dried blood and saliva.

– 70% isopropyl alcohol has become an effective agent for surface decontamination in dental office.

CHAPTER 02

INSTRUMENT PROCESSING AND STERILIZATION

- One of the most important aspect of the dental treatment is to process contaminated instruments and other patient-care items for reuse.
- Proper processing of contaminated dental instruments is a multistep process. It is as follows,

S. No.	Step	Technique
1.	Transport	Transport contaminated instruments to the processing area in a way that minimizes the risk of exposures to the persons. Use appropriate PPE and a rigid leak proof container.
2.	Cleaning	Clean the instruments with a hands-free, mechanical process such as an ultrasonic cleaner or instrument washer. If instruments cannot be cleaned immediately, use a holding solution.
3.	Packaging	In the clean area, wrap/package instruments in appropriate materials. Place a chemical indicator inside the package next to the instruments.
4.	Sterilization	Load the sterilizer according to the manufacturer's instructions. Label the packages. Do not overload the sterilizer. Place packages on their edges in single layers or on racks. Operate the sterilizer. Allow packages to cool before removing them from sterilizer. Allow packages to cool before handling.
5.	Storage	Store the instruments in a clean, dry environment in a manner that maintains the integrity.
6.	Delivery	Deliver the packages to the point of views in a way that maintains sterility of the instruments until they are used. Inspect each package for damage. Open the package aseptically.

PATIENT CARE ITEMS

– These are classified into three types based on the potential risk for infection associated with their intended use.

– It is as follows,

1. **Critical Instruments**
   – Are the things used to penetrate soft tissue or bone.
   – They have the greatest risk of transmitting infection.
   – Should be sterilized by heat.
     Ex: Forceps, Scalpels, Bone chisels, Scalers and Burs.

2. **Semicritical Instruments**
   – Are those which touch mucous membranes or nonintact skin.
   – Have a lower risk of transmitting infection.
   – Can be heat sterilized or by high-level disinfection process.
     Ex: Mouth mirrors, High volume evacuator tips, Rubberdam forceps, Amalgam instruments, etc.

3. **Noncritical Instruments**
   – Are those which contact only with intact skin.
   – Have the least risk of transmitting infection.
   – Can be cleaned and processed with an intermediate to low level disinfection.
     Ex: Dental X-ray head, Lead apron and Curing light, etc.

STERILIZATION IN OPERATIVE DENTISTRY

Methods of Sterilization

1. Autoclaving, steam pressure sterilization.
2. Chemical vapour pressure sterilization.
3. Dry heat.
4. Ethylene oxide sterilization.

1. Autoclaving

– In this apparatus the material is exposed to 121°C for 15–20 min at 15 lb pressure / sq. inch.
– It is used to sterilize—culture media, Rubber goods, Syringes, Gowns, Instruments.

Sterilization of Burs in Autoclaving

– Burs are placed in 2% Sodium nitrate containing bottles, either glass beakers or metal beakers are kept in autoclave for sterilization.

2. Chemical Vapour Pressure Sterilization

– Sterilization by chemical vapour under pressure, i.e. 131°C 20 lbs pressure sq. inch - 30 min.
– *Uses:* Sterilization of corrosion sensitive burs, metallic instruments, pliers.

3. Dry Heat Sterilization

– *Red heat:* It is directly by holding on flame. Used for needles, forceps, inoculating wires.
– *Hot air oven:* Carbon steel instruments and burs.
– *Incineration:* Hospital dressings are burnt.

4. Ethylene oxide sterilization

– Used to sterilize complex instruments and delicate materials.
– Ethylene oxide gas at high temperature below 100° C for several hours.

Sterilization of Handpieces and Related Rotary instruments

– Scrubbing with disinfectant
– Steam sterilization
– Chemical vapour pressure
– Cleaning with soap
– Wiping with alcohol

Sterilization of Impressions

– Washing the impression with disinfectant solution, such as 3% phenol, ethyl alcohol, and formaldehyde.

STERILIZATION IN ENDODONTICS

I. Chemical sterilization

– 2% benzalkonium chloride in 50% isopropylalcohol.
– Swabbing with hydrogen peroxide followed by tincture of iodine.
– Ethyl alcohol (2 parts) + formalin (1 part) to destroy spore formers.

II. Cold sterilization

– Sterilization by cold chemical solutions.
– *Quaternary ammonium compounds:* Kills vegetative organisms.
– *Ethyl alcohol and isopropyl alcohol :* Kills vegetative bacteria, TB bacilli.
– *Alcohol-formalin solution :* Kills vegetative bacteria, TB bacilli, spores.

– *Orthophenyl phenol and benzyl para chlorophenol*: Kills vegetative bacteria, TB bacilli, certain fungi and viruses but not spores.

III. Autoclaving

– Common method.
– **Method (According to Ingle)** : At 121°C at 15 psi for 15–40 minutes.
– The time depends on the items to be autoclaved, the size of the load and type of container used.

IV. Chemiclave/Chemical vapour sterilization/Harvey chemiclave

– Similar to autoclave.
– Solutions used are alcohol, acetone, formaldehyde, water.

Method

1. According to Ingle at 132°C at 20 psi for 20 min.
2. According to Grossman, at 135°C at 15 lbs for 10–15 min.

V. Dry heat sterilization

1. *Prolonged dry heat*

– It sterilizes at 160°C for 2 hours.

2. *Rapid dry heat sterilization*

– Small chamber, high speed dry heat sterilizer.
– Operated at 190°C, sterilize unpackaged instruments in 6 minutes and packaged instruments in 12 minutes.

3. *Intense dry heat*

A. Hot salt sterilizer

– Apparatus consists of a metal cup in which table salt is kept at a temperature between 425–475°F.
– A thermometer is used always to measure the temperature.
– *Root canal instruments such as broaches, files, reamers are sterilized for 5 sec.*
– *Absorbent points and cotton pellets for 10 sec.*

Advantages

– Use of ordinary salt instead of metal or beads.
– Eliminates the risk of clogging the root canal.

B. Glass bead sterilizer

– Glass beads are effectively substituted for the hot salt sterilizer provided glass beads less than 1mm diameter.

– Larger beads are not effective in transferring the heat to the endodontic treatment.

Method

Temperature : 425–475° F (218–246° C)
Time : 5 sec.

Disadvantage

– Only small instruments can be sterilized.

VI. Sterilization of some other endodontic instruments

1. Dappendish

– Swabbing thoroughly with tincture of thimerosal followed by alcohol.
– Swabbing is done under pressure with the intent of physically removing the debris and micro-organisms.

2. Long handle instruments, tip of cotton pliers, blades of scissors and other instruments

– Dipping the working point in alcohol and flaming twice.

3. Bulky instruments such as cotton pliers, and cement spatulas

– Sterilized quickly by passing the working blades through a flame several times.

4. Mixing slab (glass slab)

– By swabbing the surface with tincture of thimerosal followed by a double swabbing with alcohol.

5. Gutta-percha cones

– May be kept sterile in screw-capped vials containing alcohol.
– Sterilized by immersing in 5.2% sodium hypochlorite for 1 min then rinse the cone with hydrogen peroxide and dry it between two layers of sterile gauze.
– **Alternative method**—immersion in polyvinyl pyrolidone iodine for 6 min.

6. Silver cones

– Sterilized by slowly passing them back and forth through a bunsen flame for 2 or 4 times or by immersion in the hot salt sterilizer for 5 sec.

7. Burs

– Autoclave
– Dry heat sterilization
– Dipping in alcohol

8. Handpiece sterilization

– FDA and ADA recommend that reusable dental handpieces and related instruments should be heat sterilized between each patient use.
– Handpieces can be sterilized by steam, chemical vapour and ethylene oxide gas (ETO).

CAUSES OF STERILIZATION FAILURE

1. Improper instrument preparation.
2. Improper packaging of instruments.
3. Improper loading of the sterilizer chamber.
4. Improper temperature in the sterilization chamber.
5. Improper timing of the sterilization cycle.
6. Equipment malfunction.

MONITORING STERILIZATION

– Two methods are commonly used to monitor sterilization in office, i.e.
   1. Process indicators
   2. Biologic indicators

1. Process indicators

– Process indicators are usually strips, tape, or paper products marked with special ink that changes colour on exposure to heat, steam, chemical vapour or ETO.

– The ink changes colour when the items being processed have been subjected to sterilizing conditions.

– But a process indicator usually does not monitor how long such conditions were present.

2. Biologic indicators

– Biologic indicators are usually preparations of non-pathogenic bacterial spores that serve as a challenge to a specific method of sterilization.

– If a sterilization method destroys spore forms that are highly to that method, it is logical to assume that all other life forms have also been destroyed.

– The bacterial spores are usually attached to a paper strip within a biologically protected packet.

– The spore packet is placed between instrument packages or within an instrument packages itself.

– After the sterilizer has cycled, the spore strip is cultured for a specific time lack of culture growth indicates sterility.

CHAPTER 03

ISOLATION AND MOISTURE CONTROL

GOALS OF ISOLATION

1. Moisture Control

– Moisture in mouth can render a hinderance towards the operating procedures.

– Moisture control refers to excluding sulcular fluid, saliva and gingival bleeding from operating field.

– Effective method of moisture control is use of rubber dam, suction devices and absorbents.

2. Retraction and Access

– This is to provide maximum exposure of operating field.

– It involves, open mouth and retracting the gingival tissue, tongue, lips and cheeks.

– Rubber dam, high volume evacuators, absorbents, retraction cords, mouth prop are used.

3. Harm Prevention

– Major priority is minimal harm to patient.

– Excessive saliva and handpiece spray can alarm the patient.

– Small instruments and restorative debris can be swallowed and accidental soft tissue damage can occur.

– Rubber dam, high volume evacuators are used.

METHODS OF ISOLATION

I. To isolate from moisture

   1. *Indirect methods*

     i. Relaxed position of the patient

     ii. Local anesthesia

     iii. Drugs (Antisialogogues, antiaxiety drugs, muscle relaxants)

   2. *Direct methods*

     i. Rubber dam

     ii. Gingival retraction

     iii. Cotton rolls and cellulose wafers

     iv. Throat shields

     v. High volume evacuators and saliva ejectors

II. To isolate from soft tissues

   i. Retraction of cheeks, tongue, lips.

   ii. Gingival retraction.

1. Local anesthesia

– It plays an important role in eliminating the discomfort and controlling moisture.

2. **Cotton roll isolation and cellulose wafers**

   – Partial isolation with cotton rolls, absorbent wafers and saliva ejectors provides a rapid and effective control of the operating field.

   – *Isolation of maxillary teeth:* A medium sized cotton roll is placed in facial vestibule (Fig. 3.1 A and B).

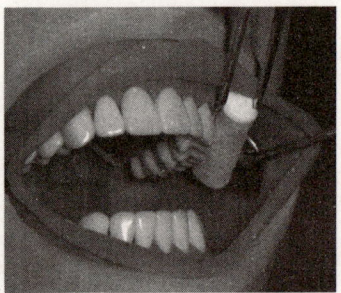

Fig. 3.1 A

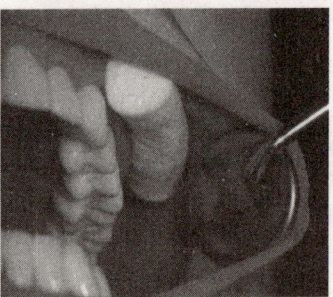

Fig. 3.1 B

   – *Isolation of mandibular teeth:* A medium sized cotton roll is placed in the facial vestibule and a larger one between the teeth and tongue (Fig. 3.2 A to C).

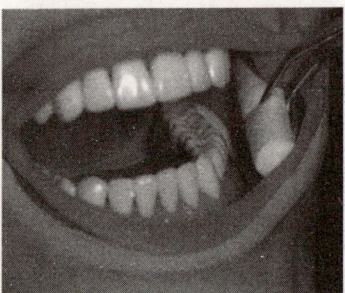

Fig. 3.2 A

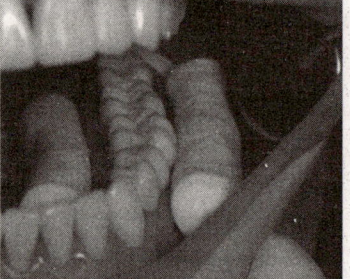

Fig. 3.2 B

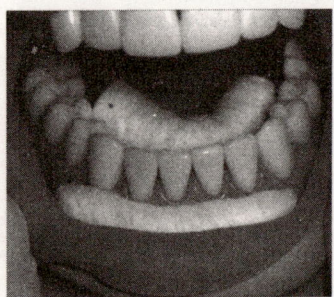

Fig. 3.2 C

   – Cellulose wafers may be used to retract the cheek and provide additional absorbency.

   – Cotton rolls and wafers must be replaced as soon as they become saturated.

   – Dry cotton rolls are moistened before they are removed to prevent the pulling of the epithelial covering of the mucosa.

3. **Throat Shields**

   – These are indicated when there is danger of aspirating or swallowing small objects.

   – A gauge sponge is unfolded and spread over the tongue and the posterior part of the mouth.

   – Used to recover small objects.

4. **High Volume Evacuators (HVE)**

   – It is used to remove saliva, blood, water and debris.

   – It works on a vacuum principle that is similar to that of a household vacuum cleaner.

Suction Tips (Fig. 3.3)

   – They are larger in circumference and are designed with a straight or slight angle in the middle.

   – Each end has a bevelled (having a surface angle that meets another angle) working end so that the tip can be positioned parallel to the site for better suction.

   – They are made of a durable plastic and are disposed after a single use. Also available in stainless steel or reusable plastic but which must be sterilized before reuse.

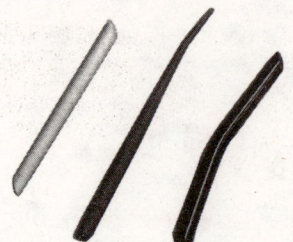

Fig. 3.3

Grasping the Evacuator (Fig. 3.4 A and B)

– The HVE may be held in the *thumb-to-nose grasp* or the *pen grasp*.

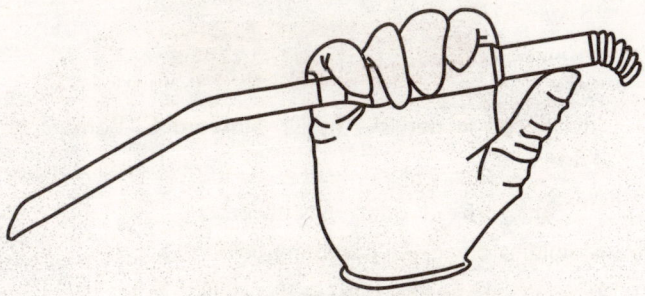

Fig. 3.4 A Thumb-to-nose grasp

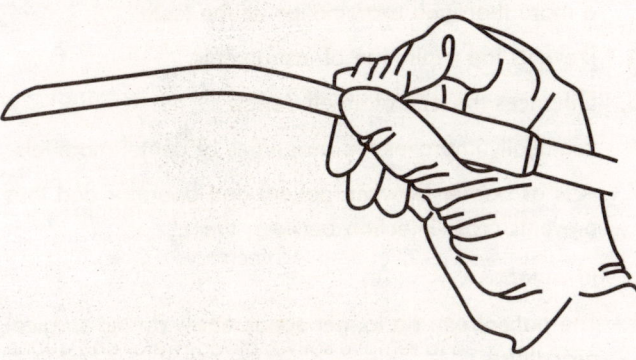

Fig. 3.4 B Pen grasp

Positioning the Evacuator

– When assisting a right handed dentist, the assistant grasps the evacuator in the right hand.

– Guide lines to be followed,

1. Place the evacuator before the dentist positions the handpiece and mouth mirror.

2. Position the suction tip on the surface of the tooth that is closest to you.

3. Position the tip close to the tooth being treated.

4. Position the bevel of the suction tip so that it is parallel to the tooth surface.

5. Keep the edge of the suction tip even with or slightly beyond the occlusal surface or incisal edge.

5. Saliva ejectors (Fig. 3.5 A and B)

– It is small, straw - shaped oral evacuator that is used during less - invasive dental procedures.

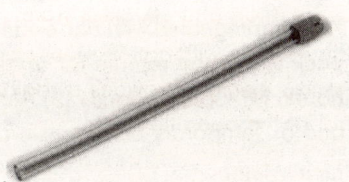

Fig. 3.5 A

– Its main function is to remove liquids from the mouth and is not enough powerful to remove solid abris.

– It is made from soft plastic tubing that can be shaped for easy placement in the oral cavity.

– It can be used by holding it throughout the procedure, using repeated sweeps of the mouth to remove fluids or by positioning the suction in the mouth during a procedure.

– To place the saliva ejector in a stationary position, bend and form the tubing into the shape of a candy cone. This shape allows it to be positioned under the tongue where most fluids will accumulate.

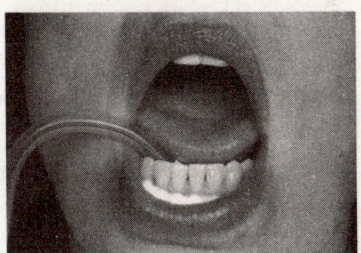

Fig. 3.5 B

6. Gingival Tissue Retraction

– Gingival tissue retraction refers to apical and lateral displacement of gingival tissue to aid in proper visibility and accessibility during subgingival tooth preparation and to aid in proper flow of impression material into the area.

Methods of gingival tissue retraction

1. Physicomechanical Method.

2. Chemicalmethod.

3. Electrosurgical method.

4. Surgical method.

1. *Physico Mechanical Methods*

– This involves mechanically forcing the gingival tissue away from tooth surface, laterally and apically.

– *Methods :* (1) Application of extraheavy weight rubber dam, (2) Replacement of cotton twigs in the gingival sulcus (3) Placement of cotton twigs impregnated with zinc oxide eugenol. This pack should be remain for a minimum of 48 hours, (4) Copper bands (5) Aluminium shell, and 6. Temporary acrylic resin copings.

2. Chemical Method

– This method involves carrying various chemicals into gingival sulcus.

– *Chemicals used are:*

1. Vasoconstrictors like epinephrine and nor-epinephrine.
2. Biologic fluid coagulants like alum, aluminium chloride, aluminium, potassium sulphate, tannic acid, etc.

– These chemicals coagulate blood and tissue fluids.

– Astringents like zinc chloride and silver nitrate.

– *Gingival retraction cords*

Available as :   Braided

Twisted

Flattened

Knitted

– They may be supplied as already impregnated with chemical.

– A suitable length of the cord is tucked into the gingival sulcus using blunt ended instrument around the tooth.

3. Electrosurgical Method

– Here 4 types of action can be produced at the electrode end namely, cutting, coagulation, fulguration and dessication.

– For gingival tissue retraction mostly cutting and rarely coagulation action are employed.

4. Surgical Method

– This involves surgical excision of interfering gingival tissue using a sharp scalpel blade or surgical knife.

– *Method:* Gingivoplasty, rotary gingival curettage (Gingettage).

Other Methods Include

Mirror and Evacuator Tip Retraction

– A secondary function of the mirror and evacuator tip is to retract cheek, lip and tongue.

Mouth Props

– Used in restorative procedures of posterior teeth.

– Maintains adequate mouth opening and permits extended or multiple operations of desired.

– Available as block type or ratchet type.

Drugs

– Drugs like atropine are used to control salivation.

– Rarely indicated.

RUBBER DAM

– Introduced to dentistry by Dr. Stanford C. Barnum in 1864.

Advantages

1. Maintains dry, clean operating field.
2. Improves the accessibility and visibility.
3. Aids in the reduction of pain (The dry fibrilla in dentin lose their ability to transmit sensations of pain). Aids in a more thorough examination of the teeth.
4. Prevents the aspiration of instruments.
5. Enhances the operators efficiency.
6. Potentially improves the properties of dental materials.
7. Acts as barrier between patient and operator and thus prevents cross-infection between them.

Disadvantages

1. The patient can no longer speak easily during surgical procedure.
2. The teeth which has been clamped may be sensitive for some hours after the clamp has been removed.
3. Time consuming for application.
4. Difficulty in applying and removal.
5. Not economic.
6. The rubber is allergic to some patients.

Contraindications

1. Teeth that are not completely erupted.
2. Procedures on third molars.
3. Extremely malposed teeth.
4. Patients suffering from asthma.
5. Patients allergic to latex.

Rubberdam Kit

– It consists of,

1. Rubberdam material
2. Rubberdam punch
3. Rubberdam stamp
4. Rubberdam clamps (Retainer)
5. Rubberdam clamp forceps

6. Rubberdam lubricant

7. Rubberdam napkin

8. Rubberdam holder or frame

9. Waxed dental floss or tape

10. Miscellaneous

1. Rubberdam Material

– It is usually latex rubber.

– Available in rolls or precut sheets of sizes 5" x 5" for children and 6" x 6" for adults.

– It is available in variety of thicknesses, i.e. *thin* (0.15 mm), *medium* (0.20 mm), *heavy* (0.25 mm), *extra heavy* (0.30 mm) and *special extra heavy* (0.35 mm)

– It is also available in colours, i.e. *green* (heavy), *blue* (medium) and *black*.

– A Dark coloured one is preferred because it contrast well with the teeth; fragments torn off and left behind are seen easily and removed.

– Rubberdam material is shiny at one side and dull on another side.

– Because dull side is less light reflective, it is placed facing the occlusal side of the isolated teeth.

– Advantages of the thinner sheet are its easy application and the comfort it provides to the patient.

– Advantages of the heavier sheet are its ability to retract soft tissue and its resistance to scuffing and tearing by the dental bur.

– Medium thickness is recommended for molar applications, heavy (or extra heavy) for anterior and bicuspid applications.

2. Anchoring Devices

– For the rubberdam to be securely attached to the area being isolated, there are several devices and methods.

A. Anchoring Clamps (Fig. 3.6 A and B)

– Each clamp consists of two jaws, one on each side carrying the tooth attachment blades (prongs) and sometimes dam engaging projections (wings), a bow which connects the two jaws and which should be elastically strainable and resistant enough to impart a gripping force on the attaching blades against the teeth.

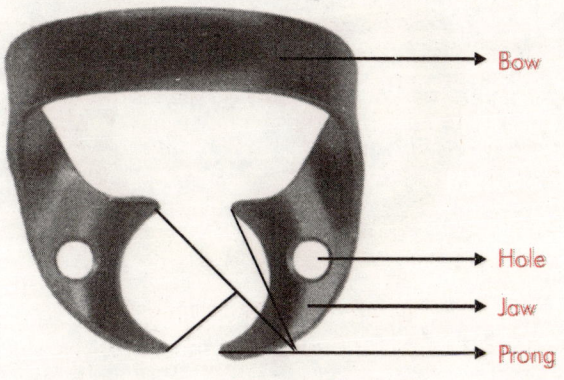

Fig. 3.6 A

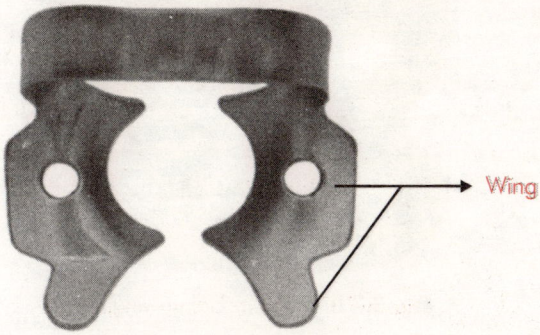

Fig. 3.6 B

– According to the type and shape of the tooth attachment blades, clamps can be, (Fig. 3.7 A to G).

1. *Clamps with four point contact blades (with wings)* : (The blade portions of the jaw point inwards at each corner, so that all the gripping forces will be applied on these four points only). They contact the axial angles of the tooth and create a very secure attachment with the tooth. It is indicated when the retaining curvature of the tooth surfaces is not present (newly erupting teeth) and in single tooth isolation. The disadvantages are that the clamp has possible traumatic effect on weakened undermined tooth structure; interference with the placement of matrix bands, retainer and wedges.

2. *Clamps with circumferential contact blades (Wingless):* The blade portion has no projections and will contact the tooth surface evenly throughout its length. It is less retentive. It is less traumatic. It is used when the axial angles are lost or do not coincide with the corners of the four point contact clamps and when the axial convexity of the tooth surface is sufficient for anchorage.

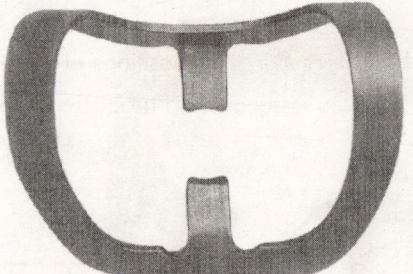

Fig. 3.7 A Anterior clamp-wingless

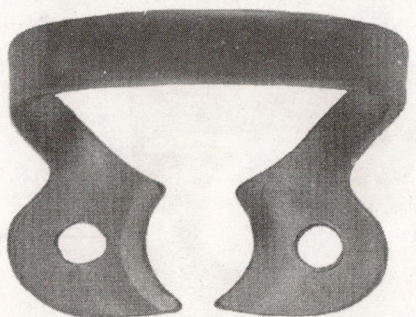

Fig. 3.7 B Premolar clamp-wingless

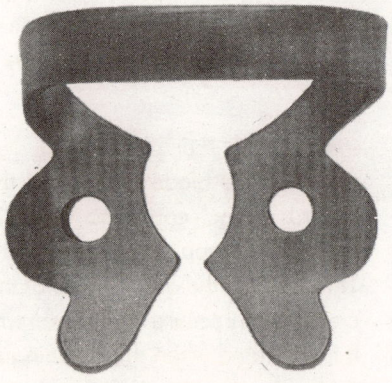

Fig. 3.7 C Premolar clamp-winged

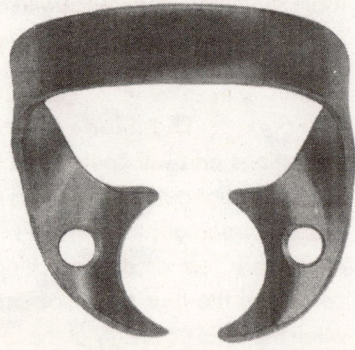

Fig. 3.7 D Maxillary clamp-wingless

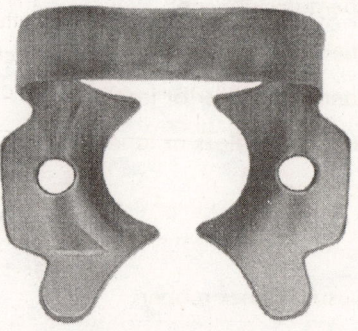

Fig. 3.7 E Maxillary clamp-winged

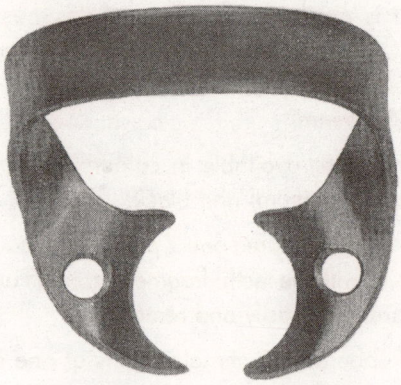

Fig. 3.7 F Mandibular clamp-wingless

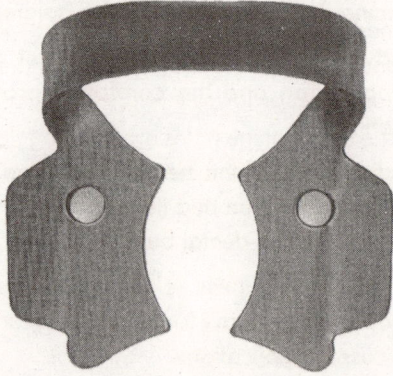

Fig. 3.7 G Mandibular molar clamp-winged

– Wings are provided to give extra retraction of rubberdam from the operating field.

– A good basic set of clamps has the following,

1. BW, JW molar clamps, wingless: Used when the clamp is positioned on the tooth before the rubber.

2. K molar clamp, winged: The wings allow the clamp and rubber to be placed simultaneously.

3. GW premolar clamp.

4. EW clamp used on any small tooth.

5. AW molar clamp, wingless used on partially erupted teeth only.

6. Cervical clamp, Ferrier pattern, for use on anterior teeth where retraction of rubber or gingivae is required to allow access to a cervical cavity.

B. *Retracting anchoring clamps*

- These are clamps especially designed to other functions besides anchoring the dam to the tooth.

i. The 212 Clamp series consists of double bowed clamps, specially designed for retracting the facial or lingual gingiva away from class - 5 cavity preparations.

ii. The Schultz clamp series resembles the 212 clamp but are split in half facio-lingually making them a gingivally retracting clamp with one bow only. Used especially when a second bow cannot be accommodated due to a lack of space or limited access.

3. Rubberdam Punch (Fig. 3.8)

- Used to cut the holes in the rubber which will encompass the teeth to be isolated.

- It has a lever type plunger and a rotatable table containing holes of different diameters.

- Usually the larger holes accommodate molars, medium size holes are for premolars, upper cuspids and sometimes for upper incisors, and the smallest holes are for lower incisors.

- The edges of the holes are very angular. The appropriate hole in the table is moved to coincide with the plunger, and the rubber is placed in between the plunger and the table and appropriate hole is punched.

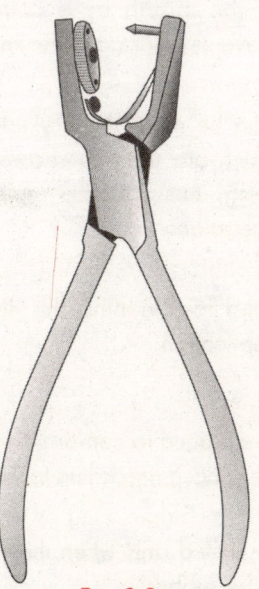

Fig. 3.8

4. Rubberdam Stamp (Fig. 3.9)

- Used for marking the positions of the holes.

- The inked rubber stamp produces a series of dots on the rubber corresponding to the average positions of the teeth.

- When the dam is in position, it should reach up to a point just below the patients nose, thus covering the mouth but not the nose.

- To achieve this when applying the rubber to the maxillary teeth or mandibular third molars, the position of the upper central incisors should be stamped about 2.5 cm (1 inch) from the top edge of the rubber sheet. For mandibular teeth the holes should be placed further up the sheet to avoid the rubber covering the nose.

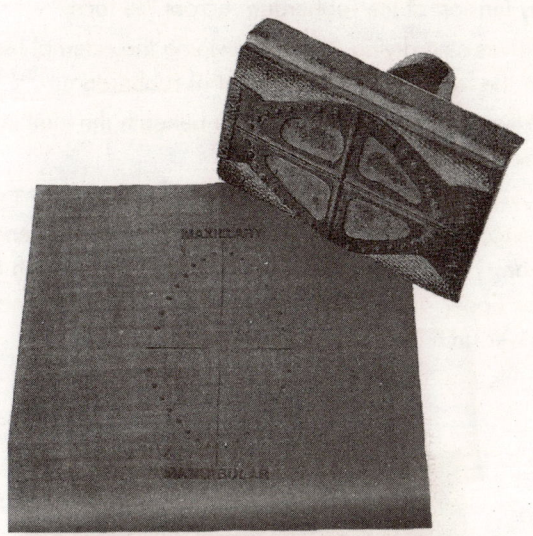

Fig. 3.9

5. Rubberdam Clamp Forceps (Fig. 3.10)

- This is a modified forceps which retracts the jaws of a clamp away from each other, allowing the clamp to overcome the occlusal diameter of the tooth and to be seated apical to the height of the axial contour.

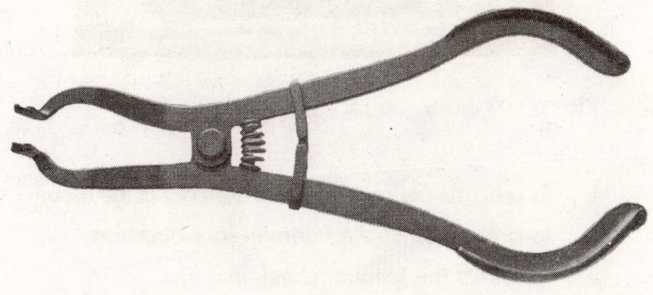

Fig. 3.10

6. Rubberdam Lubricant

- A water soluble lubricant applied on the area of the punched holes facilitates the passing of the dam septa through proximal contacts.
- It is commercially available.

7. Rubberdam Napkins

- These are absorbent paper or cloth towels that can be applied between the rubberdam and the patients face.

Advantages

1. Absorbs saliva and prevents drooling.
2. The additional comfort reduces the stimulated flow.
3. Reduces the allergic reactions by preventing the contact between rubberdam and the skin of the patient.
4. Aids in the prevention of pressure marks often created by tension of the rubberdam across the face.
5. Serves as a drying device for wiping the external tissues of the face during the removal of rubberdam.
6. Prevents the debris from falling beneath the clothing of the patient.

- Overall measurement is 9 inches square, with a 1 inch concavity at the upper border, the concavity extending from 1 inch from either end. The size of the mouth hole for upper arch is 2 inches long, 1 inch wide, and for lower arch is 3 by $1^3/_8$ inches.

8. Rubberdam Holder or Frame (Fig. 3.11)

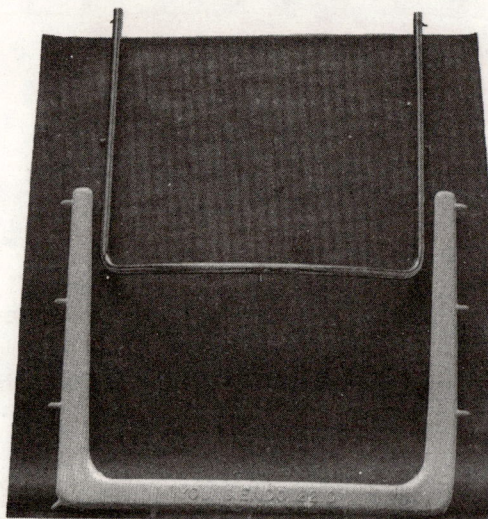

Fig. 3.11

Objectives

1. To keep the peripheries of the dam out of the mouth.
2. To stretch the applied dam in four directions.
3. To retract the tongue, cheek and lips.
4. To clear the operation field for further procedures.

Classification

- They can be classified as,

A. Strap type

- It depends on the back of the patient's head for anchorage.
- It is more convenient for the operator because they do not obstruct the field of vision in anydirection. Ex : Woodburry holder, Wizzard holder.

B. Hanging frame holders

- Are, U-shaped, elliptical or rectangular metal or plastic frames, with multiple prongs at their peripheries.
- Are most popular holders.
- Advantages are ease of application and allowance for minimal contact of the rubber with the skin.

9. Waxed Dental Floss or Tape

- Used to carry the rubber past a tight contact point; also in adjusting the septal portions of the rubber.

10. Miscellaneous

A. Rubber bands

- Frequently a small piece of rubber band may be used to retract the rubberdam comfortably and hold the gingival region to the contact point, in lieu of additional clamps.

B. Beavertail Burnisher

- Used to tuck unturned ends of the rubber under the free margin of the gingival.

C. Zinc Oxide Ointment

- A little soothing ointment placed on the corners of the mouth by a cotton roll applicator prevents cracking of the lips from long dryness.

D. Black Impression Compound

- Can be made into cylinders of varying sizes which are used to secure the clamps to the teeth, ensuring no movement during the operation.

E. 70% alcohol

- Used for cleaning the dam and teeth after application.

Placement of Holes

- The holes are placed to conform to the curvature of the arch and are spaced according to the distances between the teeth.
- Holes are punched only when they are positioned and marked on the rubber.

– To assure the uniformity of rubber borders after application, two landmarks can be used ; For maxillary applications, the incisors should lie one inch from the upper border, for mandibular applications, the most posterior hole is slightly right or left of the center of the rubber.

– Distances between the holes should be comparable to spaces between the centers of each tooth.

– The circumference of the arch is reflected in the location of the holes to space the holes so that the rubber will snugly engage each tooth without puckering.

– If the holes are placed too closely together or incorrectly aligned, they will fit over the teeth but will be stretched to the side, permitting saliva to leak by.

– If the holes are too far apart, excess rubber stock remains and is puckered between the teeth.

– *A liberal number of teeth should always be included in a dam application. An anterior application should include a minimum of seven teeth. Posterior application should usually reach from the first or second molar to the opposite cuspid.*

– Generally, clamp is attached one tooth distal to the tooth receiving treatment.

– Holes must be sharp and clean cut. Holes with ragged edges will cause the rubber to tear when tightly stretched.

Procedure of Application

1. Preparation

– *Armamentarium*

1. Basic four instruments: mirror, explorer, cotton pliers, plastic instruments.

2. Rubberdam kit

3. Saliva ejector

4. Scissors

– Gross bits of calculus and other debris are removed, contact points are checked by the passage of dental tape and sharp edges of enamel that might cut the rubber are removed.

– *For tight and broad contacts :* Open the contact slightly with pressure from a beavertail burnisher wedged for a moment just gingival to the contact point as the septal rubber dam passes.

– *For sharp cavity edges:* Smooth with chisels or hatchets or cavity is reopened and outline form is re-established.

– *For sharp or rough restoration margins:* Trim to contour with gold knife, disks or strips.

– *For foreign material between teeth:* Remove with ligature, explorer, and warm water.

2. Punch Holes

– Select the size of rubber dam needed.

– The distance of one hole to the next is equal to the distance of the center of the next tooth at the gingival third. This is the position of the rubberdam when completely placed.

– *Note :* When preparing class 2, 3 or 4 cavities, the rule on distance between the tooth centers should be modified on that septum where the cavity lies.

– Follow the arch form of the teeth (especially the irregularities of tooth position) in punching holes A hole may be punched in the upper left hand corner for identification of that corner during the placement of the upper (first) snap of the rubber dam holder on to the left border of the rubberdam.

Rubberdam for Upper Teeth

1. First holes punched are for central incisors, 1 inch from the superior border (center) of the rubberdam. *Modifications :* A. For a narrow upperlip, especially in a women or child, the holes should be a little less than 1 inch from the superior border, B. For a long upper lip or in the presence of mustache, the distance is little more than 1 inch.

2. Upper teeth to be included in the rubber dam ordinarily should be according to the following plan (FDI notation) for class 1, 2, 3 and 4 cavities.

3. *Size of holes to punch :* The punch has 5 holes, from the smallest (no.1) to the largest (no.5). No. 2 and 4 are sufficient for all purposes. no. 2 is for anterior teeth and bicuspids ; no. 4 is for molars. One size larger should be used for the tooth to receive the clamp.

4. The lines of holes should follow irregularities in teeth. The arch of the holes should not follow the incisal edges of the anterior teeth but should correspond to the position of the teeth at their cervical lines.

Rubberdam for Lower Teeth

1. The first hole punched is the one through which the holding clamp is to be placed.

A. **First Molar:** The rubberdam should be imaginarily divided into three equal portions by two vertical lines extending from the superior to the inferior (chin) border. At a point 3 inches from the superior border of the rubber dam and 1/4 inch toward the center

Cavity Teeth	Extend from ____ to ____
12, 11, 11 or 22	14 – 24
13 or 23 mesial	14 – 24
13 distal	16 – 24
23 distal	14 – 26
15 and 14	16 – 21
24 and 25	11 – 26
16 mesioocclusal	17 or 16 – 21
26 mesioocclusal	11 – 26 or 27
16 mesioocclusal	17 – 21
26 mesioocclusal	11 – 27
17 mesioocclusal	18 or 17 – 21
27 mesioocclusal	11 – 27 or 28
18 or 17 distoocclusal	18 – 21
28 or 27 distoocclusal	11 – 28

Cavity Teeth	Extend from ____ to ____
32, 31, 41 or 42	34 – 44
33 or 43 mesial	34 – 44
33 distal	36 – 42 or 32
43 distal	42 or 32 – 46
34 mesioocclusal	36 – 42 or 32
44 mesioocclusal	42 or 32 – 46
34 distoocclusal or 35	36 – 44
44 distoocclusal or 45	44 – 46
36 mesioocclusal	37 or 36 – 34
46 mesioocclusal	44 – 46 or 47
36 distoocclusal	37 – 34
46 distoocclusal	44 – 37
37 mesioocclusal	38 or 37 – 34
47 mesioocclusal	44 – 47 or 48
37 distoocclusal or 38	38 – 34
47 distoocclusal or 48	44 – 48

of the rubberdam from one of the lateral lines, is the point for punching the hole for the first molar.

B. *Second Molar :* The hole is punched about 1/8 inch chinwise from that of the first molar and slightly toward the center of the dam.

C. *Third Molar :* The hole is punched about 1/4 inch chin wise from that of the first molar and slightly towards the center of the dam.

D. *Second Bicuspid :* Use anterior rubberdam. The hole is punched about 1/8 inch nosewise or of that for a first molar.

E. *First Bicuspid :* Use anterior rubberdam. The hole is punched about 1/4 inch nosewise from the first molar point.

2. Lower teeth to be included in the rubberdam should follow the following plan for class 1, 2, 3 and 4 cavities.

3. Size of the hole may be confined to no. 2 and 4.

4. Follow the irregularities as mentioned above.

5. When punching holes for the teeth to be included in the rubberdam it is helpful to punch an additional hole in that corner of the dam which will be at the upper left position when adjusted. This is for identification since in the punching and preliminary placement, the entire dam may be twisted.

Rubberdam punching for the class 5 (gingival) cavity

1. Include only those teeth in the rubberdam to permit the modelling compound which holds the special cervical clamp in place to rest on teeth and not on the rubber dam.

2. Punch the holes in the correct position for selected teeth except the hole for the tooth having the class 5 cavity. This should be punched outside the arch.

3. Placement of Rubberdam

   – A dental floss is used to check the interproximal contacts and remove debris from the teeth to be isolated.

   – After assessing the form and tooth alignment, now punch the holes.

- Lubricate the dam on both sides. Lips and corners of the mouth are also lubricated to prevent irritation.

- Select the retainer and test the retainer's retention and stability by lifting gently in an occlusal direction. An improperly fitting retainer will rock or be easily dislodged.

- Positioning the dam over the retainer: Before placing the dam, the floss tie is threaded through the anchor hole.

  - Now stretch anchor hole of the dam over the retainer and then under the jaws.

  - The septal dam must always pass through its respective contact in single thickness.

  - If in case it does not pass through, dental tape can be used.

- Rubber dam is grasped and pulled through the napkin and position it on the patient's face.

- Unfold the dam and, hold the frame in place, attach the dam to the metal projections on the left and right side simultaneously.

- Attaching the neck strap is optional.

- If there is a tooth distal to the retainer, the distal edge of the posterior anchor hole should be passed through the contact to ensure a seal around the anchor tooth.

- If the stability of retainer is questionable, low fusing modelling compound may be applied.

- Dam is passed over the anterior anchor tooth, anchoring the anterior portion of the rubber dam.

- By stretching the septal dam faciogingivally and linguogingivally one can pass the septa through as many contacts as possible without a dental tape.

- Waxed dental tape can be used to pass the dam through the remaining contacts.

- Now invert the dam into the gingival sulcus to complete the seal around the tooth and to prevent leakage.

- Faciolingually the inversion is completed using an explorer or a beaver-tail burnisher, by moving the explorer around the neck of the tooth facially and lingually.

- Confirm the properly applied rubber dam.

- In case of proximal surface preparation a wedge is placed interproximally as final step in rubberdam application.

4. Removal of Rubberdam

- Before removal, suction away any debris thus preventing it from falling into the floor of mouth.

- Stretch the dam facially, pulling the septal rubber away from the tooth.

- Clipping each septum with blunt tipped scissor, free the dam from interproximal spaces.

- Engage the retainer with retainer forceps and remove the retainer.

- Once the retainer is removed, remove the dam and frame simultaneously.

- Wipe the lips, rinse the mouth and massage the tissues to enhance circulation around on the anchored teeth.

- Examine the dam to determine that no portion of the dam has remained between or around the teeth.

CHAPTER 04

THE OPERATING FIELD

THE DENTAL TREATMENT AREA

– The basic equipment found in each treatment area includes a patient dental chair, stools for the dentist and assistant during a procedure, dental units, cabinets for storage, an operating light, a radiograph unit, a radiograph view box and a sink for washing.

1. PATIENT DENTAL CHAIR

– It is designed to provide pateint comfort.
– Chairs are available in sizes for adult and pediatic practices (Fig. 4.1).

Parts

1. Head rest
2. Back rest
3. Chair seat
4. Foot portion
5. Arm rest
6. Chair base
7. Foot control

– **Head rest** holds the patient's head securely and comfortably in the appropriate position for the treatment being provided.
– **Back rest, chair seat and foot portion** supports the patient's lumbar region of the back, bottom and knees when properly seated.
– **Arm rest** provides the support to the arms of the patient.
– **Chair base** supports the remaining parts and permits the chair to lower or increase the height from the floor.
– **Foot control** provides operating controls for rotatory instruments.

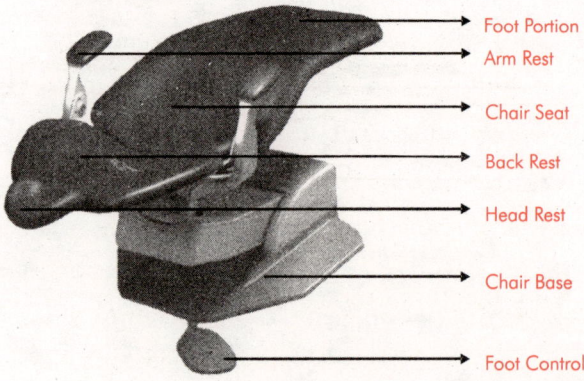

Foot Portion
Arm Rest
Chair Seat
Back Rest
Head Rest
Chair Base
Foot Control

Fig. 4.1

– Dental chair has several controls to adjust for patient comfort and flexibility in positioning during dental treatment.

– The entire chair can also be adjusted to higher and lower positions for easier patient and oral access.

Types of Chair Positions

1. Upright Position (Fig. 4.2)

– The back of the chair is positioned at 90° angle.

– This position is used for patient entry and exit.

– Provides easy access for the operator when working on the patient's lower right side.

– This position may also be used when radiographs are exposed and impressions taken.

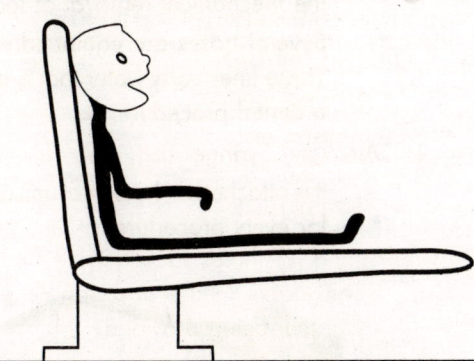

Fig. 4.2

2. Supine Position (Fig. 4.3)

– The patient is positioned as if lying down.

– The patient's head and knees will be approximately at the same level.

– Most dental treatment is completed in this position.

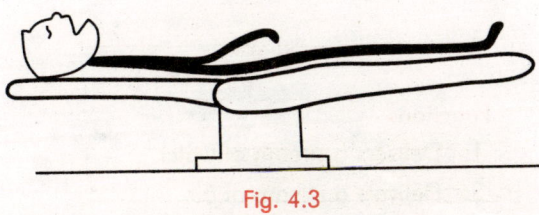

Fig. 4.3

3. Semi-Upright / Semi-Supine Position (Fig. 4.4)

– It is between supine and upright positions, i.e. approximately at 45° angle.

– This position is usually used for the pregnant women and for the patient's with respiratory or cardiovascular problems.

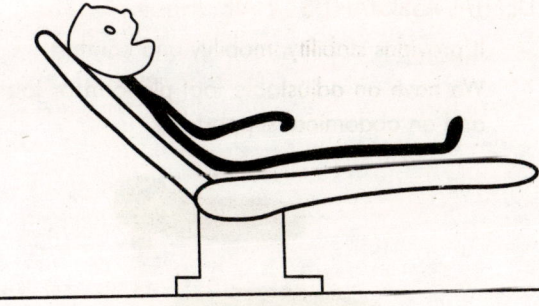

Fig. 4.4

4. Sub-supine/Trendelenburg Position (Fig. 4.5)

– In this position, pateint's head is lower than the feet.

– It is recommended for emergency situations and unconscious patient's.

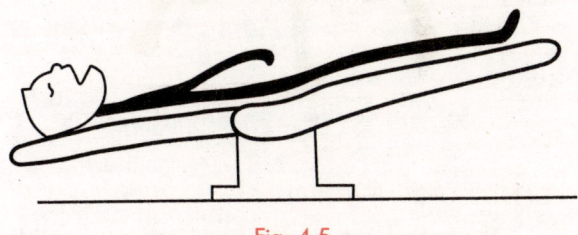

Fig. 4.5

2. OPERATOR'S CHAIR (Fig. 4.6)

– It provides a large seat and back with easily adjustable lumbar support.

– Will have provision for the adjustment of height and mobility.

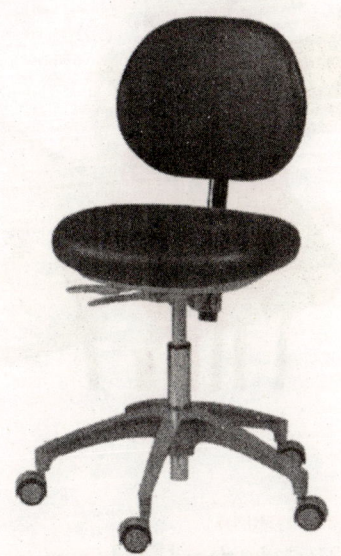

Fig. 4.6

3. DENTAL ASSISTANT'S CHAIR (Fig. 4.7)

- It provides stability, mobility and comfort.
- We have an adjustable foot platform or foot ring and an abdominal support bar.

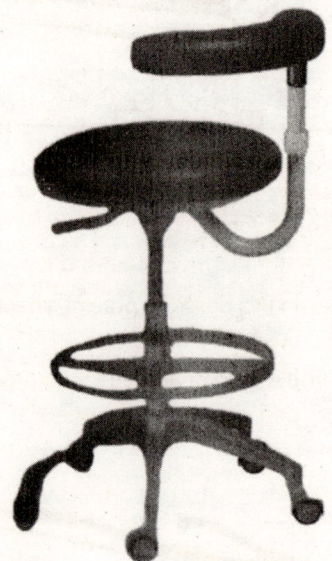

Fig. 4.7

4. DENTAL UNIT (Fig. 4.8)

- The basic function of a dental unit is to provide the necessary electrical and air-operated mechanisms to the hoses, attachments and working parts of the unit.
- The attachments and controls of the dental unit are operated by initiating a master switch.

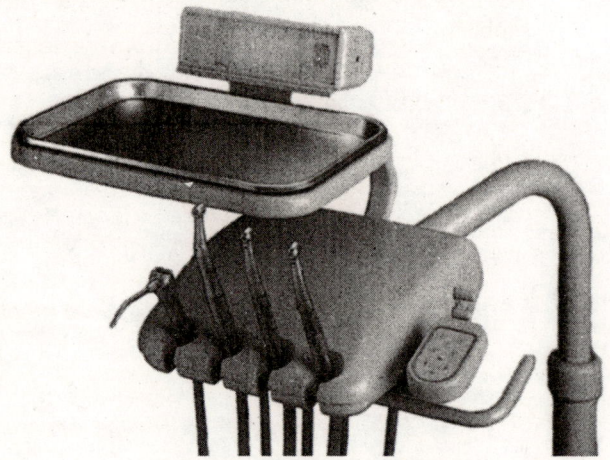

Fig. 4.8

1. Delivery Systems

- It includes dental handpieces, air water syringe, etc.

2. Rheostat

- Dental handpieces are attached to a specific hose in the dental unit.
- The dentist will use a rheostat to operate and control the speed.
- It is a foot controlled device that is placed on the floor near the operator with foot pressure, the slow-speed and high-speed handpieces can be controlled.

3. Waterlines

- Dental unit supplies the water needed for dental procedures.
- This is crucial for keeping an area clean as well as cooled against the heat resulting from the mechanical removal of tooth structure.
- Several hoses are equipped with water lines. These lines carry water that is used throughout a dental procedure.

4. Air-Water Syringe (Fig. 4.9)

- It is attached to the dental unit and is a necessity for every procedure.

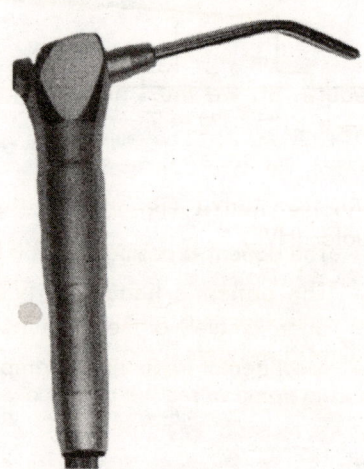

Fig. 4.9

Functions

1. Delivers a stream of water.
2. Delivers a stream of air.
3. Delivers a combined spray of air and water.
- The tip of the air-water syringe should be replaced after every procedure.

5. Operating Light (Fig. 4.10)

- It is used to illuminate the oral cavity during the treatment procedure.
- The light is very bright and care should be taken to avoid shining it into the patient's eyes.

– The light is attached to a flexible arm that is attached to the dental chair.

– First the light should be positioned on the patients's chest approximately 25 to 30 inches below the patient's chin.

– The light is turned on and then slowly adjusted upward to illuminate the oral cavity.

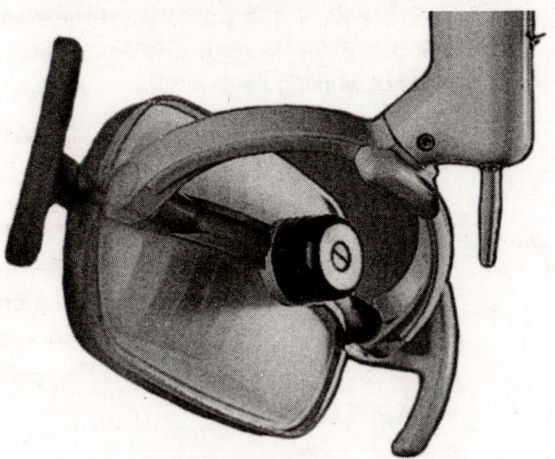

Fig. 4.10

5. ORAL EVACUATION SYSTEM

– Water is commonly used throughout a dental procedure. So we must have some means to remove it.

– To do that, the dental unit contains two evacuation system, i.e. saliva ejector and high-volume evacuator (HVE).

6. CURING LIGHT (Fig. 4.11)

– It is a wand like attachment used to 'harden or cure' light cured dental materials.

– The curing light causes the chemical reaction that allows the material to harden.

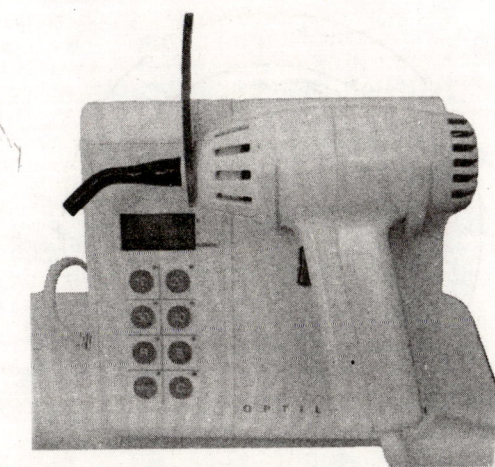

Fig. 4.11

– The components of the light are the protective shield handle and the trigger switch to turn it on and off.

7. AMALGAMATOR (Fig. 4.12)

– It is used to triturate or mechanically mix dental materials by vigorously shaking the capsule that holds the ingredients.

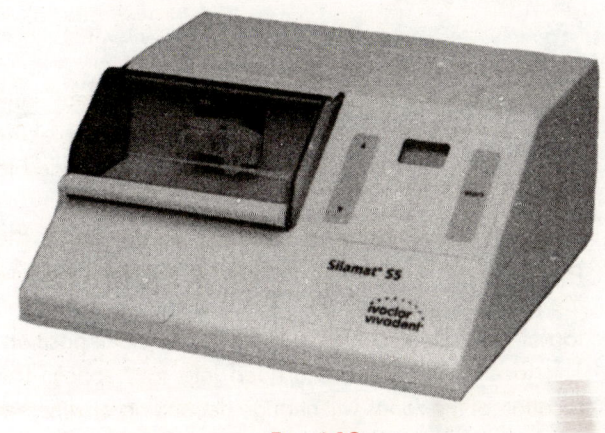

Fig. 4.12

8. DENTAL RADIOGRAPH UNIT

– It is used to take the radiographs.

9. VIEW BOX FOR RADIOGRAPHS

– A view box is used to read and diagnose radiographs.

– It consists of a bright white light source with a frosted - glass or plastic cover.

– The radiographs are mounted and then placed on the view box for evaluation.

– The light source shines through the radiograph, allowing for a better visual evaluation from the dentist.

10. MISCELLANEOUS

1. Central Vacuum Compressor

– It provides the suction needed for the oral evacuation systems.

– It consists of two parts, i.e. the compressor, which creates the flow of air and the vacuum tank, which screens the flow of air to create suction.

2. Central Air Compressor

– It provides compressed air for the air-water syringe and air - driven hand pieces.

– The capacity of the compressor depends on the number of dental units used in the practice.

– Because of the noise level and for safety reasons, the compressor system is placed outside the clinical setting.

POSITIONING OF THE DENTAL TEAM AND THE PATIENT

A. OBJECTIVES
1. Access to the operative field.
2. Visibility.
3. Comfort.
4. Patient safety.

B. ZONES OF OPERATIVE FIELD
- Operating zones are based on a "clock concept" and offer the best way to identify the working position of the dental team, dental equipment and supplies needed to perform a procedure (Fig. 4.13)
- Visualize a circle placed over the dental chair, the patient's face is in the center of the circle and the top of the patient's face is in the center of the circle and the top of the patient's head is at the 12 O' clock position. The face of the clock is divided into four zones. The location of the zones will change depending on whether the operator is right-handed a left-handed. The operator's position varies within that zone depending on the treatment to be delivered.
- This basic concept is utilized for practicing the efficient and comfortable clinical dentistry and it can be applied to any dental procedure.
- Operative field is divided into 4 zones, they are,

1. *Operator's Zone (right handed-7 O' clock to 12 O' clock)*
   - This is the zone where the operator seats and it has several common positions.

2. *Transfer Zone (right handed-4 O' clock to 7 O' clock)*
   - Located near the oral cavity where instruments and materials are transferred between the operator and the assistant.

3. *Assistant Zone (right handed-2 O' clock to 4 O' clock)*
   - It is the zone where the assistant is seated and it allows the assistant to access both the transfer zone and the static zone.

4. *Static Zone (right handed-12 O' clock to 2 O' clock)*
   - Contains auxiliary equipments and supplies for the operating team.

C. POSITIONING OF THE OPERATOR
- Operator is seated well back on the stool with feet flat on the floor, legs relaxed and relatively together and thighs parallel to the floor.
- The back is straight and supported by the back rest.
- The head and neck are slightly bent toward the patient, so that eyes are directed downward.
- An optimal eye to work distance is regarded as 16–18 inches.

D. OPERATOR'S CHAIR POSITION
- Operator seats in the operator's zone and the following are the several positions which are practiced at working field (Fig. 4.13)

For a right handed operator

1. *12 O' clock : Direct Rear Position*
   - Operator is located directly behind the patient and looks down over the patient's head.
   - Position is primarily used for operating on the lingual surfaces of mandibular anterior teeth.
   - *Disadvantage:* Severe bending of the operators back and neck.

2. *11 O' clock : Right Rear Position*
   - It is considered to be universal operating position as it provides access to all areas directly or indirectly using a mouth mirror except the more distal areas of the mandibular right quadrant, the cervical areas on the patient's right posterior quadrants.

3. *9 O' clock : Right Position*
   - The operator is directly to right of patient.
   - It provides access for operating on the facial surfaces of the maxillary and mandibular right posterior teeth. Occlusal surfaces of mandibular right posterior teeth.

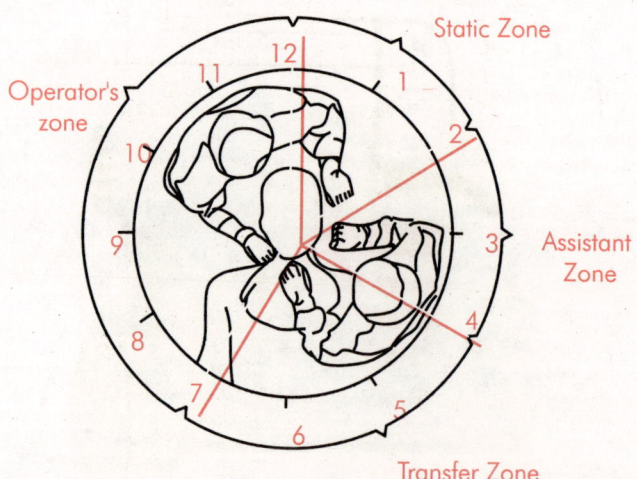

Fig. 4.13

4. *7 O' clock : Right Front Position*
- Position provides access to mandibular anterior teeth, mandibular posterior teeth and maxillary anterior teeth.

E. POSITIONING OF THE DENTAL ASSISTANT
- The assistant should be seated at a higher position (such that the assistant's head is 4 to 6 inches higher than the operator's) on his/ her stool, so his/her knees will be in level with the patient's head, with his/her feet resting on the foot rest of his/her chair.
- The assistant should be seated with his/her back straight and with an unobstructed straight line view of the field of operation.

F. OPTIMUM DISTANCE FROM OPERATOR TO PATIENT
- Acceptable position in (Fig. 414) shows the patient at the operator's elbow level and the oral cavity of the patient approximately 15 inches from the operator's eyes.

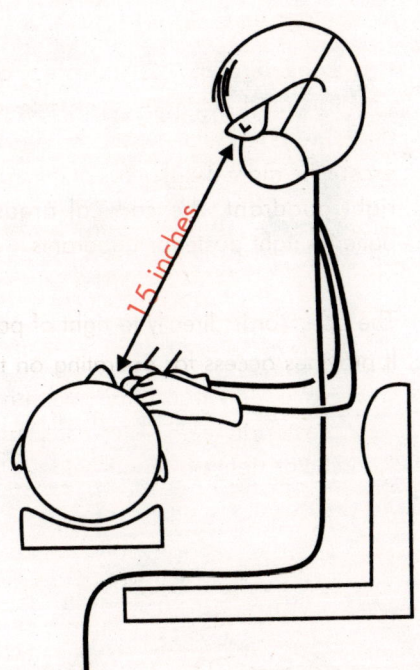

15 inches

Fig. 4.14

BASIC INSTRUMENT TRAY SETUP
- The order of arranging the instruments in the bracket tray is as follows,

1. *Diagnostic instruments:* Mouth mirror, Probe, Explorer, Tweezer.
2. *Excavating instruments:* Spoon excavator, Discoid, Cleoid.
3. *Hand cutting instruments:* Enamel Hatchet, GMT.
4. *Filling instruments:* Cement spatula, Agate spatula, Plastic filling instrument.
5. *Condensing instruments:* Round condenser, Parallelogram condenser.
6. *Burnishing instrument:* Ball burnishers.
7. *Carving instruments:* Hollenback, Ward's and Diamond carvers.
8. *Amalgam carrier.*
9. *Miscellaneous instruments:* Scissors, B.P. blade, Matrix bands and retainers, Cotton holder, Dappendish, etc.

Section VI

The Review

CHAPTER 01

THE REVIEW

- This section contains a mixture of MCQ's and one word questions. To encourage textbook reading, we have not given answers to all questions except for a few.

1. What part of instrument is located between the handle and the working end?

2. What classification of instruments is used to remove decay manually?

3. What are the four uses of mouth mirror?

4. What is the main feature of the working end of an explorer?

5. What instruments makeup the basic setup?

6. Which instrument is used to measure the sulcus of a tooth?

7. What are the two most common excavators used in restorative dentistry?

8. What instrument is used to carve anatomy back into the interproximal portion of an amalgam restoration?

9. What instrument is used to pack amalgam?

10. What type of instrument is discoid/cleiod?

11. What type of scissors is placed on the restorative tray setup?

12. What is the another term for Howe pliers?

13. What are the two most common types of dental handpieces?

14. How fast does the low-speed handpiece operate?

15. Which attachment is used to hold a latch-type bur?

16. How fast does the high-speed handpiece operate?

17. How is the tooth kept cool and clean during the use of the high-speed handpiece?

18. What type of bur locking system is used on the high-speed handpiece?

19. What type of shank fits into the contra-angle attachment?

20. Restorative burs are made from what material?

21. What design of bur is a 33 ½ ?

22. What gives the diamond bur its advantage?

23. What is used to hold a disc in the handpiece?

24. The first number in the instrument formula indicates?

25. The type of chisel with the shank and blade slightly curved is?

26. Instrument used to plane buccoproximal and linguoproximal walls in a class II cavity is?

27. In dental burs, the angle formed b/w the back of the blade and the tooth surface is called as?

28. Honing machine is used for?

29. What are the advantages of serrations on the condenser face?

30. How does the high-speed handpiece work?

    Is driven by compressed air. The head of the handpiece contains a cartridge which contain the air turbine with a central chuck. The turbine held in position by two sets of ball bearings. When air pressure turns the turbine, the central chuck also rotates along with it. The bur will be attached to the central chuck.

31. How does the bur stay in the central collect chuck?

    The central chuck is hollow. One end of the chuck is split into leaves that can be released or tightened by turning the bur chuck anticlockwise. While inserting or removing the bur, the central chuck should be open and the bur chuck is turned in a clockwise direction to tighten the central chuck.

32. What is bur chuck?

    A device used to loosen or tighten the central collect chuck to insert or remove a bur.

33. How are instruments classified?

34. What are the parts of an instrument?

35. Discuss the Black's instrument nomenclature?

36. Discuss the Black's instrument formula?

37. What are direct cutting and lateral cutting instruments?

38. What is instrument contrangling?

39. Discuss about single bevelled instruments?

40. What are the functions of mouth mirror?

41. List the types of explorers?

42. What are the diagnostic instruments?

43. How to identify the right and left GMT?

44. Classify the speeds in dentistry?

45. What are the parts of a bur?

46. List the various types of burs?

47. What is rake angle?

48. In a tooth in which the pulp has been removed, the pulpal wall becomes the axial wall.

49. What is butt joint?

50. What is lap/slip joint?

51. 'Eburnation' of dentin is seen in?

52. List the various types of cavities?

53. Define the cavity preparation?

54. List the steps in cavity preparation?

55. Define outline form and list the factors influence the outline form?

56. Define primary resistance form and list the various ways of achieving it?

57. Define primary retention form and list the various types?

58. Define secondary resistance and retention form and list the various types of it?

59. What are the functions of liners?

60. On what tooth structure is a liner placed?

61. Contraindications of varnish?

62. What does an insulating base do for a tooth?

63. What effect does eugenol have on the pulp?

64. Where is a base applied in the preparation?

65. What dental instrument is used to adapt a base into place?

66. What is the primary method of Hg contamination resulting from dentistry?
    a. Vapour release from patients
    b. Sewage contamination
    c. Cotton rolls in the trash
    d. Hg release from corpses after burial
    e. Spillage or losses in the dental office

67. What is a typical discharge limit for Hg contaminated water going into a sanitary sewer system?
    a. 5.0 ¼ g/l
    b. 3.0 ¼ g/l
    c. 1.0 ¼ g/l
    d. 0.1 ¼ g/l
    e. 0.01 ¼ g/l

68. Dental amalgam is defined as:
    a. A mixture of mercury with any metal
    b. A mixture of mercury with silver
    c. A mixture of mercury with silver and tin
    d. A mixture of mercury with any zinc alloy
    e. The alloy for mixing with mercury

69. How much mercury (by weight) is in a modern set dental amalgam?
    a. >60%
    b. 55–60%
    c. 50–55%
    d. 45–50%
    e. 40–45%

70. What is the copper content in low copper dental amalgam alloys?

   a. 0–5%
   b. 5–12%
   c. 12–30%
   d. 30–38%
   e. 38–50%

71. What COMPONENTS are typical in low copper dental amalgam alloy?

   a. Ag-Sn
   b. Ag-Sn-(Cu)-(Zn)
   c. Sn-Cu-Zn
   d. Ag-Sn-Cu-(Zn)
   e. Ag-Sn-Cu-Zn

72. What components are typical of high copper dental amalgam alloy?

   a. Ag-Sn-Cu
   b. Ag-Sn-Cu-(Zn)
   c. Ag-Sn-Zn
   d. Ag-Sn
   e. Sn-Cu-Zn

73. Which one of the following terms is not synonymous with the rest in the list?

   a. Comminuted particles
   b. Filings
   c. Lathe-cut particles
   d. Irregular particles
   e. Spherical particles

74. Comminution is:

   a. Milling or filing an ingot into powder particles
   b. Heat treatment to control the setting reaction of powder particles
   c. Decreasing the mercury content of an amalgam
   d. Eliminating the copper content of an amalgam alloy
   e. Elimination of the tarnish on an amalgam restoration

75. Spherical dental amalgam alloy particles are generally produced by:

   a. Liquid alloy atomization
   b. Flame melting of lathe cut particles
   c. Vitrification of lathe cut particles
   d. Comminution
   e. Heat treating lathe cut particles

76. Which one of the following is not a standard method of classification for dental amalgams?

   a. Particle shape
   b. Copper content
   c. Zinc content
   d. Number of powder particles
   e. Mercury content

77. Which one of the following is a high copper dental amalgam alloy?

   a. Velvalloy
   b. Caulk spherical
   c. Shofu spherical
   d. Dispersalloy
   e. New true dentalloy

78. Which one of the following is a low copper dental amalgam alloy?

   a. Tytin
   b. Sybralloy
   c. New true dentalloy
   d. Dispersalloy
   e. Aristalloy Cr

79. What is the reason Zn is used in a dental amalgam alloy?

   a. Oxygen scavenger in production
   b. Reducing mercury vapour release from the set restoration
   c. Improved hardness
   d. Controlling the setting reaction
   e. Prevent tarnishing

80. What is the reason Sn is included in a dental amalgam alloy?

   a. Corrosion protection
   b. Improved ductility
   c. Prevent tarnishing
   d. Increased tensile strength
   e. Particle dissolution during reaction

81. What is the reason Cu is included in a dental amalgam alloy?

   a. Corrosion protection
   b. Increased ductility
   c. Prevention of tarnishing
   d. Reduction in amalgamation speed
   e. Improved condensability

82. The setting reaction of dental amalgam proceeds primarily by:

   a. Dissolution of the entire alloy particle into mercury
   b. Dissolution of the Cu from the particles into mercury
   c. Mercury reaction with Ag on or in the alloy particle
   d. Formation of Zn-Hg crystals
   e. Precipitation of Sn-Hg crystals

83. What is the abbreviation for the Ag-Sn phase?

   a. Gamma
   b. Gamma 1
   c. Gamma 2
   d. Eta
   e. Epsilon

84. What is the abbreviation for the Ag-Hg phase?
    a. Gamma
    b. Gamma 1
    c. Gamma 2
    d. Eta
    e. Beta

85. What is the abbreviation for the Sn-Hg phase?
    a. Gamma
    b. Gamma 1
    c. Gamma 2
    d. Beta
    e. Epsilon

86. Which phase in a set dental amalgam contains most of the mercury?
    a. Gamma
    b. Gamma 1
    c. Gamma 2
    d. Eta
    e. Epsilon

87. Which one of the following is responsible for contraction during the dental amalgam setting reaction?
    a. Cooling of the amalgam mixture after trituration
    b. Settling of the particles in the fluid matrix
    c. Higher density of the product phases *versus* reactant phases
    d. Loss of mercury due to vaporization
    e. Mercury penetration into the pores of the powder particles

88. Which one of the following is responsible for expansion during the dental amalgam setting reaction?
    a. Lower density of the product *versus* reactant phases
    b. Impingement of Ag-Hg crystals in matrix during growth
    c. Increased temperature of the mass due to exothermic heat
    d. Dissolution of selective components out of the particles
    e. Formation of by-product gases during the reaction

89. What is the ADA limit for expansion or contraction during the setting of dental amalgam?
    a. <1 μm/cm
    b. <20 μm/cm
    c. <50 m/cm
    d. <100 m/cm
    e. <250 m/cm

90. Which one of the following variables does not influence the amount of dimensional change during setting of dental amalgams?
    a. Alloy particle size or shape
    b. Hg/alloy ratio
    c. Trituration time
    d. Condensation method
    e. Burnishing technique

91. What does the batch (or lot) number code of "040501" on an amalgam alloy mean?
    a. It was produced on January 5, 2004 (First two letters indicate *year*, next two for *day* and last two are for *month*)
    b. It was shipped on January 5, 2004
    c. It is no longer acceptable after January 5, 2004
    d. That it contains 4Sn-5Cu-1Zn in the alloy
    e. That it should not be used before January 5, 2004

92. A properly triturated dental amalgam mixture should look like a:
    a. Grainy, dull mass
    b. Coherent, smooth mass
    c. Grainy, wet mixture
    d. Fibrous, dull mass
    e. Fibrous, shiny mass

93. Which one of the following produces the most mercury-rich matrix removal?
    a. Condensation late in the working time
    b. Use of the largest condenser tip
    c. Use of the most load during condensation
    d. Non-overlapping condensing strokes
    e. Burnishing

94. What is the effectiveness for high copper dental amalgams?
    a. 1–2 years
    b. 4–5 years
    c. 8–12 years
    d. 20–25 years
    e. 30–50 years

95. Which one of the following mechanisms of failure is most common for low copper dental amalgam?
    a. Excessive tarnish
    b. Bulk fracture
    c. Intergranular corrosion of the occlusal surface
    d. Dental caries
    e. Marginal fracture

96. Which one of the following mechanisms of failure is most common for high copper dental amalgam?
    a. Excessive tarnish
    b. Bulk fracture
    c. Intergranular corrosion of the occlusal surface
    d. Enamel wall fracture from thermal expansion stresses
    e. Marginal fracture

97. What is the typical compressive strength (after 24 hrs) for high copper amalgam?
    a. 25,000 psi
    b. 35,000 psi
    c. 45,000 psi

d. 55,000 psi
e. 65,000 psi

98. What is the percentage of the final strength (24 hr) is developed by a newly placed (15 min) dental amalgam?

a. < 40 %
b. 40–60 %
c. 60–80 %
d. 80–95 %
e. 95–98 %

99. Which one of the following amalgams displays the highest early strength?

a. Irregular particle low copper amalgam
b. Spherical particle low copper amalgam
c. Irregular particle high copper amalgam
d. Irregular + spherical particle high copper amalgam
e. Spherical particle high copper amalgam

100. Marginal fracture of dental amalgam is not associated with this property.

a. Compressive strength
b. Creep
c. Mercury content
d. Electrochemical properties
e. Thermal conductivity

101. Which one of the following mechanical properties is the most important in determining the resistance to marginal fracture?

a. Compressive strength
b. Tensile strength
c. Shear strength
d. Flexural strength
e. Brittleness

102. Which one of the following does not affect the strength of dental amalgam?

a. Time between trituration and condensation
b. Mercury content
c. Zinc content
d. Condensation effectiveness
e. Porosity

103. What is the creep value for most high copper dental amalgams?

a. 10%
b. 5–10%
c. 1–5%
d. <1%
e. 0%

104. The creep value of low copper dental amalgams correlates with:

a. Marginal fracture
b. Bulk fracture
c. Tensile strength
d. Setting time
e. Burnishability

105. Which one of the following intraoral ions is primarily responsible for amalgam tarnish?

a. Cl
b. S
c. Na
d. K
e. O

106. Which one of the elements in dental amalgam in primarily responsible for tarnish?

a. Silver
b. Tin
c. Zinc
d. Mercury
e. Copper

107. What type of electrochemical corrosion is most common at the margins of dental amalgam?

a. Galvanic corrosion
b. Structure-sensitive corrosion (local galvanic corrosion)
c. Crevice corrosion (concentration cell corrosion)
d. Intergranular corrosion
e. Stress corrosion

108. In low copper dental amalgams, which phase is the most anodic?

a. Gamma
b. Gamma 1
c. Gamma 2
d. Eta
e. Epsilon

109. During electrochemical corrosion of low copper dental amalgam, which corrosion product which forms is insoluble?

a. Sn-O
b. Sn-O-Cl
c. Sn-Cl
d. Ag-Cl
e. Cu-Sn

110. During electrochemical corrosion of high copper dental amalgam, which corrosion product which forms is insoluble?

a. Sn-O
b. Sn-O-Cl
c. Sn-Cl
d. Ag-Cl
e. Cu-Sn

111. In a high copper dental amalgams, which phase is the most anodic?

a. Gamma
b. Gamma 1
c. Gamma 2
d. Eta
e. Beta

112. Which alloy pair produces the most powerful galvanic corrosion couple?
    a. Dental gold casting alloy / conventional dental amalgam
    b. Conventional dental amalgam / high copper dental amalgam
    c. Gamma phase / gamma one phase
    d. Spherical high copper amalgam / irregular high copper amalgam

113. Penetrating corrosion occurs in:
    a. Low copper dental amalgams because gamma 2 corrodes
    b. Low copper dental amalgams because gamma 1 corrodes
    c. High copper dental amalgams because gamma 2 corrodes
    d. High copper dental amalgams because gamma 1 corrodes
    e. High copper dental amalgams because eta corrodes

114. Superficial corrosion occurs in:
    a. Low copper dental amalgams because gamma 2 corrodes
    b. Low copper dental amalgams because gamma 1 corrodes
    c. High copper dental amalgams because gamma 2 corrodes
    d. High copper dental amalgams because gamma 1 corrodes
    e. High copper dental amalgams because eta corrodes

115. During the corrosion of low copper dental amalgam, which one of the following components may be lost from the restoration?
    a. Silver
    b. Tin
    c. Copper
    d. Mercury
    e. Zinc

116. During the corrosion of high copper dental amalgams, which one of the following elements may be lost from the restoration?
    a. Silver
    b. Tin
    c. Copper
    d. Mercury
    e. Zinc

117. Mercury vapour limits (TLV) are defined by OSHA as:
    a. < 1   g/m3
    b. < 10   g/m3
    c. < 25   g/m3

    d. < 50   g/m3
    e. < 90   g/m3

118. Mercury vapour produces hypersensitivity reactions in:
    a. < 1/1,000,000 people
    b. < 1/500,000 people
    c. < 1/100,000 people
    d. < 1/1,000 people
    e. < 1/100 people

119. Spherical high copper dental amalgams (vs low copper types) have:
    a. Better edge strength
    b. Better condensability
    c. Better ductility
    d. Higher initial strength
    e. Lower corrosion resistance

120. What are the two major goals for luting cements?
    a. Retention and sealing
    b. Hybrid layer formation and pulpal medication
    c. Stress distribution and chemical bonding to the restoration
    d. Minimal chemical irritation of the pulp and high strength
    e. Thermal insulation and chemical bonding to tooth structure

121. Which one of the following situations causes pulpal inflammation?
    a. Fluid movement in dental tubules
    b. High acidity of dental cements
    c. Long-term decomposition of cement reactions products
    d. Diffusion of endotoxins to the pulp
    e. High concentrations of sucrose in saliva near open tubules

122. Which one of the following is the most important property for dental cement to guarantee long-term clinical success?
    a. Compressive strength
    b. Resistance to solubility and disintegration
    c. Low coefficient of thermal expansion
    d. Radiopacity similar to tooth structure
    e. Setting contraction

123. Microleakage of bacterial endotoxins will result in:
    a. Pulpal inflammation
    b. Sensitivity
    c. Cement dissolution
    d. Loss of adhesion to dentin
    e. Plaque formation under the cement

124. Which one of the following dental cements does not contain zinc oxide as part of its powder composition?
    a. Zinc phosphate cement
    b. Zinc silico-phosphate cement

c. ZOE cement
d. Durelon cement
e. Silicate cement

125. Which one of the following dental cements does not contain water as part of the composition of the liquid component?
    a. ZP
    b. ZOE
    c. PCC
    d. SC
    e. GI

126. Which one of the following has an extremely important effect on the final properties of a dental cement?
    a. P/L ratio
    b. Temperature at mixing
    c. Relative humidity
    d. Rate of mixing
    e. Amount of ambient light

127. What is the effect of 10% porosity on the strength of dental cement?
    a. 10% increase
    b. 10% decrease
    c. 20% decrease
    d. 50% decrease
    e. None

128. Phosphoric acid solutions which are used as the liquid component of zinc phosphate and silico-phosphate cements have an initial pH value of:
    a. 0.1 to 1.0
    b. 1.0 to 2.0
    c. 2.0 to 3.0
    d. 3.0 to 5.0
    e. 5.0 to 7.0

129. Which one of the following cements uses a liquid that is an aqueous solution of polymer?
    a. ZP
    b. ZOE-EBA
    c. GI
    d. SPC
    e. SC

130. During the initial setting reaction for dental cements, approximately what percentage of powder is reacted?
    a. 10 to 25%
    b. 25 to 50%
    c. 50 to 75%
    d. 75 to 90%
    e. 90 to 100%

131. Approximately what level of cement setting reaction is complete after the first hour?
    a. 0–25%
    b. 25–50%

c. 50–75%
d. 75–90%
e. 90–100%

132. What is the method of determining the setting time for dental cement reactions?
    a. Peak exotherm of the reaction
    b. Time interval to 150 psi strength
    c. Large Gilmore needle
    d. Loss of gloss
    e. None of the above

133. Which one of the following cements should be mixed on a chilled glass slab?
    a. ZOE cement
    b. ZOE reinforced cement
    c. ZOE-EBA cement
    d. Zinc phosphate cement
    e. Polycarboxylate cement

134. For which one of the following dental cement types is the incremental addition of powder to the liquid extremely important during the mixing of the cement?
    a. CP
    b. PCC
    c. ZP
    d. ZOE
    e. GI

135. Which one of the following zinc phosphate cement components primarily controls the reactivity of the powder and the liquid during mixing?
    a. Zinc oxide powder particle size
    b. Magnesium oxide additives
    c. Aluminum phosphate buffers
    d. Zinc phosphate buffers
    e. Water content of the liquid

136. Which one of the following mixing methods is correct for zinc phosphate cement manipulation?
    a. 6 incremental additions of P over 90–120 sec with stropping on chilled glass slab.
    b. 3 incremental additions of P over 90–120 sec using a chilled glass slab.
    c. Rapid combination of all P into all L at the outset.
    d. 3 incremental additions over 120 sec using a paper mixing pad.
    e. None of the above.

137. Which one of the following dental cement phas not crystalline?
    a. Zinc eugenolate
    b. Tertiary zinc phosphate
    c. Zinc oxide
    d. Magnesium oxide
    e. Zinc polyacrylate

138. Which one of the following methods is acceptable for retarding the polycarboxylate cement reaction during mixing?
    a. Use a chilled glass slab
    b. Use chilled components
    c. Add water to the liquid components
    d. Decrease the powder-to-liquid ratio
    e. Use incremental addition of powder to liquid

139. Fluoride release from silicate cement involves:
    a. Fluoride ion dissolution from particles and diffusion through the matrix
    b. Fluoride uptake from saliva and re-release at other times
    c. Hydrogen ion substitution from saliva for fluoride ion in the matrix
    d. Visible light acceleration of ionization of components in residual powder
    e. Precipitation of fluoride by calcium ions in saliva

140. The setting reaction of polycarboxylate cement creates which one of the following reaction products in the matrix?
    a. Zinc ethoxybenzoate
    b. Zinc eugenolate
    c. Tertiary zinc phosphate
    d. Zinc polyacrylate gel
    e. Calcium phosphate

141. Which one of the following acids have not been copolymerized into PCC liquid?
    a. Acrylic acid
    b. Maleic acid
    c. Itaconic acid
    d. Tartaric acid
    e. Phthallic acid

142. Traditional glass ionomer cements are a hybrid of:
    a. ZP and PCC
    b. SC and SPC
    c. ZOE-EBA and SC
    d. SC and PCC
    e. HV-EBA and ZP

143. The final reaction product matrix of a traditional GI cement is composed of:
    a. Ca acrylate gel
    b. Al acrylate gel
    c. Tertiary zinc phosphate
    d. Crystalline zinc ethoxybenzoate
    e. BIS-GMA polymer

144. Which one of the following does not include a glass ionomer reaction product?
    a. MM-GIC
    b. Compomer
    c. RM-GIC

d. RR-GIC
e. Giomer

145. Fluoride is released from glass ionomer cements by:
    a. Saliva reaction with residual glass particles
    b. Diffusion out of the matrix
    c. K and Na exchange reactions with CaF2
    d. Secondary chemcial reactions of saliva with the matrix
    e. Dissolution of fluoroapatite filler particles in the cement

146. After 1 week the typical fluoride release levels for a glass ionomer are:
    a. 20–25 ppm
    b. 15–20 ppm
    c. 10–15 ppm
    d. 5–10 ppm
    e. 1–2 ppm

147. Which one of the following vehicles cannot be used to recharge glass ionomer cement?
    a. Toothpastes
    b. Mouthwashes
    c. Topical fluorides
    d. HF

148. What is the powder component in GICs (traditional glass ionomers)?
    a. Zinc oxide
    b. Silica
    c. Lithium aluminosilicate
    d. Aluminosilicate glass
    e. Alumina

149. What is the liquid component in GICs (traditional glass ionomers)?
    a. Polyacrylic acid
    b. Polymethacrylic acid
    c. Polymethyl methacrylate
    d. BIS-GMA polymer
    e. Phosphoric acid

150. Which one of the following has not been used as part of the GIC liquid composition?
    a. Acrylic acid
    b. Tartaric acid
    c. Maleic acid
    d. Citric acid
    e. Itaconic acid

151. Which one of the following has not been used to modify the GIC powder composition?
    a. Aluminosilicate glass
    b. Amalgam alloy particles
    c. Ag-Pd particles
    d. TiO_2 particles
    e. Alumina

152. How is F ion released from a cured GIC?
    a. Intraoral fluids dissolve it out of the glass particles
    b. CaF$_2$ salts dissolve and release the fluoride
    c. Fluoride ions in the matrix are released
    d. Sodium fluoride salts release the fluoride
    e. Acid in the oral environment dissolves the residual glass

153. What causes the initial setting reaction in a GIC?
    a. Release of fluoride ions from the aluminosilicate glass
    b. Crosslinking of polyacrylic acid polymer chains by aluminum ions
    c. Loss of water from the matrix phase
    d. Crosslinking of polyacrylic acid polymer chains by calcium ions
    e. Crystallization of the dissolved salts from the powder particles

154. What causes the final setting reaction of in a GIC?
    a. Release of fluoride ions from the aluminosilicate glass
    b. Crosslinking of polyacrylic acid polymer chains by calcium ions
    c. Crosslinking of polyacrylic acid polymer chains by aluminum ions
    d. Loss of water from the matrix phase
    e. Crystallization of the dissolved salts from the powder particles

155. What produces chemical adhesion to tooth structure for a GIC?
    a. Chelation of polyacrylic acid with calcium ions
    b. Chelation of polyacrylic acid with aluminum ions
    c. Reactions of the fluoride ions with hydroxyapatite
    d. Precipitation of calcium phosphate from the dissolved powder
    e. Precipitation of calcium oxide

156. Contaminated or overly wet tooth surfaces interfere with the:
    a. Adaptation of the cement for chemical bonding
    b. Initial setting reaction
    c. Final setting reaction
    d. Release of fluoride ion
    e. Colour of the final cement

157. Which one of the following is key during the first 24 hours for conventional GIs?
    a. Protection against contact with moisture
    b. Protection against intraoral acid contact
    c. Protection from ultraviolet radiation
    d. Protection against salivary protein contact
    e. Protection against fluoride release

158. What is the time of maximum fluoride release RATE out of the cement?
    a. During the first a few minutes
    b. During the first 24 hours
    c. During the first month
    d. During the first year
    e. After the first year

159. Which one of the following is not a major use for glass ionomers?
    a. Class V filling material
    b. Liner
    c. Base
    d. Cement
    e. Tunnel preparations

160. Which application takes best advantage of chemical adhesion of glass ionomers?
    a. Class V filling material
    b. Liner
    c. Base
    d. Cement
    e. Tunnel preparations

161. Which application takes best advantage of the fluoride release of glass ionomers?
    a. Liner
    b. Base
    c. Root caries restorations
    d. Retrograde filling material
    e. Core

162. Which one of the following has the most influence on the final mechanical and chemical properties of conventional GI cements?
    a. Fluoride content of the aluminosilicate glass
    b. Mixing technique
    c. Powder-to-liquid ratio
    d. Acidity of the mixture
    e. Reaction exotherm

163. What is the mechanism of reinforcement of metal-modified GIs?
    a. Addition of stronger powder particles
    b. Addition of particles which can be chelated by matrix
    c. Addition of particles which can dissolve and affect reaction
    d. Addition of particle that accelerate fluoride release
    e. Addition of insoluble particles

164. What is the major difference between chemically-cured and light-cured (LC) GIs?
    a. LC produces second matrix
    b. LC version has no acid–base reaction
    c. LC versions accelerate release of F from alumino-silicate glass
    d. LC eliminates all moisture sensitivity of material
    e. LC version increases adhesion to tooth structure

165. Which one of the following is not part of a "multiple-curing" GI system?
    a. Ca++ ion crosslinking of acid-functional polymer chains
    b. Al+++ ion replacement of Ca++ crosslinking
    c. Visible light polymerization of matrix monomers into polymer
    d. Chemical curing of matrix monomers into polymer
    e. F ion crosslinking of polymer chains

166. What is the term used for glass ionomers that are very similar to composites?
    a. Hybrid ionomers
    b. Compomers
    c. Hybrid composites
    d. Giomers
    e. Glass ionomer modified composites

167. Which one of the following is not an objective for pulp protection?
    a. Adhesion to amalgam
    b. Chemical protection
    c. Mechanical protection
    d. Thermal protection
    e. Pulpal medication

168. Pulpal sensitivity is caused primarily by:
    a. Vibration from cavity preparation
    b. Thermal trauma
    c. Electrical trauma
    d. Fluid flow in tubules
    e. Chemical irritation from bacteria

169. Fluid flow is detected by:
    a. Mechanoreceptors on the edge of the pulp
    b. C-axis nerve fibers that penetrate into the tubules
    c. Odontoblast cells
    d. Odontoblastic processes
    e. Fibroblasts

170. Chronic inflammation is caused primarily by:
    a. Mechanical inflammation
    b. Fluid flow in tubules
    c. Thermal trauma
    d. Microleakage of endotoxins
    e. Chemical irritation from dental materials

171. The dentin smear layer increases:
    a. Chemical adhesion for varnishes
    b. Mechanical adhesion for liners
    c. Thermal insulation for the pulp
    d. Coverage of tubule openings
    e. Formation of reparative dentin

172. Reduction in tooth sensitivity with decreased fluid flow in tubules is related to the:
    a. Number of tubules above a critical size
    b. Square of the tubule radius
    c. Cube of the tubule diameter
    d. Fourth power of the tubule radius
    e. Surface energy at the tubule opening

173. Copalite is classified as:
    a. Solution liner
    b. Suspension liner
    c. Cement liner
    d. Cement base
    e. Cement filling material

174. Suspension liners [e.g. Ca(OH)$_2$ in H$_2$O] harden intraorally by the:
    a. Physical reaction of drying
    b. Physical reaction of a sol-gel transformation
    c. Chemical reaction of acids and bases
    d. Chemical reaction involving polymerization
    e. Chemical reaction involving chelation

175. What is the typical thickness range for varnishes?
    a. 2–5 μm (0.002–0.005 mm)
    b. 10–50 μm (0.010–0.050 mm)
    c. 50–100 μm (0.050–0.100 mm)
    d. 100–200 μm (0.100–0.200 mm)
    e. 200–1000 μm (0.200–1.000 mm)

176. What is the thickness of thermal insulation required for pulpal protection?
    a. 2–5 μm (0.002–0.005 mm)
    b. 10–50 μm (0.010–0.050 mm)
    c. 50–200 μm (0.050–0.100 mm)
    d. 200–1000 μm (0.200–0.500 mm)
    e. 1000–2000 μm (1.000–2.000 mm)

177. Varnishes should be applied in:
    a. 1 thin coat
    b. 1 thick coat
    c. 2 thin coats
    d. 2 thick coats
    e. 1 thin and 1 thick coat

178. How much tubule coverage is produced by 1 thin coating of varnish?
    a. 25%
    b. 50%
    c. 75%
    d. 90%
    e. 100%

179. The chemical composition of copalite includes all of the following, except:
    a. Organic resin
    b. Chloroform solvent
    c. Acetone solvent
    d. Alcohol solvent
    e. Calcium hydroxide

180. What is the average lifetime for the integrity of a varnish film?
    a. 1 hour
    b. 1 day
    c. 1 month
    d. 1 year
    e. 10 years

181. DYCAL is classified as a:
    a. Solution liner
    b. Suspension liner
    c. Cement liner
    d. Cement base
    e. Cement filling material

182. Dental materials that are designed as pulpal medicaments contain:
    a. Calcium hydroxide or eugenol
    b. Calcium phosphate or eugenol
    c. Calcium hydroxide or methyl salicylate
    d. Zinc oxide or eugenol
    e. Calcium hydroxide or zinc oxide

183. The pH of concentrated calcium hydroxide solutions is:
    a. pH = 1–3
    b. pH = 3–5
    c. pH = 5–7
    d. pH = 7–9
    e. pH = 9–11

184. Which intraoral component is required to start the setting of DYCAL?
    a. Ca ions from tooth structure
    b. Higher temperatures of the intraoral tissues
    c. Denatured proteins in the smear layer
    d. Monovalent ions from saliva
    e. Moisture for calcium hydroxide dissociation

185. What is the key ionic species for the setting of DYCAL and life?
    a. Zn^{++}
    b. Ca^{++}
    c. Sn^{++}
    d. K^+
    e. Na^+

186. Which factor is least important to thermal protection of the pulp?
    a. Thickness of the insulating material
    b. Temperature gradient from the mouth to the pulp
    c. Time period of thermal imbalance
    d. Coefficient of thermal conductivity
    e. Copper content in the overlying dental amalgam

187. Thermal transients in the mouth are typically:
    a. 5–10s in the range of 37–95 °C
    b. 5–10s in the range of 5–95 °C
    c. 30–60s in the range of 5–60 °C
    d. 60–90s in the range of 0–100 °C
    e. 60–90s in the range of 10–45 °C

188. The rate of change of temperature in the pulp depends on:
    a. Thermal conductivity of overlying materials
    b. Thermal diffusivity of overlying materials
    c. Thermal contraction of overlying materials
    d. Thermal expansion of overlying materials
    e. Electrical conductivity of overlying materials

189. Which one of the following is false about a cement liner?
    a. The setting reaction is accelerated by moisture
    b. The liner should be placed in relatively thin layers
    c. It has sufficient strength in 6–7 mins to support amalgam condensation
    d. It releases constituents for pulpal medication
    e. It provides adequate mechanical strength to replace existing dentin

190. Dental materials to be used at bases should have compressive strengths of:
    a. 1000– 5000 psi [7–35 MPa]
    b. 5000–12000 psi [35–80 MPa]
    c. 12000–15000 psi [80–100 MPa]
    d. 15000–30000 psi [100–200 MPa]
    e. 30000–60000 psi [200–400 MPa]

191. Which one of the following statements is false about bases?
    a. An intermediate base is between the restoration and dentin
    b. A primary base is adjacent to the dentin
    c. A secondary base is next to the restoration
    d. A dental cement base is used to transfer stresses to sound dentin
    e. A dental cement base is mixed at low powder-to-liquid ratios.

192. What stresses must be supported during amalgam condensation?
    a. 50–170 psi [0.3–1.2 MPa]
    b. 170–500 psi [1.2–3.5 MPa]
    c. 500–1000 psi [3.5–7 MPa]
    d. 1000–5000 psi [7–35 MPa]
    e. 5000–7000 psi [35–70 MPa]

193. Which one of the following cements are typically used as bases?
    a. SPC, ZP, ZOE
    b. ZP, PC, GI, RMGI
    c. ZOE-EBA, ZP, GI
    d. CH, ZP, PC
    e. ZP, PC, COM

194. Which one of the following is not a stage in chain reaction polymerization?
    a. Activation
    b. Initiation
    c. Configuration
    d. Propagation
    e. Termination

195. Which one of the following monomers produces a linear polymer matrix?
    a. BIS-GMA
    b. MMA
    c. TEGDM
    d. Urethane dimethacrylate

196. Which one of the following species is comparatively high concentration in the average composite composition?
    a. Colorants
    b. Initiator
    c. Accelerator
    d. UV stabilizer
    e. Low MW monomer

197. Which of the following is false about chain reaction polymerization reactions during the setting of composite materials?
    a. Fast
    b. Involves double bonds
    c. Endothermic
    d. Requires initiation
    e. Involves acrylic monomers

198. The linear coefficient of thermal expansion for BIS-GMA polymer is which one of the following values?
    a. 2 ppm/°C
    b. 11 ppm/°C
    c. 45 ppm/°C
    d. 81 ppm/°C
    e. 90 ppm/°C

199. The BIS-GMA monomer unit is:
    a. Mono-functional
    b. Di-functional
    c. Tri-functional
    d. Tetra-functional
    e. Penta-functional

200. The reactive end groups of BIS-GMA monomer are most similar to which one of the following structures?
    a. Bisphenol-A
    b. Methyl methacrylate
    c. Benzoyl peroxide
    d. Methyl acrylate
    e. Urethane

201. Which one of the following categories of material will not be found in a visible light cured composite formulation?
    a. Reinforcing filler
    b. Visible light initiator
    c. Inhibitor
    d. PEMA
    e. BISGMA

202. All of the following are true about BIS-GMA monomer, except:
    a. Includes a bisphenol-A nucleus in the backbone
    b. Is high viscosity
    c. Is highly volatile
    d. Is called Bowen's resin
    e. Is impossible to purify by crystallization

203. Which of the following is not present in an auto-polymerizing dental composite?
    a. BIS-GMA
    b. BPO
    c. DHPT
    d. Silane
    e. PMMA

204. For silane coupling agents to effectively bond filler particles to matrices, which chemical species must be present on the filler particle surfaces?
    a. Si-O
    b. Zn-O
    c. Ba-O
    d. Zr-O
    e. H_2O

205. The three major components of composite restorative materials are:
    a. Resin — silane — filler
    b. Silane — filler — bonding system
    c. Bonding system — filler — acrylic resin
    d. Acid etchant — bonding agent — acrylic resin
    e. Acid etchant — bonding agent — filler

206. What is the role of silane in composite?
    a. Coupling agent
    b. Bonding agent
    c. Conditioning agent
    d. Acid etchant
    e. Polishing agent

207. Which one of the following is not a component of bonding agents used with composite restorations?
    a. Reinforcing filler
    b. Inhibitor
    c. Initiator
    d. Low MW monomer
    e. BIS-GMA

208. Which one of the following methods is not used to categorize composite restorations?
    a. Weight percent filler level
    b. Volume percent filler level
    c. Method of matrix activation
    d. Filler particle size (or distribution)
    e. Composite shade

209. Earlier generations of composites (macrofills) contained which one of the following volume percent levels of filler?
    a. 30 v/o
    b. 40 v/o
    c. 50 v/o
    d. 60 v/o
    e. 70 v/o

210. Which one of the following products contains the most filler?
    a. Macrofill composites
    b. Pit-and-fissure sealants
    c. Microfill composites
    d. Heterogeneous microfills
    e. Hybrid composites

211. Which one of the following products contains only very small filler particles?
    a. Macrofill composites
    b. Midifill composites
    c. Minifill composites
    d. Microfill composites
    e. Hybrid composites

212. Which one of the following materials is not a commercial composite?
    a. Delton
    b. Filtek Z250
    c. Prodigy condensable
    d. Heliomolar
    e. Revolution

213. Which of the following hybrid filler systems would not be clinically practical?
    a. Macrofill + microfill
    b. Midifill + microfill
    c. Minifill + microfill
    d. Minifill + nanofill
    e. Microfill + nanofill

214. What does a heterogeneous filler contain?
    a. Organic and inorganic phases
    b. Two different inorganic phases
    c. Porosity within the filler particle
    d. Crystalline and non-crystalline ceramic phases

215. Which one of the following systems is currently not used for curing composites?
    a. Ultraviolet-light curing
    b. Visible-light curing
    c. Chemical curing
    d. Dual curing
    e. Very high intensity light curing

216. Which one of the following produces the least depth-of-cure?
    a. Laser curing
    b. Very high intensity light curing
    c. Chemical curing
    d. Visible-light curing
    e. Dual curing

217. Microfilled composites are retained principally by:
    a. Resin tags
    b. Gross mechanical retention
    c. Chemical bonding to enamel
    d. Chemical bonding to dentin
    e. Chemical bonding to enamel and dentin

218. Which one of the following acids is generally recommended for etching?
    a. Maleic acid
    b. Polyacrylic acid
    c. Tartaric acid
    d. Phosphoric acid
    e. EDTA

219. In which of the following categories is dentin bonding of critical importance?
    a. Class III and IV restorations
    b. Class V and Erosion-Abrasion restorations
    c. Class I and II restorations

220. Which one of the following does not affect the depth-of-cure of double bonds incomposites?
    a. Method of activation
    b. Incremental addition
    c. Post-curing
    d. Composite color
    e. Finishing procedure

221. What is the reason for choosing a self-curing (or dual curing) composite rather than light-curing one?
    a. Large size of the restoration
    b. Poor access for the curing light
    c. High level of filler content
    d. Type of filler in the composite
    e. Ease of finishing

222. Which one of the following materials is not a retarders or inhibitors of chain reaction polymerization?
    a. Eugenol
    b. Calcium hydroxide
    c. Water
    d. Air
    e. Hydroquinone

223. Which one of the following materials should not be used as a base or liner below a composite resin restoration?
    a. Zinc oxide eugenol cement
    b. Calcium hydroxide cement
    c. Zinc phosphate cement
    d. EBA modified ZOE cement
    e. Polycarboxylate cement

224. What is the main reason for avoiding the use of green stones, white stones, or coarse diamond burs for finishing a composite?
    a. Heat generation
    b. Battering of enamel margins
    c. Poor abrasivity
    d. Scratch width
    e. Discoloration of the composite

225. What is the primary problem resulting from polymerization shrinkage?
    a. Marginal gap formation and microleakage/staining
    b. Separation of the filler and matrix phases
    c. Markedly increased water absorption
    d. More rapid occlusal wear
    e. Matrix discoloration

226. What is the typical level of polymerization shrinkage for most dental composites?
    a. < 0.25 %
    b. 0.25–2.0%
    c. 2.5–4.0 %
    d. 6.0–10 %
    e. 10–12 %

227. What do dental composites produce when they undergo superficial decomposition over long times?
    a. Monomers
    b. Formaldehyde and water
    c. Acrylic acid
    d. Bisphenol A
    e. Oligomers

228. What type of appearance will the area of a tooth have that has been etched, washed, and dried?
    a. Smooth
    b. Frosted
    c. Pitted
    d. Dark

229. Operative dentistry is concerned with the prevention and treatment of defects of what tooth surfaces?
    a. Enamel and cementum
    b. Enamel and dentin
    c. Dentin and cementum
    d. Cementum only

230. Which of the following instruments is used primarily to remove debris from tooth cavities?
    a. Hoes
    b. Chisels
    c. Hatchets
    d. Spoon excavators

231. An even-numbered gingival margin trimmer is designed for use on which of the following tooth surfaces?
    a. Mesial
    b. Distal
    c. Facial
    d. Lingual

232. An odd-numbered gingival margin trimmer is designated for use on which of the following tooth surfaces?
    a. Mesial
    b. Distal
    c. Facial
    d. Lingual

233. What type of working end does an amalgam carrier have for transportation?
    a. Solid
    b. Layered
    c. Pointed
    d. Hollow

234. An amalgam condenser is often referred to as which of the following instruments?
    a. Carvers
    b. Burnishers
    c. Pluggers
    d. Carriers

235. Which of the following instruments is designed for carving proximal tooth surfaces?
    a. Tanner #5
    b. 2. #1/2 Hollenback
    c. Frahm 2/3
    d. Cleoid-discoid

236. Which of the following advantages will occur to composite restorations when using a plastic instrument?
    a. Will not discolour
    b. Will not bend
    c. Will not melt
    d. Will not break

237. A "W" prefix on a rubber dam clamp indicates which of the following designs?
    a. Without clamp
    b. Without wrapper
    c. Without slipping
    d. Without wings

238. Which of the following rubber dam frames is the most popular?
    a. "A" frame
    b. Young
    c. Wizard
    d. Woodbury

239. What type of material is always tied around a rubber dam clamp before placement in the mouth?
    a. Floss
    b. Dental chain
    c. Rubber latex
    d. Clamp retriever

240. Which of the following types of matrix bands is most commonly used in restorative dentistry?
    a. Wide #2
    b. Junior #13
    c. Precontoured
    d. Straight #1

241. Which of the following is the most commonly used matrix retainer?
    a. Universal #1
    b. Universal adult
    c. Universal straight
    d. Universal contra-angled

242. Wood or clear plastic wedges measure about how long in length?
    a. 1 inch
    b. 1/2 inch
    c. 3/4 inch
    d. 1/4 inch

243. The operator's zone for a right handed dentist is located between which of the following positions?
    a. 1 and 3 O'clock
    b. 2 and 4 O'clock
    c. 5 and 8 O'clock
    d. 8 and 11 O'clock

244. The assistant's zone for a right handed dentist is located between which of the following positions?
    a. 1 and 3 O'clock
    b. 2 and 4 O'clock
    c. 5 and 8 O'clock
    d. 8 and 11 O'clock

245. The transfer zone is located between which of the following positions?
    a. 8 to 11 O'clock
    b. 2 to 4 O'clock
    c. 3 to 6 O'clock
    d. 4 to 8 O'clock

246. The static zone is located between which of the following positions?
    a. 8 to 11 O'clock
    b. 11 to 1 O'clock
    c. 4. 11 to 2 O'clock
    d. 4 to 8 O'clock

247. How many inches should the dentist's eyes be from the treatment site if the patient is properly positioned?
    a. 5 to 12
    b. 14 to 16
    c. 18 to 36
    d. None of the above

248. In what zone will the instrument exchange between the dentist and the assistant take place?
    a. Operator's
    b. Assistant's
    c. Transfer
    d. Static

249. Dental materials are exchanged between the dentist and the assistant in what zone?
    a. Operator's
    b. Assistant's
    c. Transfer
    d. Static

250. What device is used to remove blood, pus, saliva, and debris from the oral cavity?
    1. Low-volume ejector
    2. High-volume ejector
    3. High-volume evacuator
    4. High-volume aspirator

251. What type of cavity is present when three or more surfaces are involved?
    a. Large
    b. Small
    c. Medium
    d. Complex

252. When the dentist has finished removing the tooth structure in a cavity preparation, what type of feeling will the dentin have when felt by an explorer?
    a. Firm
    b. Loose
    c. Brittle
    d. Semi-hard

253. What is the last cutting step in the preparation of the cavity?
    a. Finishing the tooth walls
    b. Finishing the dentin walls
    c. Finishing the enamel walls
    d. Finishing the occlusal walls

254. Stubborn particles of debris may be removed from a cavity preparation by which of the following materials?
    a. Alcohol
    b. 2 × 2 gauze
    c. 4 × 4 gauze
    d. Small cotton pellet

255. What two materials are used in a cavity preparation to protect the pulp?

    a. Bases and resins
    b. Fluoride and amalgam
    c. Bases and cavity liners
    d. Cavity liners and amalgam

256. What material is used to seal the dentinal tubules to help prevent microleakage in a cavity preparation?

    a. Bases
    b. Cements
    c. Amalgam
    d. Cavity varnish 17

257. When the dentist is making the final adjustment to the matrix, which of the following steps should the dental assistant be preparing?

    a. Changing the bur in the handpiece
    b. Placing the precapsulated amalgam in the amalgamator
    c. Charting the completed restoration in the dental record
    d. All of the above

258. What instrument will the dentist use to bring any excess mercury from the amalgam to the top of the restoration?

    a. Carver
    b. Hatchet
    c. Burnisher
    d. Mouth mirror

259. Which of the following materials may be used to remove any roughness or overhang of an amalgam restoration in the proximal area?

    a. Dental tape
    b. Dental floss
    c. Metal filing strip
    d. Plastic filing strip

260. Which of the following composite resins is available for use in operative dentistry?

    a. Hybrid
    b. Microfilled
    c. Macrofilled
    d. All of the above

261. What composite shade will appear if the tooth becomes dehydrated?

    a. Darker
    b. Lighter
    c. Transparent
    d. Chalky white

262. What type of matrix may be placed on the tooth before the acid etching procedure begins?

    a. Wood
    b. Metal

    c. Rubber
    d. Celluloid

263. Glass ionomer cement will bond directly with which of the following tooth surfaces?

    a. Enamel
    b. Dentin
    c. Cementum
    d. All of the above

264. Endodontic treatment is also known as what type of therapy?

    a. Pulp
    b. Nerve
    c. Root canal
    d. Apicoectomy

265. What is the primary purpose of endodontics?

    a. To relieve pain
    b. To extract teeth
    c. Preserve the pulp and periapical tissues
    d. Treatment of diseases of the pulp and periapical tissues

266. If injured pulpal tissue undergoes necrosis, which of the following situations occur?

    a. Pulp dies
    b. Pulp lives
    c. Pulp is transplanted
    d. Pulp is irritated

267. Which, if any, of the following is not a cause of an injured dental pulp?

    a. Traumatic blows
    b. Thermal irritation
    c. Chemical irritation
    d. None of the above

268. The diagnosis of pulp and periapical conditions occur in what phase of treatment?

    a. During the treatment only
    b. After the treatment only
    c. Both 1 and 2 above
    d. Before the treatment

269. Signs of discoloured teeth, crown fracture, and gross caries can be found during which of the following procedures?

    a. Dental history exam
    b. Clinical examination
    c. Thermal sensitivity test
    d. Percussion test

270. The presence of a dark area on a radiograph surrounding the apex of the root is also referred to by what other term?

    a. Dental caries
    b. Periodontal abscess

c. Type I fracture

d. Radiolucency

271. The sensation of a slight tingling or warm feeling is felt during which of the following diagnostic tests?

a. Cold test

b. Percussion

c. Pulp testing

d. Selective anesthesia

272. During a cold test, if the pulp is inflamed, the patient will experience what type of sensation to the cold?

a. Sharp

b. Tingling

c. Lingering

d. Violent pain

273. If a patient experiences no response to a heat or cold test, the pulp is considered to have which of the following conditions?

a. Vital

b. Mobile

c. Inflamed

d. Necrotic

274. A percussion test determines which of the following conditions?

a. Periapical inflammation

b. Vitality

c. Pulpitis

d. Mobility

275. What type of application is used for palpation?

a. Anesthesia

b. Pulp tester

c. Mouth mirror

d. Finger pressure

276. Which of the following tests involves the movement of tooth between the handles of two instruments?

a. Mobility

b. Palpation

c. Percussion

d. Transillumination

277. Transillumination is most effective on which of the following teeth?

a. Anterior

b. Posterior

c. Deciduous

d. Permanent

278. Placing a pulp cap over a layer of remaining dentin is referred to by what term?

a. Pulpotomy cap

b. Direct pulp cap

c. Partial pulp cap

d. Indirect pulp cap

279. What type of therapy consists of internal debridement, cleaning, shaping, and permanent filling?

a. Pulpotomy

b. Pulpectomy

c. Root canal

d. Apicoectomy

280. The surgical removal of the pulp chamber is known by which of the following terms?

a. Pulpectomy

b. Pulpotomy

c. Apicoectomy I

d. Incision and drainage

281. What is the procedure called when the entire pulp is removed?

a. Completed pulpotomy

b. Pulpal removal

c. Pulpectomy

d. Apicoectomy

282. What method is used to seal the apical end of the root canal in conjunction with an apicoectomy?

a. Periapical curettage

b. Calcified root canal filling

c. Root amputation

d. Retrograde filling

283. Paper points are used in endodontics for which of the following reasons?

a. To deliver medications to the canal

b. To dry out the root canals

c. To measure working distance

d. To remove the pulp

284. Which of the following is not an advantage for using gutta-percha points for root canal restorative materials?

a. Poor heat conductor

b. High thermal expansion

c. Radiopaque

d. Shrinks when used with a solvent

285. Endodontic explorers are used for which of the following reasons?

a. Locate canal openings

b. Lateral condensation

c. Enlarge pulp canal

d. Pulp removal

286. What is the major difference between endodontic and cotton forceps?

a. Size

b. Made of rubber

c. Ends are grooved

d. Angle of the working end

287. What symbol is used to identify barbed broaches?
   a. Six-pointed star
   b. Eight-pointed star
   c. Ten-pointed star
   d. Six-rings

288. Which of the following instruments is used to enlarge the pulp canal?
   a. Broaches
   b. Endodontic explorer
   c. Paper points
   d. Reamers

289. Which of the following are types of root canal files?
   a. G and H
   b. H and F
   c. H and K
   d. K and J

290. What are the two types of endodontic condensers?
   a. Plugger/woodsen
   b. Woodsen/vertical condenser
   c. Plugger/spreader
   d. Spreader/woodsen

291. Which of the following materials prevents injury to the apex of the root and periapical tissues?
   a. Rubber dam
   b. Lentulo spiral
   c. Stops
   d. K files

292. Which of the following solutions is most frequently used for irrigation of the root canal?
   a. Sterile saline
   b. Hydrogen peroxide
   c. Root canal solution
   d. Sodium hypochlorite

293. The length of an endodontic treated tooth is measured using which of the following rulers?
   a. Standard
   b. Endodontic millimeter
   c. Endodontic centimeter
   d. Endodontic inch

294. How are rubber stops placed on files and reamers?
   a. Right angle
   b. Oblique angle
   c. Vertical angle
   d. Horizontal angle

295. What portion of the master cone is coated with cement?
   a. Apical first
   b. Apical second
   c. Apical third
   d. Apical fourth

296. The excess length of the gutta-percha is removed by which of the following instruments?
   a. Scalpel
   b. Heated file
   c. Iris scissors
   d. Heated instrument

297. The principal goal(s) of bonding are:
   a. Sealing and retention
   b. Esthetics and reduction of postoperative sensitivity
   c. Retention and reduction of tooth flexure
   d. Strengthening teeth and esthetics
   e. Sealing and thermal insulation

298. Which one of the following applications does not involve an adhesive joint?
   i. Enamel bonding system
   ii. Pit-and-fissure sealant
   iii. Dentin bonding system
   iv. Amalgam bonding system
   v. Composite cement

299. Which one of the following applications does not involve an adhesive joint?
   i. Surface sealant
   ii. Composite resin cement
   iii. Dentin bonding system
   iv. Amalgam bonding system
   v. Orthodontic bonding system

300. Which one of the following is not a major requirement for development of good adhesion?
   i. Clean adherend
   ii. Calcium ions present for bonding
   iii. Good wetting
   iv. Intimate adaptation
   v. Good curing

301. Dentin bonding systems involve which of the following exclusive joint components?
   i. Adhesive only
   ii. Adherend only
   iii. Adhesive/adherend
   iv. Adhesive/adherend/adhesive
   v. Adherend/adhesive/adherend

302. What is the typical shear bond strength range for enamel bonding systems?
   i. 2–6 MPa
   ii. 6–12 MPa
   iii. 12–18 MPa
   iv. 10–22 MPa
   v. 22–35 MPa

303. What is the typical shear bond strength range for newer dentin bonding systems?
   i. 2–6 MPa
   ii. 6–12 MPa

iii. 12–18 MPa
iv. 18–22 MPa
v. 22–35 MPa

304. Which of the following variables is least important for bonding?

   i. Substrate
   ii. Tooth
   iii. Material
   iv. Patient
   v. Fluoride history

305. Which category of factors is most important in determining clinical performance?

   i. Operator factors
   ii. Tooth factors
   iii. Location factors
   iv. Material factors
   v. Patient factors

306. Which of the following correctly describes the shape of hydroxyapatite crystals?

   i. Cylindrical
   ii. Parallelopipeds
   iii. Dodecahedrons
   iv. Hexagonal rods
   v. Keyhole shaped tubes

307. At which location in enamel is the density of enamel crystals the lowest?

   i. Prismless enamel
   ii. DEJ
   iii. Center of enamel prisms
   iv. Edges of enamel prisms
   v. Facial enamel

308. Which of the following is not a conditioner?

   i. Phosphoric acid
   ii. EDTA
   iii. Maleic acid
   iv. Citric acid
   v. BIS-GMA

309. What is the principal mechanism for enamel bonding?

   i. Physical bonding
   ii. Primary chemical bonding
   iii. Hydrogen bonding
   iv. Micromechanical bonding
   v. Incoherent bonding

310. In normal dentin, how far does an odontoblastic process extend from the cell?

   i. 10–20 μm
   ii. 0.5 mm
   iii. 1 mm
   iv. Half way to the DEJ
   v. Most of the way to the DEJ

311. What is the typical volume of dentin occupied by dentinal tubules in the outer third of dentin?

   i. 50%
   ii. 40%
   iii. 25%
   iv. 14%
   v. 5%

312. What is the principal mechanism for dentin bonding?

   i. Physical bonding
   ii. Primary chemical bonding
   iii. Hydrogen bonding
   iv. Micromechanical bonding
   v. Chelation bonding

313. Which one of the following is most important event for dentin bonding?

   i. Smear layer removal
   ii. Smear plug removal
   iii. Peritubular dentin decalcification
   iv. Intertubular dentin decalcification
   v. Collagen denaturation

314. What is the hybrid zone?

   i. Decalcified peritubular dentin
   ii. Embedded smear layer
   iii. Embedded smear plugs
   iv. Bonding agent/composite interface
   v. Embedded smear layer and intertubular dentin

315. Which of the following terms is not associated with the "hybrid zone" ?

   i. Bonding agent
   ii. Interpenetration zone
   iii. Resin impregnation zone
   iv. Pseudo-chemical bonding
   v. Micromechanical bonding

316. What is the principal monomer in the bonding agent of "amalgam bonding systems" that is responsible for wetting and promoting micromechanical bonding?

   i. 4-META
   ii. HEMA
   iii. BIS-GMA
   iv. UDM
   v. TEGDMA

317. What is the most important clinical variable affecting "amalgam bonding" system strength?

   i. Conditioning time for enamel
   ii. Bonding agent thickness
   iii. Type of dental amalgam
   iv. Moisture control
   v. Age of the tooth structure

318. How can you detect small amounts of Hg in the dental operatory?

   i. Hg vapour is a slightly yellow gas

ii. Hg vapour has a sweet taste

iii. Hg vapour causes itching around the eyes

iv. Hg liquid tends to stain the skin

v. Hg must be measured with instruments

319. Which phase in set dental amalgam restoration contains almost all the Hg?

   i. Gamma

   ii. Gamma 1

   iii. Gamma 2

   iv. Eta

   v. Epsilon

320. During dental amalgam polishing or removal operations, at what temperature does the first liquid mercury-rich phase appear?

   i. 128 °C

   ii. 211 °C

   iii. 320 °C

   iv. 355 °C

   v. 580 °C

321. Which one of the following individuals is at the least risk for mercury toxicity in the dental office?

   i. Dentist

   ii. Assistant

   iii. Hygienist

   iv. Patient

   v. Housekeeping personnel

322. What is the main reason for slow polishing with cooling during dental amalgam polishing?

   i. To minimize melting of the Ag-Hg phase

   ii. To increase the cutting efficiency of the abrasive

   iii. To slowly dissolve the tarnish layers

   iv. To smear material into the marginal openings

   v. To avoid cutting enamel

323. Which one of the following forms of mercury is present in dental amalgam as a hazard?

   i. Elemental mercury

   ii. Inorganic mercury

   iii. Organic mercury

   iv. Chelated mercury

   v. Catalytic mercury

324. Which one of the following pathways is the route for the most rapid absorption of mercury coming from dental amalgam restorations?

   i. Skin

   ii. Lungs

   iii. Gastrointestinal tract

   iv. Dentinal tubules

   v. Oral mucosa

325. What is the TLV for mercury safety as established by OSHA?

   i. 0.03 mg/m³

   ii. 0.50 mg/m³

   iii. 0.20 mg/m³

   iv. 50 mg/m³

   v. 500 ppb

326. Which one of the following Sources contributes the greatest amount of mercury to the body each day?

   i. Air

   ii. Water

   iii. Diet

   iv. Dental sources

   v. Medical sources

327. Which one of the following incidents involving mercury problems represents the greatest number of human deaths?

   i. Mercury mining

   ii. Minamata Bay accident

   iii. Iraq accident

   iv. Alamogordo accident

   v. Sweden pollution

328. Which one of the following tissues in the body is the most deleteriously affected by mercury toxicity?

   i. Brain

   ii. Liver

   iii. Lungs

   iv. Circulatory system

   v. Lymph system

329. What is the half-life of Hg in the human body?

   i. 1 day

   ii. 21 days

   iii. 43 days

   iv. 55 days

   v. 98 days

330. Which of the following is not a normal pathway of Hg excretion?

   i. Hair and fingernails

   ii. Feces

   iii. Urine

   iv. Lungs

   v. Saliva

331. What is the main symptom for Hg hypersensitivity?

   i. Multiple sclerosis symptoms

   ii. Headaches

   iii. Ringing in the ears

   iv. Localized erythema

   v. Swelling of lymph nodes

332. Mercury toxicity from dental amalgams is detected by:

   i. Intra-oral air samples

   ii. Urine samples

   iii. Hair samples

   iv. Blood samples

   v. No known methods

333. Mercury hypersensitivity from dental amalgams is detected by:

    i. Intraoral air samples
    ii. Intraoral voltage measurements
    iii. Blood samples
    iv. Muscle strength measurements
    v. No known methods

334. Mercury hypersensitivity in general can be measured:

    i. Inaccurately by patch tests
    ii. Accurately by immune system tests
    iii. Kinesiology tests
    iv. Blood assays
    v. Chelation tests

335. What is the ADA recommendation for individuals suspected of hypersensitivity to mercury?

    i. Removal of all amalgams
    ii. Placement of sealants over the amalgams
    iii. Patch test to confirm the suspicion
    iv. Blood tests for mercury toxicity
    v. Referral to an allergist or dermatologist

336. How is mercury released during electrochemical corrosion of low copper dental amalgams?

    i. Formation of soluble Hg-Cl
    ii. Release of Hg ions
    iii. Formation of soluble HgS
    iv. Dissolution of Ag-Hg
    v. It is not released

337. How is mercury released during electrochemical corrosion of high copper dental amalgams?

    i. Formation of soluble Hg-Cl
    ii. Release of Hg ions
    iii. Formation of soluble HgS
    iv. Dissolution of Ag-Hg
    v. It is not released

338. What is the most active route of release of mercury from dental amalgam restorations?

    i. Corrosion of the gamma 2 phase
    ii. Tarnish of the restoration
    iii. Wear and abrasion of the surface
    iv. Liquid diffusion from the surface
    v. Stimulated vapour pressure release

339. What are the highest levels of mercury release measured under the "worst scenario" conditions of 12–16 occlusal amalgams and active surface stimulation during chewing?

    a. 1 mg/m^3
    b. 10 m/m^3
    c. 30 m/m^3
    d. 50 m/m^3
    e. 100 m/m^3

340. On a timely basis, mercury levels in the office should be:

    i. Eliminated by vacuuming the carpets and cleaning the floors
    ii. Eliminated by employees using chelation drugs
    iii. Dusting all floor areas with sulfur
    iv. Monitored by submitting employee hair samples for Hg analysis
    v. Monitored by annual blood samples for Hg analysis

341. The occlusal isthmus of an MO dental amalgam restoration is more resistant to fracture if the

    a. Pulpal depth is 1 mm
    b. Occlusal dovetail is present
    c. Axiopulpal line angle is rounded
    d. Unsupported enamel at the gingivocavosurface margin is planed

342. Which of the following statements correctly describes the relationship between marginal leakage of an amalgam restoration and age of the restoration?

    a. Marginal leakage increases as the restoration ages
    b. Marginal leakage decreases as the restoration ages
    c. Marginal leakage is severe throughout the life of the restoration
    d. Marginal leakage does not exist throughout the life of the restoration

343. Which of the following is a fundamental guideline that governs the outline form of a class II cavity prepartion?

    a. Avoid angles in the proximal outline
    b. Extend the gingival margin beneath the free margin of the gingival
    c. Extend the margins until sound enamel is obtained within the cavity outline
    d. Include pits and fissures in the occlusal surface if the patient is very susceptible to caries

344. Direct pulp capping is indicated when there is

    a. A large exposure
    b. Pain response to cold
    c. No hemorrhage from the exposure
    d. An accidental mechanical exposure in clean, dry field
    e. All of the above

345. A large carious lesion on the distal surface of maxillary central incisor involving the incisal angle is a

    a. Class I lesion
    b. Class II lesion
    c. Class III lesion
    d. Pit and fissure lesion
    e. Smooth surface lesion
        1. (a) only
        2. (b) or (e)
        3. (c) or (e)
        4. (d) only
        5. (e) only

346. Resistance to proximal displacement in the ideal class II restoration is provided by

    a. The adjacent tooth
    b. Occlusal dovetail
    c. Converging proximal walls
    d. Retention grooves proximoaxial line angles
    1. (a), (b) and (c)
    2. (a), (b) and (d)
    3. (a) and (c) only
    4. (b) and (c) only
    5. (b) and (d) only
    6. (c) and (d)

347. The bur should be titled lingually when preparing the occlusal aspect of a class II dental amalgam preparation on a mandibular first premolar inorder to

    A. Remove all carious tooth structure
    b. Prevent encroachment on the facial pulp horn
    c. Prevent encroachment on the lingual pulp horn
    d. Maintain dentinal support of the lingual cusp
    1. (a) and (b)
    2. (a) and (c)
    3. (b) and (d)
    4. (c) and (d)
    5. (d) only

348. The specific purposes of acid etching enamel before insertion of a composite restoration or a sealant are provided

    a. A dry surface
    b. Less surface area
    c. More surface area
    d. A clean surface
    e. A roughened surface
    1. (a), (b), and (d)
    2. (a), (c), and (d)
    3. (a), (c), and (e)
    4. (b), (d) and (e)
    5. (b) and (e) only
    6. (c) and (e) only

349. Before inserting amalgam into an MOD cavity prepartion, a matrix is placed around the tooth. Which of the following procedures should be accomplished next?

    a. The band should be burnished into contact with adjacent teeth
    b. The matrix retainer should be tightened as much as possible and reinforced facially and lingually with compound
    c. Tapered wedges should be placed interproximally to obtain close adaption of the matrix at gingival margins
    d. Tapered wedges should be placed carefully to hold the band in close adaption to the gingival margin without separating the teeth

    1. (a), (b) and (c)
    2. (a) and (c) only
    3. (a), (c), and (d)
    4. (a) and (d) only
    5. (b) and (c) only

350. A deficient margin at a proximogingival cavosurface angle of a freshly packed class II amalgam restoration may have been caused by

    a. Poor condensation of the amalgam
    b. Neglecting to wedge the matrix band
    c. Use of too large an initial increment of amalgam
    d. Debris in the corner of the proximal box
    e. Use of hand condensaton rather than mechanical
    f. Condensation
    1. (a), (b) and (c)
    2. (a), (b), (c) and (e)
    3. (a), (c) and (e) only
    4. (a), (c) and (d)
    5. (b), (d) and (e)
    6. All of the above

351. How should the margins of a dental amalgam restoration be trimmed?

    a. By carving along the margins with a sharp instrument that rests on the
    b. Tooth surface
    c. By carving from the restoration to the tooth with a sharp instrument
    d. By carving from the tooth to the restoration with a sharp instrument
    e. By burnishing from the tooth to the restoration until the amalgam is trimmed to the margin

352. In preparing a class I cavity for dental amalgam, the dentist will diverge the mesial and distal walls toward the occlusal surface. This divergence serves to

    a. Prevent undermining of the marginal ridges
    b. Provide convenience form
    c. Resist the forces of mastication
    d. Extend the preparation into areas more readily cleansed

353. A patient presents with an amalgam restoration fractured at the isthmus six months after placement. The most likely cause is

    a. Recurrent caries
    b. Inadequate depth of the preparation
    c. Excessive width of the preparation
    d. Premature occlusal contact

354. Why is a matrix for a class II dental amalgam restoration extended occlusally to the cavity preparation?

    a. It serves as a guide to determine the completed restoration
    b. It allows for overfilling the amalgam

c. It prevents escape of the amalgam during condensation

355. A bevel contraindicated on the cavosurface angles of a class I dental amalgam cavity preparation. Which of the following best explains why?

    a. This type of margin is prone to microleakage
    b. The cavosurface bevel makes burnishing are difficult
    c. A thin flange of the amalgam restorative material might fracture
    d. As the tooth undergoes natural attrition, the amalgam margin can abrade

356. An MO amalgam restoration is more resistant to fracture if

    a. An occlusal dovetail is present
    b. The axiopulpal line angle is beveled or rounded
    c. Pins are placed in the dentin of the cavity preparation
    d. The unsupported enamel at the gingivocavosurface margin is planed

357. The outline form of a cavity preparation is the

    a. Shape or form of the preparation after carious dentin has been excavated
    b. Shape or form the preparation assumes after retention form has been completed
    c. Shape or form of the preparation on the surface of the tooth
    d. First step to be accomplished in cavity preparation after carious dentin has been removed
    e. Next step to be accomplished in cavity preparation after resistance form has been established

358. It is preferable to prepare narrow cavities rather than wide cavities in order to

    a. Reduce operating time
    b. Conserve tooth strength
    c. Avoid undermining the enamel
    d. Avoid overheating the pulpal tissues

359. Most detrimental to the strength of a posterior tooth in a cavity preparation is an increase in

    a. Axial depth
    b. Pulpal depth
    c. Gingival depth
    d. Faciolingual width
    e. Mesiodistal dimension of the cavity

360. Preparations of class I cavities for the reception of amalgam, direct filing gold and gold inlay have in common

    a. Undercutting mesial and distal walls
    b. Divergence of mesial and distal walls occlusally
    c. Divergence of facial and lingual walls occlusally
    d. Converge of facial and lingual walls occlusally

361. Which of the following hand instruments is the most applicable for placing the retention grooves in the distal box of class II amalgam preparation on a mandibular left second premolar?

    a. 10-17-14
    b. 15-8-8
    c. 15-8-14
    d. 13-80-8-14
    e. 13-95-8-14

362. In radiographs of an incipient carious lesion limited to the enamel on proximal surfaces of a prosterior tooth, the lesion appears

    a. As a radiopaque area
    b. As a triangle with the apex at the tooth surface
    c. Larger in the radiograph than actually exists clinically
    d. All of the above
    e. None of the above

363. A deficient margin at a proximogingival cavosurface angle of a freshly condensed class II amalgam restoration may have been caused by

    a. Poor condensation of the amalgam
    b. Neglecting to wedge the matrix band
    c. Use of too large an initial increment of amalgam
    d. Debris in the corner of the proximal box
    e. Use of hand condensation rather than mechanical condensation
        1. a, b, and c only
        2. a, b, c, and e
        3. a, c, and d
        4. a, c, and e only
        5. b, d, and e

364. Proper proximal contour is given to an amalgam restoration placed in a class II cavity preparation by

    a. Carving restoration
    b. The matrix retainer
    c. Adapting a contoured matrix
    d. Restorative material
    e. Overfilling the cavity preparation with the restorative material
        1. a and b
        2. a and c
        3. b and c
        4. b and d
        5. c and d
        6. c and e
        7. All of the above

365. Beveling the enamel margin of a composite resin preparation is accomplished in order

    a. Improve esthetics
    b. Improve wettability of the surface during bonding
    c. Smooth the enamel and cavosurface margins
    d. Expose the ends of the enamel rods for acids attack

1. a and b
2. a and c
3. a and d
4. b and c
5. b and d
6. c and d

366. The bur should be titled lingually when preparing the occlusal aspect of a class II preparation on a mandibular first premolar in order to

    a. Remove unsupported enamel
    b. Prevent encroachment on the facial pulp horn
    c. Prevent encroachment on the lingual pulp horn
    d. Maintain dentinal support of the lingual cusp
    1. a and b
    2. a and c
    3. b and d
    4. c and d
    5. d only

367. Threaded pins used in a dental amalgam restoration should be placed at the dentinoenamel junction

    a. Approximately 1 mm. In depth at a position axial to the
    b. Approximately 2 mm. In depth at a position axial to the dentino enamel junction
    c. Parallel to the external surface between the pulp and the tooth surface
    d. Occlusal to the bifurcation to avoid entering the pulp
    1. a, b, and e
    2. a, c, and d
    3. a, c, and e
    4. b and d
    5. c and d only

368. Inclusion of pins in an amalgam restoration results in an increase in

    a. Retention
    b. Reinforcement
    c. Tensile strength
    d. Compressive strength
    1. a only
    2. a and b
    3. a, c, and d
    4. a and d only
    5. b only
    6. All of the above

369. Resistance to proximal displacement in the ideal class II restoration is provided by

    a. The adjacent tooth
    b. Occlusal dovetail
    c. Converging proximal walls
    d. Retention grooves in proximoaxial line angles
    1. a, b, and c
    2. a, b, and d

3. a and c only
4. b and c only
5. b and d only
6. c and d

370. Which of the following faults in class II restorations may be predisposing factors to periodontal disease?

    a. Gingival overhang
    b. Weak proximal contact
    c. Broad contact faciolingually
    d. Contact in the gingival third
    e. Improperly shaped occlusal embrasure
    1. a, b, c and d
    2. a, b, c and e
    3. a, c and e only
    4. b, d and e
    5. All of the above

371. The periapical film is the film of choice in evaluating

    a. Root surfaces
    b. Occlusal caries
    c. Proximal caries
    d. Supporting bone
    e. The periodontal ligament space
    1. a, b and e
    2. a, c and d
    3. a, d and e
    4. b, d and e
    5. All of the above

372. Which component of amalgam will cause contraction?

    a. Copper
    b. Tin
    c. Zinc
    d. Silver

373. How is scrap amalgam stored?

    a. Under water
    b. Under sulfide
    c. Glycerin

374. Side effect of interaction with mercury

    a. Xerostomia
    b. Slurred speech
    c. Nausea
    d. Glaucoma

375. Which metal is added to amalgam to prevent expansion?

    a. Chromium
    b. Nickel
    c. Zinc
    d. Cobalt
    e. Silver

376. Which of the following is the composition of water based glass ionomer?

    a. Zinc oxide powder and poly acrylic acid

b. Aluminosilicate glass and polyacrylic acid
c. Aluminosilicate glass and polyacrylic acid
d. Zinc oxide powder and polycarboxylic acid

377. You can decrease the strength of zing oxide eugenol cement by adding
a. Ethoxybenzoic acid
b. Acrylic
c. Petrolatum
d. Cotton

378. Which of the following is not recommended under a composite?
a. Zinc phosphate
b. Glass ionomer
c. Zoe
d. Calcium hydroxide

379. ZoE is a good temporary restoration because
a. Less irritant
b. Increased strength
c. Good seal
d. Antibacter

380. What is the composition of a composite?

381. For adequate curing of composite what wave length do you need
a. 275–375
b. 400–475
c. 500–600
d. 600–700

382. Which component of amalgam will cause contraction?
a. Copper
b. Tin
c. Zinc
d. Silver

383. How is scrap amalgam stored?
a. Under water
b. Under sulfide
c. Glycerin

384. Side effect of interaction with mercury
a. Xerostomia
b. Slurred speech
c. Nausea
d. Glaucoma

385. The greatest potential hazard of chronic mercury toxicity comes from
a. Skin contact with mercury
b. Inhalation of mercury vapour
c. Amalgam restorations in a patient
d. Ingestion of amalgam scrap during removal of an old restoration

386. Many instruments have three measurements in their formulas. The number 12 in formula 12-5-6 indicates that the blade is
a. 0.12 mm in width
b. 1.2 mm in width
c. 1.2 mm in length
d. At a 12° angle with the shaft

387. The property of amalgam that makes it undesirable to bevel occlusal margins of an amalgam cavity preparation is its
a. Flow
b. Ductility
c. Brittleness
d. Malleability
e. High edge strength

388. Which of the following dental materials is easily confused with caries when viewed radiographically?
a. Zinc oxide-eugenol
b. Zinc phosphate cement
c. Polycarboxylate cement
d. Calcium hydroxide, USP

389. According to microleakage studies, which of the following restorative materials shows the best initial seal when placed in a cavity preparation, and thereby protects the pulp from the effects of microleakage?
a. Dental amalgam
b. Unfilled resin
c. Direct filling gold
d. Glass ionomer cement
e. Acid-etched composite resin

390. Which of the following components could replace eugenol in a zinc oxide paste?
a. Oil of cloves
b. Acetic acid
c. Alginic acid
d. Carboxylic acid
e. Ortho-ethoxybenzoic acid

391. Which of the following chemical phenomena is common to zinc oxide eugenol and polycarboxylate cements
a. Chelation
b. Crosslinking
c. Esterification
d. Saponification
e. Copolymerization

392. Glass ionomer cements are composed of
a. Zinc oxide powder and polycarboxylic
b. Zinc oxide powder and phosphoric acid liquid
c. Aluminosilicate powder and phosphoric acid liquid
d. Aluminosilicate powder and polycarboxylic liquid

393. On a carbide bur, a greater number of cutting blades results in
    a. Less efficient cutting and a smoother surface
    b. Less efficient cutting and a rougher surface
    c. More efficient cutting and a smoother surface
    d. More efficient cutting and a rougher surface

394. Improved zinc oxide-eugenol materials serve as good temporary restorations pending placement of a permanent restoration because they
    a. Have excellent marginal
    b. Have a therapeutic palliative effect on the dental pulp
    c. Have thermal insulation qualities comparable to those of dentin
    d. Maintain opposing and adjacent teeth in their respective positions
    e. All of the above

395. Examination of a patient with a hypersensitive tooth reveals an obviously leaking temporary restoration that, when removed, discloses a good cavity preparation of average depth with no carious debris and no pulpal exposure. Suspecting a possible hyperemic pulp, the dentist should place an anodyne dressing of
    a. Zinc oxide-eugenol
    b. Zinc phosphate cement
    c. A varnish followed by zinc oxide-eugenol
    d. A varnish followed by zinc phosphate cement
    e. Calcium hydroxide followed by zinc phosphate cement

396. The thickness of a good class II matrix should be approximately
    a. 0.5 mm
    b. 0.002 mm
    c. 0.002 inches
    d. 0.0002 inches

397. Materials contraindicated for placement under and in contact with a composite resin include
    a. Varnish
    b. Calcium hydroxide
    c. Zinc oxide-eugenol
    d. Zinc phosphate cement
    1. a and b only
    2. a, b, and c
    3. a, b and d
    4. a and c only
    5. b and c only
    6. b, c and d
    7. c and d only

398. Prolonged vigorous mixing of zinc phosphate powder into the liquid on a cooled slab promotes a higher powder-liquid ratio and a superior cementation medium by providing a
    a. Higher viscosity
    b. Lower viscosity
    c. Weaker final set
    d. Stronger final set
    e. Higher solubility of set cement
    f. Lower solubility of set cement
    1. a, c and f
    2. a, d, and e
    3. a, d, and f
    4. b, d and e
    5. b, d and f

399. Compared with zinc phosphate cement, poly-carboxylate cement
    a. Has lower compressive strength
    b. Has equivalent tensile strength
    c. Elicits less pulp response
    d. Can bond to tooth structure
    1. a and c
    2. b and d
    3. c and d
    4. All of the above

400. In addition to maintaining a dry field, the rubber dam functions to
    a. Retract soft tissue
    b. Protect the patient
    c. Protect the operator
    d. Save time
    e. Improve access
    1. a, b, and c
    2. a, b, and e
    3. a, c and d
    4. b, c and d
    5. b, d and e
    6. c, d and e
    7. all of the above

401. Moisture contaminated zinc-containing amalgam manifests
    a. Grossly delayed expansion
    b. Higher setting expansion
    c. Reduced compressive strength
    d. An increase in the amount of gamma phase
    1. a and b
    2. a and c
    3. a and d
    4. b and c
    5. b and d
    6. c and d

402. Calcium hydroxide is generally the material-of-choice in vital pulp capping because it
    a. Is less irritating to the pulp
    b. Encourages dentin bridge formation
    c. Seals the cavity better than most other materials

403. To ensure better thermal and protective insulation of the pulp during a capping procedure, calcium hydroxide should be
    a. Applied to a thickness of 3.0 mm
    b. Placed in all cavity preparations
    c. Covered with a stronger base
    d. Preceded by application of a cavity varnish
    e. Preceded by application of a zinc phosphate cement

404. The copal resin varnish that is placed in the cavity preparation before the amalgam is condensed provides
    a. Sealing the margins for the lifetime of the restoration
    b. Long-term sealing of several years duration
    c. Short-term sealing of the margins
    d. No sealing of the margins

405. Each of the following describes the properties of improved zinc oxide eugenol materials except one. Which one is this exception?
    a. They provide an excellent marginal seal
    b. They have palliative effect on the dental pulp
    c. They have thermal insulation qualities
    d. They are easily removed from the cavity preparation

406. To prevent physical injury most effectively when using pickling solutions, dentists should wear which of the following?
    a. Safety goggles
    b. Utility gloves
    c. A face mask

407. A practitioner pickles gold alloy restorations by heating them to redness and plunging them into an acid bath. **This procedure can result in which of the following?**
    a. Oxidation of the metal
    b. Porosity in the casting
    c. Warpage of the restoration
    d. Surface roughness of the restoration

408. Handpiece stones can be used primarily to sharpen which of the following operative instruments?
    a. Curved chisels
    b. Enamel hatchets
    c. Binangle chisels
    d. Spoon excavators

409. The reduction of which of the following represents the most significant advantage of the acid-etch technique?
    a. Microleakage
    b. Pulpal irritation
    c. Setting shrinkage of the matrix
    d. Coefficient of thermal expansion

410. In selecting a dental base, the dentist should give greatest consideration to which of the following?
    a. The biocompatibility of the base
    b. The strength of the base
    c. The thickness of the remaining dentin

411. A newly condensed amalgam restoration seems to chip away when being carved. What is the likely cause of this problem?
    a. A low-copper alloy was used
    b. Moisture contamination occurred
    c. The alloy was incompletely wetted with mercury
    d. The amalgam was not condensed with the recommended pressure
    e. The amalgam was condensed after its working time elapsed

412. Which of the following most affects curing of a light-activated composite resin?
    a. Increment thickness
    b. Shade of composite
    c. Length of exposure

413. Before adhesion can take place between a liquid and a solid, it is essential that the liquid surface
    a. Provide some mechanical interlocking with the solid
    b. Exhibit a large contact angle with the solid
    c. Enter into some form of chemical reaction with the solid
    d. Exhibit a small contact angle with the solid

414. Visible light curing units are MOST hazardous to the
    a. Retina
    b. Lens
    c. Cornea
    d. Iris

415. A properly trimmed wooden wedge will do each of the following except one. Which one is this exception?
    a. Protect the gingival tissue
    b. Provide space for the matrix band
    c. Prevent overcontouring of the contact area
    d. Reduce moisture leakage into the cavity preparation

416. Amalgam scrap should be stored in a tightly-sealed container and covered with which of the following?
    a. Water
    b. Glycerin
    c. Sulfide solution
    d. Sodium hypochlorite solution

417. Which of the following best explains how high-copper amalgam restorations differ from conventional amalgam restorations? The high-copper restorations
    a. Have little or no tin–mercury phase
    b. Require less mercury, so there is more matrix formed
    c. Corrode at an accelerated rate due to increased copper content

d. Are unaffected by moisture contamination in the presence of zinc

418. A practitioner who is restoring a tooth with composites wishes to be sure that the matrix has adhered to the filler. Which of the following agents adheres the resin matrix to the filler?
    a. Wetting
    b. Coupling
    c. Catalyzing
    d. Activating

419. Which of the following do polycarboxylate and glass ionomer have in common?
    a. Zinc oxide
    b. Polysiloxane
    c. Phosphoric acid
    d. Polyacrylic acid
    e. Ion-leachable glass

420. The setting time of zinc phosphate cement can retarded by
    a. Increasing the ratio of powder to liquid
    b. Diluting the liquid with a small amount of water
    c. Accelerating the rate of addition of powder to liquid
    d. Decreasing the rate of addition of powder to liquid

421. Which of the following is most related to turbulence of molten gold in the casting process?
    a. Venting
    b. Volume of metal
    c. Placement of sprue
    d. Position in the ring
    e. Temperature of the ring

422. The proper zone of a gas-air blowpipe flame used for melting casting gold alloys is
    a. The reducing zone
    b. The oxidizing zone
    c. The zone closest to the nozzle
    d. A combination of oxidizing and reducing zones

423. Mercury vapourization in an amalgam restorative procedure utilizing wellsealed, premeasured capsules is most likely to occur during
    a. Mulling
    b. Carving
    c. Trituration
    d. Condensation
    e. High-speed evacuation

424. Creep of a metal indicates that the metal
    a. Lacks edge strength
    b. Has excessive flexibility
    c. Has insufficient retention
    d. Will deform under static load
    e. Has insufficient crushing strength

425. Cavity varnish is indicated for use under amalgam restorations to
    a. Prevent galvanic currents from reaching the pulp
    b. Improve the marginal seal of the restoration
    c. Seal the dentinal tubules completely
    d. Act as an effective thermal insulator
    e. All of the above

426. The discoloured, corroded superficial layer frequently seen on the surface of a dental amalgam restoration is most likely
    a. Mercury
    b. A sulfide
    c. Gamma 2
    d. Copper oxide

427. In mixing zinc phosphate cement, which clinical variable has the greatest effect on the strength of the cement?
    a. Spatulation time
    b. Liquid–powder ratio
    c. Temperature of the mixing slab
    d. Number and size of powder increments

428. Which of the following agents may be used on dentin as a cavity medicament because it does not irritate the dental pulp?
    a. Alcohol
    b. Calcium hydroxide
    c. Ethyl chloride
    d. Silver nitrate
    e. 10% hydrogen peroxide
    f. None of the above

429. On a carbide bur, a greater number of cutting blades results in
    a. Less efficient cutting and smoother surface
    b. Less efficient cutting and rougher surface
    c. More efficient cutting and a smoother surface
    d. More efficient cutting and a rougher surface

430. The rotary instrument that produces the roughest tooth surface after use is a:
    a. 3/8 inch fine garnet disk at slow speed
    b. Cross-cut tapered fissure bur at slow speed
    c. Plane tapered fissure bur at high speed
    d. 12-fluted carbide fissure bur at high speed

431. Examination of a patient with a hypersensitive tooth reveals an obviously leaking temporary restoration that, when removed, discloses a good cavity preparation of average depth with no carious debris and no pulpal exposure. Suspecting a possible hyperemic pulp, the dentist should place an anodyne dressing of
    a. Zinc oxide-eugenol
    b. Zinc phosphate cement

c. A varnish followed by zinc oxide-eugenol
d. A varnish followed by zinc phosphate cement
e. Calcium hydroxide followed by zinc phosphate cement

432. A patient returns to the dentist two weeks after a gold onlay was cemented with zinc phosphate cement. The patient complains of moderate sensitivity to cold. Occlusion is evaluated and the onlay is not in hyperocclusion. The dentist should
a. Take the restoration out of occlusion
b. Remove the onlay and place a sedative dressing
c. Take and evaluate a periapical radiograph
d. Advise the patient to avoid extreme temperatures and that the sensitivity to
e. Cold will gradually decrease

433. A zinc oxide-eugenol cement base is contraindicated for use with self-curing resin restorative materials because
a. The compressive strength of the cement is too low
b. Cement interferes with the polymerization of the resin
c. Zinc oxide and Bis-GMA form a soluble compound
d. The cement increases the polymerization shrinkage of the resin

434. Which of the following factors govern the rate of set of a zinc phosphate cement?
a. Powder-liquid ratio
b. Rate of powder incorporation
c. Particle size of the powder
d. Manner of spatulation
e. Water content in the liquid
1. a, b and d
2. a, b, c and e
3. a, b, d and e
4. a, c, d and e
5. b, c, d and e
6. All of the above

435. Which of the following apply when using a light to cure light activated composite resin?
a. The light should be held as close to the resin surface as possible
b. The light should be held at least 5.0 mm from the resin surface
c. A shield should be placed between the light tip and the operator's eyes
d. Curing time should be increased with darker resin shades
e. Curing time should be increased with lighter resin shades
1. a, c and d
2. a, c and e
3. a and d only

4. b, c and d
5. b, c and e
6. b and e only

436. Pure gold can be contaminated when it comes in contact with
a. Moisture
b. Sulfur vapours
c. Eugenol vapours
d. Oxygen rich flame
1. a, b and c
2. a, b and d
3. a, c and d
4. b, c and d
5. All of the above

437. The high copper dental amalgams are superior to other amalgams because high copper dental amalgams
a. Are less likely to corrode
b. Have less marginal breakdown
c. Are workable at lower Hg-alloy ratios
d. Generally have higher compressive strength
1. a and b only
2. a, b and d
3. a and c only
4. a and d only
5. b only
6. b, c and d

438. Which of the following influence tooth temperature during a cutting procedure?
a. Diameter of the bur
b. Sharpness of the bur
c. Bur/tooth contact time
d. Type of coolant used
e. Amount of force applied to the bur
1. a, b, c and d
2. a, b, c and e
3. a, b and d only
4. b, c and e only
5. c, d and e
6. All of the above

439. The dangers of using air as a coolant while cutting with ultra-high speed are that it may
a. Dehydrate the tooth
b. Cool the pulp below the danger point
c. Cause the tooth to be hypersensitive
d. Allow the cutting to proceed too quickly
e. Draw the odontoblasts into the dentinal tubules
1. a, c and e
2. a and d only
3. b and c only
4. c and e only
5. All of the above

440. Use of water spray and high volume evacuation is recommended when removing old amalgam or polishing dental amalgam restorations because mercury vapour is released during these procedures
    a. Both statement and reason are correct and related
    b. Both statement and reason are correct but not related
    c. The statement is correct but the reason is not
    d. The statement is not correct but the reason is an accurate statement
    e. Neither statement nor reason is correct

441. Which of the following dental cements is a luting agent that provides adhesion to calcified dental tissue?
    a. EBA-ZOE cement
    b. Silicate cement
    c. Zinc phosphate cement
    d. Polycarboxylate cement

442. Describe the Federation Dentaire Internationale system for tooth numbering?

443. What are the 2 different strokes used in the use of hand cutting instruments?

444. Which portions of a Class II dental amalgam restoration will be mechanically the weakest?

445. Should dental amalgams be polished during oral prophylaxes? Why?

446. What special precautions should be taken during the removal of a corroded dental amalgam restoration?

447. Why do Class V amalgams seem to be more tarnished that Class I amalgams?

448. A patient complains of ringing in his ear due to the contact of a new crown with an adjacent Class II amalgam. Explain what you would do to test whether this was true and how you would manage the situation?

449. Explain why spherical dental amalgams tend to have higher strengths than those based on irregular particles?

450. Explain the dilemma for using a small diameter condenser with a spherical alloy amalgam?

451. On a D-O amalgam restoration, explain the relative susceptibility of the margins to marginal fracture?

452. In a relatively shallow dental amalgam cavity preparation, what would be the result of not using cavity varnish, bonding agent, or dentin sealer before amalgam placement?

453. Why should not the smear layer be removed from the dental amalgam cavity preparation in order to produce more intimate adaptation of the amalgam and the supporting enamel and dentin structures?

454. In a moderately deep cavity preparation with one portion of the floor that is close to a pulp horn, what is the best selection of varnishes, liners, and bases to use, and what is the order and coverage of application?

455. What is the reason that calcium hydroxide is included in compositions if the odontoblasts will produce reparative or secondary dentin on their own without stimulation in 5-to-7 more days?

456. Explain the special requirements for cavity preparation for a carious lesion that has penetrated within 0.5 mm of the pulp?

457. What are the advantages of utilizing a rubber dam?

458. What are the burs numbered 55½ to 60?

459. What is the difference between cohesive and adhesive bond types?

460. From which side of the tooth should the wooden wedge be placed when using a Tollflemire matrix system?

461. List three advantages of using the dental mirror for indirect vision during operative procedures.

462. What special technique must be used to sharpen a round bladed cutting instrument such as the cleoid-discoid carver?

463. What techniques can be used to assure proper lateral condensation of the amalgam against the walls of the preperation?

464. What methods can be used to aid in avoiding and identifying "flash" when placing an amalgam?

465. Cavity varnish is indicated for use under amalgam restorations to
    a. Prevent galvanic currents from reaching the pulp
    b. Improve the marginal seal of the restoration
    c. Seal the dentinal tubules completely
    d. Act as an effective thermal insulator
    e. All of the above

466. The discoloured, corroded superficial layer frequently seen on the surface of a dental amalgam restoration is most likely
    a. Mercury
    b. A sulfide
    c. Gamma 2
    d. Copper oxide

467. In mixing zinc phosphate cement, which clinical variable has the greatest effect on the strength of the cement?
    a. Spatulation time
    b. Liquid-powder ratio
    c. Temperature of the mixing slab
    d. Number and size of powder increments

468. Which of the following agents may be used on dentin as a cavity medicament because it does not irritate the dental pulp?
    a. Alcohol
    b. Calcium hydroxide
    c. Ethyl chloride
    d. Silver nitrate
    e. 10% hydrogen peroxide
    f. None of the above

469. On a carbide bur, a greater number of cutting blades results in
    a. Less efficient cutting and smoother surface
    b. Less efficient cutting and rougher surface
    c. More efficient cutting and a smoother surface
    d. More efficient cutting and a rougher surface

470. The rotary instrument that produces the roughest tooth surface after use is a
    a. 3/8 inch fine garnet disk at slow speed
    b. Cross cut tapered fissure bur at slow speed
    c. Plane tapered fissure bur at high speed
    d. 12-fluted carbide fissure bur at high speed

471. Examination of a patient with a hypersensitive tooth reveals an obviously leaking temporary restoration that, when removed, discloses a good cavity preparation of average depth with no carious debris and no pulpal exposure. Suspecting a possible hyperemic pulp, the dentist should place an anodyne dressing of
    a. Zinc oxide-eugenol
    b. Zinc phosphate cement
    c. A varnish followed by zinc oxide-eugenol
    d. A varnish followed by zinc phosphate cement
    e. Calcium hydroxide followed by zinc phosphate cement

472. A patient returns to the dentist two weeks after a gold onlay was cemented with zinc phosphate cement. The patient complains of moderate sensitivity to cold. Occlusion is evaluated and the onlay is not in hyperocclusion. The dentist should
    a. Take the restoration out of occlusion
    b. Remove the onlay and place a sedative dressing
    c. Take and evaluate a periapical radiograph
    d. Advise the patient to avoid extreme temperatures and that the sensitivity to
    e. Cold will gradually decrease

473. A zinc oxide-eugenol cement base is contraindicated for use with self-curing resin restorative materials because
    a. The compressive strength of the cement is too low
    b. Cement interferes with the polymerization of the resin
    c. Zinc oxide and Bis-GMA form a soluble compound

    d. The cement increases the polymerization shrinkage of the resin

474. Which of the following factors govern the rate of set of a zinc phosphate cement?
    a. Powder-liquid ratio
    b. Rate of powder incorporation
    c. Particle size of the powder
    d. Manner of spatulation
    e. Water content in the liquid
    1. a, b and d
    2. a, b, c and e
    3. a, b, d and e
    4. a, c, d and e
    5. b, c, d and e
    6. all of the above

475. Which of the following apply when using a light to cure light activated composite resin?
    a. The light should be held as close to the resin surface as possible
    b. The light should be held at least 5.0 mm from the resin surface
    c. A shield should be placed between the light tip and the operator's eyes
    d. Curing time should be increased with darker resin shades
    e. Curing time should be increased with lighter resin shades
    1. a, c and d
    2. a, c and e
    3. a and d only
    4. b, c and d
    5. b, c and e
    6. b and e only

476. Pure gold can be contaminated when it comes in contact with
    a. Moisture
    b. Sulfur vapours
    c. Eugenol vapours
    d. Oxygen rich flame
    1. a, b and c
    2. a, b and d
    3. a, c and d
    4. b, c and d
    5. all of the above

477. The high copper dental amalgams are superior to other amalgams because high copper dental amalgams
    a. Are less likely to corrode
    b. Have less marginal breakdown
    c. Are workable at lower Hg-alloy ratios
    d. Generally have higher compressive strength
    1. a and b only
    2. a, b and d

3. a and c only
4. a and d only
5. b only
6. b, c and d

478. Which of the following influence tooth temperature during a cutting procedure?
   a. Diameter of the bur
   b. Sharpness of the bur
   c. Bur/tooth contact time
   d. Type of coolant used
   e. Amount of force applied to the bur
      1. a, b, c and d
      2. a, b, c and e
      3. a, b and d
      4. b, c and e
      5. c, d and e
      6. All of the above

479. The dangers of using air as a coolant while cutting with ultra-high speed are that it may
   a. Dehydrate the tooth
   b. Cool the pulp below the danger point
   c. Cause the tooth to be hypersensitive
   d. Allow the cutting to proceed too quickly

   e. Draw the odontoblasts into the dentinal tubules
      1. a, c and e
      2. a and d
      3. b and c
      4. c and e
      5. all of the above

480. Use of water spray and high volume evacuation is recommended when removing old amalgam or polishing dental amalgam restorations because mercury vapour is released during these procedures
   a. Both statement and reason are correct and related
   b. Both statement and reason are correct but not related
   c. The statement is correct but the reason is not
   d. The statement is not correct but the reason is an accurate statement
   e. Neither statement nor reason is correct

481. Which of the following dental cements is a luting agent that provides adhesion to calcified dental tissue?
   a. EBA-ZOE cement
   b. Silicate cement
   c. Zinc phosphate cement
   d. Polycarboxylate cement

INDEX